T0181001

# Pediatric Demyelinating Diseases of the Central Nervous System and Their Mimics

Emmanuelle Waubant • Timothy E. Lotze
Editors

# Pediatric Demyelinating Diseases of the Central Nervous System and Their Mimics

A Case-Based Clinical Guide

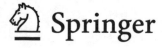 Springer

*Editors*
Emmanuelle Waubant
Clinical Neurology and Pediatrics
Regional Pediatric MS Clinic at UCSF
University of California San Francisco
San Francisco, CA, USA

Timothy E. Lotze
Division of Neurology and
Developmental Neuroscience
Department of Pediatrics
Baylor College of Medicine
Texas Children's Hospital
Houston, TX, USA

ISBN 978-3-319-87074-8      ISBN 978-3-319-61407-6   (eBook)
DOI 10.1007/978-3-319-61407-6

Printed on acid-free paper

This Springer imprint is published by Springer Nature
The registered company is Springer International Publishing AG
The registered company address is: Gewerbestrasse 11, 6330 Cham, Switzerland

# Preface

While multiple sclerosis was once considered to be strictly an adult disease, its occurrence in pediatric populations has been clearly demonstrated over the past two decades. Diagnostic criteria were initially developed in 2007 and subsequently revised in 2013 to aid clinicians in diagnosing the condition and initiating disease-modifying therapy. While many patients present with classic features of multiple sclerosis, clinicians can struggle to reach a diagnosis if they have not encountered a pediatric patient with the disease. In addition, a unique spectrum of diseases affecting the white matter of the central nervous system in pediatric populations to include acute disseminated encephalomyelitis, neuromyelitis optica, inborn errors of metabolism, leukodystrophies, and vasculopathies can further broaden the considered differential diagnosis leading to an expansive and expensive workup that can overwhelm patients, families, and clinicians.

In 2006, the National Multiple Sclerosis Society recognized the inconsistencies in the management of patients with onset of multiple sclerosis under the age of 18 and the need for improved diagnosis and care. As a result, a national pediatric MS Network was created with an initial emphasis on promoting clinical care of patients with the disease and mimics thereof. Rapidly, the network recognized the critical need for more broadly sharing difficult cases so as to improve physician education and care of such patients in light of the limitations in and access to the global knowledge of these diseases.

In 2010, under the auspices of the US Pediatric Multiple Sclerosis Network, a monthly teleconference was initiated to discuss challenging or informative cases and to help clinicians benefit from each other's experience and wisdom, as well as expose more junior physicians to the care of patients with CNS demyelinating disorders. These monthly calls would not exist without the tenacity of Dr. Jayne Ness and "our mother of all," Deborah Hertz, who worked at the National MS Society, who, from the very beginning, has been the strongest advocate for children with MS and related disorders (http://www.usnpmsc.org).

Based upon these teleconferences, this book is the product of a collection of passionate care providers who work tirelessly together to improve diagnosis and treatment of young patients with demyelinating disorders of the central nervous system.

The range of clinical cases presented herein reflects years of observations and sharing, illustrating the challenges in the diagnosis and management of these disorders. We have carefully chosen a series of representative clinical cases ranging from typical multiple sclerosis, neuromyelitis optica, and acute disseminated encephalomyelitis to mimics of these disorders with the hope to fill a major gap in the care of such patients as most of these disorders are reasonably rare and challenging to diagnose and treat. We are deeply indebted to the many authors who have volunteered their time to put these chapters together, often working in teams. We dedicate this book to the improved care of children with rare (but not that infrequent) inflammatory disorders of the central nervous system.

San Francisco, CA, USA                                              Emmanuelle Waubant
Houston, TX, USA                                                        Timothy E. Lotze

# Contents

# Contributors

**Sonika Agarwal, M.D.** Division of Neurology and Developmental Neuroscience, Department of Pediatrics Baylor College of Medicine, Texas Children's Hospital, Houston, TX, USA

**Gulay Alper, M.D.** Division of Child Neurology, Department of Pediatrics, Children's Hospital of Pittsburgh, University of Pittsburgh School of Medicine, Pittsburgh, PA, USA

**E. Ann Yeh, M.D.** Department of Pediatrics, Division of Neurology, The Hospital for Sick Children, University of Toronto, Toronto, ON, Canada

**Joshua J. Bear, M.D., M.A** Assistant Professor of Pediatrics and Neurology, University of Colorado Denver and Children's Hospital Colorado, San Francisco, CA, USA

**Sara Vila Bedmar, M.D.** Department of Neurology, Hospital Universitario 12 de Octubre, Madrid, Spain

**Leslie Benson, M.D.** Department of Pediatric Neurology, Harvard Medical School, Boston Children's Hospital, Boston, MA, USA

**Vikram V. Bhise, M.D.** Pediatrics, Neurology, Rutgers – Robert Wood Johnson Medical School, Child Health Institute, New Brunswick, NJ, USA

Division of Child Neurology, Department of Pediatrics, New Brunswick, NJ, USA

**Dorlyne M. Brchan, M.D.** Tanana Valley Clinic, Foundation Health Partners, Fort Wainwright, AK, USA

**Aaron L. Cardon, M.D., M.Sc** Division of Neurology and Developmental Neuroscience, Department of Pediatrics, Baylor College of Medicine, Texas Children's Hospital, Houston, TX 77030, USA

**Hsiao-Tuan Chao, M.D., Ph.D.** Jan and Dan Duncan Neurological Research Institute, Texas Children's Hospital, Houston, TX, USA

Division of Neurology and Developmental Neuroscience, Department of Pediatrics, Baylor College of Medicine and Texas Children's Hospital, Houston, TX, USA

**Hardeep Chohan, M.D.** Department of Neurology, University of California San Francisco, San Francisco, CA, USA

**Katherine DeStefano, M.D., M.S.** Department of Neurology, Yale University School of Medicine, New Haven, CT, USA

**Ian Ferguson, M.D.** Division of Pediatric Rheumatology, Department of Pediatrics, Yale University School of Medicine, New Haven, CT, USA

**Carla Francisco, M.D.** Multiple Sclerosis and Neuroinflammation Center, University of California, San Francisco, San Francisco, CA, USA

**Jason S. Gill, M.D., Ph.D.** Division of Neurology and Developmental Neuroscience, Department of Pediatrics Baylor College of Medicine, Texas Children's Hospital, Houston, TX, USA

**Sabrina Gmuca, M.D.** Division of Pediatric Rheumatology, The Children's Hospital of Philadelphia, Philadelphia, PA, USA

Department of Pediatrics, Perelman School of Medicine, University of Pennsylvania, Philadelphia, PA, USA

**Jennifer S. Graves, M.D., Ph.D., M.A.S** Clinical Neurology and Pediatrics, Regional Pediatric MS Clinic at UCSF, University of California San Francisco, San Francisco, CA, USA

**Seanna Grob, M.D., M.A.S** Department of Ophthalmology, Harvard Medical School, Boston, MA, USA

Department of Ophthalmology, Massachusetts Eye and Ear Infirmary, Boston, MA, USA

**Gena Heidary, M.D., Ph.D.** Department of Ophthalmology, Harvard Medical School, Boston Children's Hospital, Boston, MA, USA

**Jason Helis, M.D., M.S.** Maine Medical Partners Neurology, Scarborough, ME, USA

**Rebecca L. Holt, M.D.** Department of Neurology, Lucile Packard Children's Hospital at Stanford, Palo Alto, CA, USA

**William Hong, M.D., M.S.E** Division of Neurology and Developmental Neuroscience, Department of Pediatrics, Baylor College of Medicine, Houston, TX, USA

**Kimberly M. Houck** Division of Neurology and Developmental Neuroscience, Department of Pediatrics, Baylor College of Medicine and Texas Children's Hospital, Houston, TX, USA

**Katherine Kedzierski, M.D.** Waterbury Neurology, Middlebury, CT, USA

**Young-Min Kim, M.D.** Department of Pediatrics, Loma Linda University School of Medicine, St. Loma Linda, CA, USA

**Michael A. Lopez, M.D., Ph.D.** Developmental Neuroscience and Department of Pediatrics, Baylor College of Medicine, Texas Children's Hospital, Houston, TX, USA

**Timothy E. Lotze, M.D.** Division of Neurology and Developmental Neuroscience, Department of Pediatrics, Baylor College of Medicine, Texas Children's Hospital, Houston, TX, USA

**Dana Marafie, B.M.B.Ch** Department of Neurology, Baylor College of Medicine, Houston, TX, USA

**Elizabeth A. McQuade, M.D.** Division of Neurology and Developmental Neuroscience, Department of Pediatrics, Baylor College of Medicine, Texas Children's Hospital, Houston, TX, USA

**Bittu Majmudar, M.D.** Department of Neurology, Washington University School of Medicine in St. Louis, St. Louis, MO, USA

**Naila Makhani, M.D., M.P.H** Yale University School of Medicine, Yale New Haven Hospital, New Haven, CT, USA

**Jennifer Martelle Tu, M.D., Ph.D.** Children's National Health System, Department of Neurology, Washington, DC, USA

**Soe S. Mar, M.D.** Department of Neurology, Washington University School of Medicine in St. Louis, St. Louis, MO, USA

**Stephanie Morris, M.D.** Department of Neurology, Washington University School of Medicine in St. Louis, St. Louis, MO, USA

**Sona Narula, M.D.** Division of Neurology, The Children's Hospital of Philadelphia, Philadelphia, PA, USA

Department of Pediatrics and Neurology, Perelman School of Medicine, University of Pennsylvania, Philadelphia, PA, USA

**Jayne M. Ness, M.D., Ph.D.** The Division of Neurology, University of Alabama at Birmingham, Birmingham, AL, USA

**Bardia Nourbakhsh, M.D., M.A.S** University of California San Francisco, San Francisco, CA, USA

Department of Neurology, Johns Hopkins University, Baltimore, MD, USA

**Maryam Nabavi Nouri, M.D.** Department of Pediatrics, Division of Neurology, The Hospital for Sick Children, University of Toronto, Toronto, ON, Canada

**Yulia Y. Orlova, M.D., Ph.D.** University of Florida College of Medicine, McKnight Brain Institute, Neurology Department, Gainesville, FL, USA

**Sita Paudel, M.D.** Pediatric Neurology, Sanford Children's Hospital, Sioux Falls, SD, USA

**Carlos Quintanilla Bordás, M.D.** Department of Neurology, Consorcio Hospital General Universitario de Valencia, Valencia, Spain

**Juan Ramos Canseco, M.D.** Neurology, Rutgers – Robert Wood Johnson Medical School, New Brunswick, NJ, USA

**Geetanjali Singh Rathore, M.B.B.S., M.D.** Pediatric Neurology, University of Nebraska Medical Center, Children's Hospital and Medical Center, Omaha, NE, USA

**Jennifer P. Rubin, M.D.** Ann and Robert H. Lurie Children's Hospital of Chicago, Chicago, IL, USA

**Robert Rudock, M.D., M.B.A.** Division of Pediatric and Developmental Neurology, Department of Neurology, Washington University in St. Louis School of Medicine, St. Louis, MO, USA

**Parisa Sabetrasekh, M.D.** Department of Neurology, Children's National Medical Center, Washington, DC, USA

**Tristan T. Sands, M.D., Ph.D.** Division of Child Neurology, Columbia University Herbert and Florence Irving Medical Center, New York, NY, USA

**Teri L. Schreiner, M.D., M.P.H** Department of Neurology and Pediatrics, Children's Hospital Colorado, University of Colorado-Denver, Aurora, CO, USA

**Robert I. Thompson-Stone, M.D.** University of Rochester Medical Center, Rochester, NY, USA

**Y. Daisy Tang, M.D.** Advocare Sinatra and Peng Pediatrics, West Orange, NJ, USA

**Stuart Tomko, M.D.** Division of Neurology and Developmental Neuroscience, Department of Pediatrics, Baylor College of Medicine, Texas Children's Hospital, Houston, TX, USA

Division of Neurology and Developmental Neuroscience, Department of Pediatrics, Baylor College of Medicine/Texas Children's Hospital, Houston, TX, USA

**Nicole Ulrick, B.A** Department of Neurology and Center for Genetic Medicine Research, Children's National Medical Center, Washington, DC, USA

**Adeline Vanderver, M.D.** Children Hospital of Pennsylvania, Philadelphia, PA, USA

**Keith Van Haren, M.D.** Department of Neurology, Lucile Packard Children's Hospital and Stanford University School of Medicine, Palo Alto, CA, USA

**Wendy Vargas, M.D.** Department of Child Neurology, Morgan Stanley Children's Hospital of New York, Columbia University Medical Center, New York, NY, USA

**Amy T. Waldman, M.D., M.S.C.E.** Division of Neurology, The Children's Hospital of Philadelphia, Philadelphia, PA, USA

**Adam D. Wallace, M.D.** Department of Neurology and Pediatrics, Children's Hospital Colorado, University of Colorado-Denver, Aurora, CO, USA

**Emmanuelle Waubant, M.D., Ph.D.** Clinical Neurology and Pediatrics, Regional Pediatric MS Clinic at UCSF, University of California San Francisco, San Francisco, CA, USA

**Bianca Weinstock-Guttman, M.D.** Department of Neurology, State University of New York at Buffalo, Buffalo, NY, USA

**Pamela F. Weiss, M.D., M.S.C.E** Division of Pediatric Rheumatology, The Children's Hospital of Philadelphia, Philadelphia, PA, USA

Department of Pediatrics, Perelman School of Medicine, University of Pennsylvania, Philadelphia, PA, USA

**Anusha K. Yeshokumar, M.D.** Mount Sinai in NYC, Jamaica, NY, USA

# Part I
# Diseases That Affect the Brain

# Chapter 1
# Acute Disseminated Encephalomyelitis

Gulay Alper

## Case Presentation

A 4-year-old boy with no past medical history presented to the emergency room with a 4-day history of progressive weakness and sleepiness. His parents initially noticed drooling followed by weakness and difficulty walking. On the day of admission, he was noted to have asymmetry of the face and left-sided arm and leg weakness. In addition, he had altered mental status alternating between lethargy and aggressive behaviors. There was no history of recent illness, immunization, or trauma. No family history of autoimmune disorders was reported.

Upon admission he was lethargic with intermittent irritability but responded to simple commands. There were no meningeal signs. His cranial nerve examination showed flattening of the nasolabial fold on the left side. There was no afferent pupillary defect. He demonstrated left-sided weakness of the upper and lower extremities with an ipsilateral extensor plantar response. Strength in the right arm and leg was normal. Due to the weakness, the patient had difficulty performing finger-to-nose testing on the left and was unable to walk. No sensory deficits were noted, and there was no truncal or appendicular ataxia.

An initial head CT showed parenchymal hypodensities in the thalamus and some gray and white matter involvement. An MRI brain was then performed and showed extensive T2 hyperintense white matter lesions extending from the subcortical white matter of bilateral peri-rolandic areas to the centrum semiovale. There was a large right hemispheric white matter lesion extending from the internal capsule to the brainstem involving the right cerebral peduncle as well as the ventral portion of the pons and tegmentum (Fig. 1.1). This lesion additionally extended across the splenium of the corpus callosum. There was expansion of the right cerebral peduncle

G. Alper, M.D. (✉)
Division of Child Neurology, Department of Pediatrics, Children's Hospital of Pittsburgh,
University of Pittsburgh School of Medicine, 4401 Penn Avenue, Pittsburgh, PA 15224, USA
e-mail: Gulay.Alper@chp.edu

© Springer International Publishing AG 2017                                                    3
E. Waubant, T.E. Lotze (eds.), *Pediatric Demyelinating Diseases of the Central
Nervous System and Their Mimics*, DOI 10.1007/978-3-319-61407-6_1

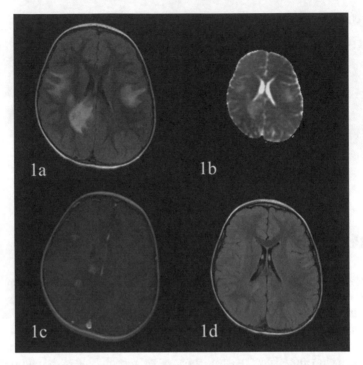

**Fig. 1.1** (**a**) Axial T2-weighted FLAIR image reveals extensive white matter signal hyperintensity extending from the subcortical white matter of the peri-rolandic areas to the centrum semiovale, with T2 prolongation also seen across the corpus callosum. (**b**) Diffusion studies show increased diffusivity of the involved areas. (**c**) T1-weighted imaging demonstrates heterogeneous enhancement pattern. (**d**) Follow-up T2-weighted FLAIR image obtained 3 months after onset shows almost-complete resolution of lesions

and the right thalamus with some mass effect seen in the right centrum semiovale. However, there was no midline shift or effacement of the ventricles. There was no diffusion restriction to suggest ischemic injury. MRA of the circle of Willis and neck arteries did not show any evidence for vasculopathy or stenosis. After the administration of gadolinium, there were areas of ill-defined nonhomogeneous enhancement in the lesions affecting the right parietal juxtacortical and periventricular white matter, right cerebral peduncle, and left temporal region. Gadolinium-enhanced MRI of the entire spine was normal. An EEG demonstrated background slowing with no epileptiform discharges.

Cerebrospinal fluid (CSF) examination showed a white cell count of $11/mm^3$ (with lymphocyte predominance), protein of 40 mg/dL, glucose of 47 mg/dL, normal IgG index (0.44), and no oligoclonal bands. CSF PCR for herpes simplex virus was negative.

Peripheral white cell count, comprehensive metabolic panel, erythrocyte sedimentation rate, and CRP were normal. Serology was negative for Lyme disease. Serum meningoencephalitis panel was unremarkable. NMO-IgG (aquaporin-4 antibody), antinuclear antibody, thyroid antibodies, anticardiolipin antibodies, and autoimmune markers for systemic rheumatological disorders were negative. Serum levels of ACE, ferritin, LDH, lactate, and pyruvate were normal.

The patient was diagnosed with acute disseminated encephalomyelitis (ADEM) and was treated with IV methylprednisolone 30 mg/kg/day for 5 days followed by an oral corticosteroid taper over 5 weeks. Through the hospital course, his condition significantly improved. At discharge, 5 days after his presentation, his facial weakness had nearly completely resolved; he had regained the ability to perform fine motor tasks with his left hand, and he was able to ambulate independently without signs of left lower extremity weakness.

Follow-up MRI obtained 3 months later showed significant improvement (Fig. 1.1). The patient has been relapse-free for over 7 years, and serial MRIs obtained during the follow-up did not show any new lesions.

## Clinical Questions

1. What are the current diagnostic criteria for ADEM?
2. How does the acuity of symptom development help to distinguish ADEM from other diseases of the central nervous system?
3. What are typical MRI features of ADEM, and how do these distinguish ADEM from other diseases of the central nervous system?
4. How does CSF examination help with the differential diagnosis?
5. What is the treatment for ADEM?
6. Why is it important to obtain serial follow-up MRIs to establish the diagnosis of ADEM?

## Diagnostic Discussion

1. ADEM is better considered as a syndrome, rather than a specific disorder, as the presentation is heterogeneous. In 2013, the International Pediatric Multiple Sclerosis Study Group (IPMSSG) published revisions to the initial 2007 diagnostic criteria for various acquired demyelinating diseases of childhood to include ADEM [1]. The diagnostic criteria for ADEM are:

   - A first polyfocal, clinical CNS event with presumed inflammatory demyelinating cause.
   - Encephalopathy (persistent alteration in consciousness or behavior change) that cannot be explained by fever, systemic illness, or postictal symptoms.
   - No new clinical and MRI findings emerge 3 months or more after the onset.
   - Brain MRI is abnormal during the acute (within the first 3 months) phase.
   - Typical findings on brain MRI:

- Diffuse, poorly demarcated, large (>1–2 cm) lesions involving predominantly the cerebral white matter.
- T1 hypointense lesions in the white matter are rare.
- Deep gray matter lesions (e.g., thalamus or basal ganglia) can be present.

Rarely, children with ADEM have an isolated relapse of the syndrome, which occurs beyond the initial 3 months of the first presentation and must again meet the above diagnostic criteria to determine a multiphasic ADEM diagnosis. Further relapses are exceedingly rare and should prompt consideration for an alternate diagnosis.

2. This child presented with acute neurological symptoms, which continued to progress over 4–5 days. Onset was gradual over a period of days rather than abrupt and, therefore, not highly suggestive of acute ischemic stroke. Neoplasms of the central nervous system usually present with a subacute course, meaning that symptoms worsen gradually over a few weeks or months, rather than days. Leukodystrophies more often present over even longer periods with no acute exacerbations. Acute inflammatory demyelination should be considered in any child presenting with acute onset of focal or multifocal neurological findings.

The time course of a first attack would not necessarily be able to distinguish ADEM from other forms of acquired demyelination, such as MS or NMO. In this regard, the clinical history, examination findings, and ancillary diagnostic studies can better discern between these various conditions. A principal and required diagnostic feature of ADEM is encephalopathy. While encephalopathy is less often encountered in the acute presentation of MS or NMO, pediatric MS patients under the age of 10 years may uncommonly present with an ADEM phenotype as their initial attack. Likewise, the expanding phenotypic spectrum of NMO can present with cerebral and/or brainstem symptoms causing altered mental status and mimicking ADEM. Therefore, initial investigation results of serum antibody studies and CSF as well as long-term follow-up are needed to best assure a final diagnosis of ADEM

3. In a child presenting with focal or multifocal neurological signs and symptoms, imaging studies should be obtained immediately. Magnetic resonance imaging is the best diagnostic tool for acquired demyelinating disorders. Although this patient presented with unilateral weakness, his encephalopathy suggested a more extensive involvement, and brain imaging demonstrated bilateral and multifocal abnormalities (Fig. 1.1a). Symptomatic and asymptomatic lesions are frequently seen on imaging studies in acute demyelination. Symptoms are determined mainly by the location and/or the size of the lesion(s). ADEM predominantly affects white matter tracts of the brain but, in contrast to MS, also commonly involves the deep gray matter of the thalami, and basal ganglia are also frequently involved [2]. The lesions in ADEM typically involve the cortex, juxtacortical, and central white matter as well as the cerebellum, brainstem, and spinal cord [2]. Although the lesions are bilateral, they are characteristically asymmetric. Lesions in ADEM tend to be larger than those seen in multiple

sclerosis, and their borders are less well defined in contrast to MS lesions, which are well circumscribed, ovoid, and oriented perpendicular to the ventricular margin. Occasionally, MS can present with an "ADEM-like" clinical and MRI phenotype in very young children [3]. However, in the case presented, the complete resolution of T2 hyperintense lesions and the absence of any further attacks or new lesions in the 7 years following the isolated event support a diagnosis of ADEM over MS.

Gadolinium enhancement is reported in up to 30% of ADEM lesions and may have an ill-defined, nonhomogeneous appearance [2]. In contrast, with multiple sclerosis, there is either homogenous lesion enhancement or a "broken ring" of enhancement at the rim of the lesion. Cerebral abscesses show a complete ring of enhancement around the rim of the lesion and often show diffusion restriction within the lesion.

In NMO, lesions often follow the distribution of aquaporin-4 (AQP4)-rich areas in the brain [4]. NMO lesions are often longitudinally extensive in their course along the optic nerves, corticospinal tracts, or spinal cord. They can have an amorphous appearance with ill-defined contrast enhancement, similar to ADEM. NMO might be considered less likely for the case presented in the absence of optic nerve and spinal cord disease, but the emerging spectrum of this disease to include cerebral and brainstem syndromes requires serologic testing for AQP4 antibodies as well as clinical and neuroimaging follow-up to rule out this diagnosis.

Although not common, white matter lesions have been reported in some cases of lupus cerebritis and autoimmune encephalitis with neuronal antibodies (such as anti-NMDA receptor encephalitis). The child had negative markers for rheumatological disorders and no systemic symptoms, as would typically be expected in these diseases. At the time this child presented, NMDA-receptor antibodies associated with autoimmune encephalitis were not clinically available, but the clinical presentation was not typical for this condition, as it lacked symptoms of psychosis, movement disorder, and seizures. In addition, the presence of such dramatic lesions involving both the gray and white matter on MRI would be unusual for NMDA-receptor antibody encephalitis.

Absence of restricted diffusion and normal vascular imaging on MRA in this case helps to rule out ischemic stroke. Vasogenic edema with increased diffusivity on ADC sequence is frequently found in ADEM lesions (Fig. 1.1b) [5]. Less frequently, restricted diffusion is seen in the hyperacute phase and in tumefactive demyelination with rapidly developing and enlarging lesions.

Spinal cord involvement has been described in up to 1/3 of ADEM patients, often demonstrating large confluent lesions extending over multiple segments, sometimes associated with cord swelling. As previously noted, longitudinally extensive spinal cord involvement is typical of NMO, and antibody testing plus follow-up are needed to discount this diagnosis. Imaging of the spinal cord should be performed routinely in ADEM, as a severe encephalopathy may mask underlying signs and symptoms of an underlying myelopathy, which can be associated with complications to include urinary retention and hemodynamic instability. In addition, it helps to define the burden of disease and guide rehabilitation.

4. While there was no fever or meningeal signs to suggest meningitis in this child, these symptoms may occur in ADEM, and CNS infection must be ruled out in the early course of evaluation. Encephalopathy, particularly mild irritability or somnolence, is a required (but nonspecific) diagnostic criterion for ADEM. While encephalopathy is a useful clinical feature to distinguish ADEM from the first attack of multiple sclerosis, it would not help to differentiate from encephalitis. CSF should be obtained to rule out encephalitis and meningoencephalitis. In this child, CSF findings do not support bacterial meningitis. CSF typically shows a lymphocytic pleocytosis in ADEM. It would be unusual to have pleocytosis in metabolic or neoplastic disorders, aside from CNS lymphoma. HSV encephalitis should be ruled out, and empirical treatment with acyclovir is frequently recommended in children presenting with focal neurological findings until CSF HSV PCR returns negative results. CSF oligoclonal bands are uncommon in ADEM, occurring in a small percentage of such patients, unlike pediatric multiple sclerosis, in which their presence is nearly ubiquitous.

5. There have been no randomized controlled trials for the treatment of ADEM. High-dose intravenous methylprednisolone is the first-line treatment choice for acute disseminated encephalomyelitis. The aim is to abbreviate the CNS inflammation to achieve and accelerate clinical improvement. Most physicians use 20–30 mg/kg/day (maximum 1000 mg/day) for 3–5 days, and this regimen often results in dramatic improvement. An oral prednisone taper over 2–6 weeks is usually administered. The prednisone taper is typically started at a lower initial dose compared with the intravenous regimen. Typically oral prednisone is started at a dosing of 1 mg/kg per day up to a maximum of 60 mg per day, and then the dose is reduced by 10 mg every 5 days to allow for a total tapering duration of 4–6 weeks.

   Other anti-inflammatory and immunosuppressive treatments such as intravenous immunoglobulin (2 g/kg divided over 5 days) have been reported with beneficial effects. Plasma exchange is recommended for severe or fulminant cases refractory to initial steroid treatment. Additional supportive treatment during the acute phase includes airway support, seizure management, and monitoring for complications of neurogenic bladder with urinary retention.

6. Serial MRIs demonstrating complete or near-complete resolution of lesions in the absence of new foci are the best confirmation of an ADEM diagnosis in retrospect. Patients may have residual gliosis from the initial event, but they should not develop new lesions beyond 3 months from the initial attack. The development of new lesions on repeat MRI should prompt the clinician to reconsider the diagnosis of a possible relapsing acquired demyelinating disease.

## Clinical Pearls

1. In a child presenting with acute neurological findings with an MRI brain demonstrating multifocal, bilateral asymmetric lesions, acute demyelination is the most likely diagnosis.
2. A diagnosis of ADEM requires the presence of specific clinical criteria to include encephalopathy. Neuroimaging of the brain and spinal cord is supportive of the diagnosis, and the clinical symptoms are determined by the location of the lesions in the central nervous system.
3. Acute management of ADEM with corticosteroids hastens recovery of neurologic deficits. Refractory cases may benefit from additional treatment with either IVIG or therapeutic plasma exchange.
4. As ADEM is a diagnosis of exclusion, patients should be investigated for alternate diagnoses to include infection, vascular disease, and autoimmune disease. More extensive investigations may be needed for metabolic disorders in patients with atypical presentations.
5. Serial MRIs obtained during follow-up are important to rule out relapsing inflammatory disorders of the CNS. Complete lesion resolution or residual gliosis from the original attack with no new lesions further confirms ADEM. The development of new lesions beyond 3 months is not a characteristic of ADEM and should prompt investigation for an alternate diagnosis.

## References

1. Krupp LB, Tardieu M, Amato MP, et al. International pediatric multiple sclerosis study group criteria for pediatric multiple sclerosis and immune-mediated central nervous system demyelinating disorders: revisions to the 2007 definitions. Mult Scler. 2013;19;1261–7.
2. Tenembaum S, Chitnis T, Ness J, Hahn JS, for the International Pediatric MS Study Group. Acute disseminated encephalomyelitis. Neurology. 2007;68(Issue 16, Supplement 2):S23–36.
3. Chabas D, Krupp LB, Tardieu M. Chapter 2: controversies around the current operational definitions of pediatric MS, ADEM, and related disorders. In: Chabas D, Waubant E, editors. Demyelinating disorders of the central nervous system in childhood. New York: Cambridge University Press; 2011. p. 10–7.
4. McKeon A, Lennon VA, Lotze T, et al. CNS aquaporin-4 autoimmunity in children. Neurology. 2008;71:93–100.
5. Zuccoli G, Panigrahy A, Laney EJ IV, et al. Vasogenic edema characterizes pediatric acute disseminated encephalomyelitis. Neuroradiology. 2014;56:679–84.

# Chapter 2
# Acute Necrotizing Encephalopathy Mimicking ADEM

Gulay Alper

## Case Presentation

A 3-year-old girl presented in status epilepticus. At the time of presentation, she had no notable past medical history and was well until 1 day prior to admission when she awoke with an elevated temperature (39.4 °C). At that time, she also had rhinorrhea and cough. Throughout the day, her parents noted decreased energy and physical activity. In the evening of the first day of her illness, the patient's father found her unresponsive and noted generalized muscle rigidity with both arms extended. She was taken to an outside hospital where examination noted decerebrate posturing, rotatory nystagmus, and urinary incontinence. Initial evaluation with brain CT showed bilateral thalamic hypodensities. Cerebrospinal fluid was reportedly normal. For initial stabilization, she was intubated, treated with intravenous phenytoin and ceftriaxone, and transferred to a tertiary care center where she was admitted to the pediatric intensive care unit.

Initial evaluation showed a comatose child with decerebrate posturing after stimulation. Deep tendon reflexes were brisk in all extremities, and plantar response was extensor bilaterally. EEG obtained on admission showed numerous electrographic seizures without clinical correlate occurring independently from bilateral posterior regions. The background electrographic activity was slow and disorganized.

Gadolinium-enhanced brain MRI obtained on admission was most notable for diffuse hyperintense T2 signal and marked swelling in the thalami bilaterally (Fig. 2.1). There was also hyperintense T2 signal in the cortex of the frontal, posterior parietal, and occipital lobes. Additional hyperintense T2 signal was seen within the brainstem involving the midbrain and the pons. There was no enhancement of the lesions. The diffusion-weighted images delineated small foci of restricted

G. Alper, M.D. (✉)
Division of Child Neurology, Department of Pediatrics, Children's Hospital of Pittsburgh,
University of Pittsburgh School of Medicine, 4401 Penn Avenue, Pittsburgh, PA 15224, USA
e-mail: Gulay.Alper@chp.edu

© Springer International Publishing AG 2017                                                    11
E. Waubant, T.E. Lotze (eds.), *Pediatric Demyelinating Diseases of the Central Nervous System and Their Mimics*, DOI 10.1007/978-3-319-61407-6_2

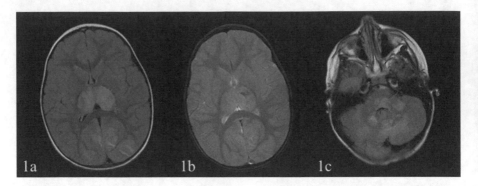

**Fig. 2.1** (**a**) T2-weighted FLAIR image demonstrates marked swelling and diffuse symmetric signal abnormality of bilateral thalami and occipital cortex. (**b**) The MPGR sequence delineates patchy foci of hypointensity in the left thalamus suggesting microhemorrhage. (**c**) The T2-weighted FLAIR image demonstrates multiple signal abnormalities in the brainstem and cerebellum

diffusion in the thalami and bilateral occipital lobes. The multiple planar gradient recalled (MPGR) sequence demonstrated small patchy foci of hypointensity in the left thalamus suggesting microhemorrhage. Brain MRA and MRV studies were normal.

Repeat CSF examination on admission showed zero white cells, one red blood cell, elevated protein 77 mg/dL, and normal glucose 70 mg/dL. IgG index was elevated at 0.78 (normal < 0.7), and no oligoclonal bands were seen. She had normal serum lactate, ammonia, amino acids, acylcarnitine, LDH, ACE, and ferritin as well as normal urine organic acids. Antibody studies for ANA, ANCA, SSA, SSB, NMO-IgG, thyroid peroxidase, and thyroglobulin were negative. Mutation analysis of mtDNA polymerase (*POLG*) was normal.

The patient was initially treated with high-dose intravenous corticosteroids for a presumed diagnosis of ADEM. After consulting with neuroimmunology, acute necrotizing encephalopathy (ANE) was alternatively suspected, and testing for influenza and other respiratory viruses was recommended. Nasopharyngeal swab PCR testing was positive for influenza A. There was otherwise no bacterial or fungal growth in the blood and cerebrospinal fluid cultures. Based upon the clinical history, MRI findings, and positive influenza A test, she was diagnosed to have ANE. In addition to corticosteroids, she received IVIG 2 g/kg as well as antiviral treatment with oseltamivir.

Throughout her hospitalization, she remained quite somnolent and developed generalized spasticity with dystonia. Her EEG obtained 3 weeks from her presentation showed severe background slowing but no epileptiform features. Following her acute treatment, she spent several months in the inpatient rehabilitation unit and continued to make some improvements in her neurological function. By 6 months from the time of her presentation, her speech was fluent, but she remained with intellectual deficits, right hemiparesis, and generalized dystonia and was not able to ambulate without assistance.

## Clinical Questions

1. What is acute necrotizing encephalopathy?
2. What are the similarities and differences of clinical presentation between ADEM and ANE?
3. What are the atypical imaging features for ADEM in this case?
4. How does the prognosis differ between ANE and ADEM?

## Diagnostic Discussion

1. Acute necrotizing encephalopathy (ANE) is a rare but distinctive disorder characterized by fever, seizures, and rapid progression to coma just after the onset of a viral infection. The first cases were initially reported in Asia by Mizuguchi et al. with several additional cases subsequently described worldwide [1]. The MRI hallmark is represented by symmetrical lesions in the thalami, brainstem tegmentum, cerebellum, and periventricular white matter. Marked involvement of bilateral thalami is a distinctive feature of ANE and is often accompanied by microhemorrhages. Additional lesions may involve the cortical and deep gray matter as well as the deep white matter and spinal cord [2]. Another distinguishing feature of ANE is the presence of deep and cortical gray matter microhemorrhages, which tend to spare the white matter [3]. The T2-weighted gradient echo imaging or the susceptibility-weighted imaging (SWI) is particularly useful in demonstrating these petechial hemorrhages in ANE.

   Although the exact pathogenesis of ANE remains obscure, the most prevalent hypothesis is that individuals suffering from ANE often have an exaggerated immune response to various viral infections by producing elevated pro-inflammatory cytokines resembling systemic inflammatory response syndrome (SIRS) [2]. The "cytokine storm" results in systemic symptoms, such as liver dysfunction, acute renal failure, shock, and disseminated intravascular coagulation. In the central nervous system, it leads to brain injury through alteration of blood vessel wall permeability without wall disruption [2].

   Most cases of ANE are sporadic; however, the observation of multiple cases in the same family with recurrent episodes of ANE led to the identification of a genetic form of the disorder, called ANE1, and to the discovery of the causative mutation in *RANBP2* [4]. A nuclear pore protein, Ran-binding protein 2, is encoded by the gene and has numerous roles throughout the cell cycle. In neurons, it is detected in association with microtubules and/or mitochondria, suggesting roles in intracellular trafficking or energy metabolism [4]. It may also affect other processes including viral entry, antigen presentation, cytokine signaling, immune responses, and blood-brain barrier maintenance [4].

2. Although ANE and ADEM both occur in children, there are some differences. ANE tends to have a higher occurrence in infants compared to ADEM. Whereas

ADEM typically develops during the postinfectious period up to several days after the initial signs and symptoms of infection have resolved, ANE occurs during the early febrile period of the viral infection and runs a fulminant course with the rapid development of coma, as demonstrated in the presented case. Further distinction of ANE from entities such as viral encephalitis can be clinically difficult. However, in contrast to CNS infection and most cases of ADEM, ANE tends not to have a CSF pleocytosis [2, 5].

3. The necrotizing nature of the lesions reflected by the presence of petechial or microhemorrhages in the deep and cortical gray matter and symmetric involvement of bilateral thalamic structures should be considered as atypical for ADEM in this patient. Bi-thalamic involvement is seen in 100% of the patients with ANE. In contrast, it only occurs in 30–50% of ADEM patients and is usually asymmetric [6]. Another distinguishing feature of ANE, rarely seen in ADEM, is the presence of microhemorrhages on MRI. These are consistent with the pathophysiological cascade from edema to petechial hemorrhage and resulting cell necrosis and cavitation [2]. It is uncommon for lesions in ADEM to have such a degree of necrosis, as most of the lesions in this disease do not have hemorrhage and tend to demonstrate complete resolution on follow-up MRI.

4. ADEM overall has a favorable prognosis with a complete recovery rate reported in 57–94% of patients [6]. In contrast to ADEM, the neurological outcome of ANE has been reported to be very poor. It has an estimated mortality rate of about 30%, and less than 10% of patients recover completely [2]. The genetic form of acute necrotizing encephalopathy is fatal in some patients. However, the majority recovers but may experience varying degrees of neurodevelopmental impairments to include cognitive and motor difficulties [7]. Approximately 50% of patients will experience a recurrent encephalopathy that often results in further neurodevelopmental disabilities.

## Clinical Pearls

1. In ANE, CSF analysis typically shows no pleocytosis, but CSF protein can be markedly elevated.
2. Microhemorrhages and symmetric bi-thalamic lesions are frequently seen in ANE, which are not typical of ADEM.
3. While ADEM has near-complete resolution with a favorable clinical prognosis, ANE lesions usually leave significant sequela characterized by severe neurological deficits.
4. It is important to consider the relapsing genetic form of ANE secondary to pathologic mutations in *RANBP2*, particularly in infants who continue to have relapses without recovering completely.

# References

1. Mizuguchi M, Abe J, Mikkaichi K, et al. Acute necrotising encephalopathy of childhood: a new syndrome presenting with multifocal, symmetric brain lesions. J Neurol Neurosurg Psychiatry. 1995;58:555–61.
2. Wu X, Wu W, Pan W, et al. Acute necrotizing encephalopathy: an underrecognized clinicoradiologic disorder. Mediat Inflamm. 2015;1–10.
3. Wong AM, Simon EM, Zimmerman RA, et al. Acute necrotizing encephalopathy of childhood: correlation of MR findings and clinical outcome. AJNR Am J Neuroradiol. 2006;27:1919–23.
4. Neilson DE, Adams MD, Orr CMD, et al. Infection-triggered familial or recurrent cases of acute necrotizing encephalopathy by mutations in a component of the nuclear pore, RANBP2. Am J Hum Genet. 2009;84:44–51.
5. Bergamino L, Capra V, Biancheri R, et al. Immunomodulatory therapy in recurrent acute necrotizing encephalopathy ANE1. Brain and Development. 2012;34:384–91.
6. Tenembaum S, Chitnis T, Ness J, for the International Pediatric MS Study Group. Acute disseminated encephalomyelitis. Neurology. 2007;68(Suppl 2):S23–36.
7. Neilson DE, Heidi S, Feiler HS, et al. Autosomal dominant acute necrotizing encephalopathy maps to 2q12.1-2q13. Ann Neurol. 2004;55:291–4.

# Chapter 3
# Pediatric Multiple Sclerosis Manifesting with Primary Psychiatric Symptoms

Stuart Tomko and Timothy E. Lotze

## Case Presentation

A 14-year-old boy with a history of attention-deficit/hyperactivity disorder (ADHD) diagnosed in the first grade with good response to methylphenidate and recent-onset headaches presented with acute-onset behavioral changes. Per his mother, he initially displayed symptoms of depression and paranoia around age 10 years old, though it did not impact his functioning, and he did not seek treatment or receive formal diagnoses at that time. At 13 years old, he developed headaches and was diagnosed with migraine with aura, which was managed with over-the-counter pain medication. An MRI brain done at that time demonstrated two non-enhancing hyperintense T2 lesions (Fig. 3.1). No further work-up was performed.

He presented for an initial psychiatric evaluation at 14 years old with acute onset of an overwhelming preoccupation of hell, salvation, and sinfulness after visiting a place of worship. At the time of initial presentation, he was rambling with nonsensical speech, tearful, paranoid, and preoccupied with death and was not eating or sleeping. He was admitted to an inpatient psychiatric unit with a diagnosis of bipolar disorder with psychosis. He was started on risperidone and paroxetine. During

S. Tomko, M.D. (✉) • T.E. Lotze, M.D.
Division of Neurology and Developmental Neuroscience, Department of Pediatrics, Baylor College of Medicine, Texas Children's Hospital, 6701 Fannon CC 1250, Houston, TX 77030, USA
e-mail: sttomko@gmail.com; tlotze@bcm.edu

© Springer International Publishing AG 2017
E. Waubant, T.E. Lotze (eds.), *Pediatric Demyelinating Diseases of the Central Nervous System and Their Mimics*, DOI 10.1007/978-3-319-61407-6_3

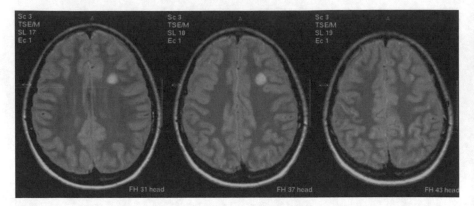

**Fig. 3.1** Selected axial fluid-attenuated inversion recovery sequences demonstrating increased T2 signal consistent with demyelinating plaques

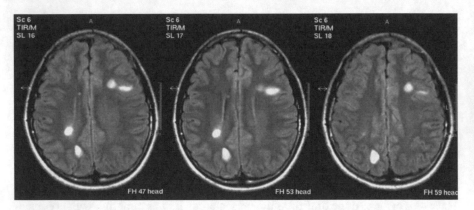

**Fig. 3.2** Selected axial fluid-attenuated inversion recovery sequences demonstrating increased T2 signal consistent with demyelinating plaques

the admission he began complaining of blurry vision, numbness in his face, drooling, and his "legs giving out." The risperidone was discontinued, and he became elated, sleepless, irritable, destructive, and convinced that God was touching him and speaking directly to him. Quetiapine was started, but his behaviors progressed to threats of killing classmates and blowing up his school and sexually provocative statements toward women, all of which were markedly different from his previous affect. Quetiapine was increased, but behaviors deteriorated further, and he endorsed seeing horns and wings growing out of his head and back and feeling God walking in his feet and started cutting crosses into his own trunk.

Approximately 5 months after his psychiatric symptoms began, he presented for neurological evaluation. A complete neurological examination at the time of presentation was normal. Given the prior history and MRI findings suggestive of an acquired demyelinating syndrome, a lumbar puncture was performed which revealed a white blood cell count of 1 cell/μL, red blood cell count of 288 cells/μL, protein

24 mg/dL, glucose 56 mg/dL, and more than two oligoclonal bands. A repeat MRI later demonstrated new hyperintense T2 lesions (Fig. 3.2). Rheumatologic studies to include testing for lupus cerebritis and antiphospholipid antibodies were negative. He was diagnosed with relapsing-remitting multiple sclerosis (MS) based on McDonald criteria, to include his previous facial sensory and leg symptoms and MRI findings (dissemination in time).

Given the apparent relationship between the onset of his psychiatric symptoms and the diagnosis of multiple sclerosis, consideration was given for his mood disorder to relate to an acute inflammatory attack. In addition, he had a poor initial response to psycho-pharmacotherapy with ziprasidone and valproic acid. As such, a course of intravenous methylprednisolone 1000 mg IV daily for 4 days was attempted. His psychosis only worsened with this treatment, and it had to be discontinued.

Glatiramer acetate 20 mg daily was chosen as a first-line therapy secondary to concerns for an interferon potentially worsening his mood disorder. Over the subsequent 4 years of follow-up, his psychiatric disorder was further stabilized with the addition to his regimen of lithium by his psychiatrist. His multiple sclerosis symptoms had good control with a total of two relapses in that interval to include one episode of optic neuritis and a second event characterized by right hemisensory loss. These were effectively treated with intravenous gamma globulin 2 g/kg divided over 5 days. He recovered well from both events and did not acquire any fixed disability. Follow-up imaging studies also showed good control of his disease with accrual of only two new lesions in the cerebral white matter over the 4 years.

## Clinical Questions

1. How often are primary psychiatric symptoms seen at MS presentation?
2. In what ways might MS present with primary psychiatric symptoms?
3. In what types of patients with psychiatric symptoms should MS be considered?
4. Are there special considerations in the work-up of patients presenting with psychiatric symptoms in whom there is concern for an organic etiology?
5. What are considerations in the management and prognosis of patients with primary psychiatric MS?

## Diagnostic Discussion

1. Though the rate of neuropsychiatric comorbidity in MS is higher than in other chronic or neurological conditions [1], the number of MS patients with primary psychiatric symptoms preceding physical symptoms has not been clearly defined. Most information at the time of publishing is limited to case reports or small case series. Available case reports include both adults and children in whom MS presented initially with psychiatric symptoms suggesting that this presentation is not

limited to a certain age group. A retrospective study reported 2.3% of patients had a comorbid psychiatric condition before or at the time of initial MS diagnosis suggesting that primary psychiatric presentation is relatively rare [2]. Another study, however, reported 63% of patients meet diagnostic criteria for a mood disorder before or soon after initial MS diagnosis, suggesting that these comorbidities may be quite common on initial presentation of MS, though they may not directly lead to diagnosis [3]. Notably, in patients with an initial psychiatric presentation, worsening of their psychiatric symptoms may represent relapse, and immune therapy in addition to psychiatric management should be considered.

2. Theoretically, any psychiatric symptom associated with MS may be the presenting symptom of MS. In general, MS patients are much more likely to experience mood disorders such as depression, bipolar disorder, and anxiety than psychotic symptoms, but psychosis seems to be overly represented in the literature as a presenting psychiatric phenotype. The higher frequency of MS presenting with psychosis, however, may in part be due to patient with dramatic new-onset psychotic features receiving more thorough evaluation than those presenting with depression or anxiety. A "cognitive presentation" of MS including prominent amnesia, often accompanied by dysphasia, dysgraphia, or dyslexia, has also been reported in a small cohort of patients [4]. In addition, a wide variety of mood disorder, pseudobulbar affect, frank psychosis, confabulations, paranoid ideas, irritability, pathologically increased libido, alcohol and substance abuse, and dementia have been reported sporadically in MS patients and may be presenting symptoms.

3. As psychiatric symptoms are not usually attributed to an organic etiology, a high index of suspicion in patients presenting with new onset of such symptoms is required. Also, most of the time, the exact nature of the relationship between a psychiatric comorbid condition and MS remains unclear (i.e., whether related in terms of pathogenesis or unrelated). Of those reported patients with a primary psychiatric presentation of MS, several additional symptoms suggested an organic etiology. Perhaps the most obvious is an abnormal neurological examination or history of symptoms suggestive of organic pathology, even if these are "soft" neurological signs not classically associated with MS. For example, our patient presented with new-onset severe headaches, blurry vision, and facial numbness in conjunction with his psychiatric symptoms. Some medical conditions that present with psychiatric symptoms are associated with specific laboratory abnormalities. For example, hyponatremia is often seen in encephalitis associated with antibodies directed toward VGKC complex proteins [5]. Eliciting these findings requires a thorough and targeted history and physical examination, as patients may not offer this information. Other features include acute onset of psychotic or demented features in an otherwise healthy individual with no prodromal phase, atypical features of the considered psychiatric diagnosis, poor response to treatment, and abnormally young age at onset.

4. Initial evaluation is similar to any patient for whom MS or another organic neurological condition is considered. The first step is a very thorough history and physical examination. A brain MRI with and without gadolinium enhancement

should be obtained to evaluate for evidence of previous or active demyelinating lesions. A lumbar puncture to evaluate CSF for oligoclonal bands, elevated IgG index, or pleocytosis is indicated. In addition, CSF may be tested for other possible etiologies such as autoimmune encephalitis including antibodies directed toward NMDAR, GAD, and VGKC, including LGI1 and CASPR2. Serological evaluation for other rheumatologic conditions that can present with neuropsychiatric features, such as systemic lupus erythematosus, Sjögren's syndrome, sarcoidosis, and celiac disease, among others, may be considered. Inborn metabolic conditions such as urea cycle disorders, porphyria, adrenoleukodystrophy, Niemann-Pick type C, and Wilson disease can also present with neuropsychiatric symptoms and should be considered. Regardless of cause, a formal neuropsychiatric evaluation by an experienced evaluator is necessary to determine the pattern of neuropsychiatric dysfunction, which can be helpful in diagnosis, academic modifications, and long-term follow-up after treatment.

5. The mainstay of treatment for acute MS is high-dose intravenous steroids. While high-dose steroids can precipitate or worsen depressive, manic/hypomanic, and psychotic symptoms, the association between worsening psychiatric symptoms and disease-modifying therapies is less clear [6]. Interferons, however, should be used with caution and are relatively contraindicated in patients with psychotic symptoms. In patients with an acute psychiatric presentation of MS, careful monitoring while using steroids is prudent. The psychiatric symptoms are best managed in conjunction with psychiatry services. Though evidence is lacking, both pharmacological and non-pharmacological treatments may be effective in managing neuropsychiatric features of MS and are often used [7]. Atypical antipsychotics, selective serotonin reuptake inhibitors (SSRI) and similar medications for mood disorder, dextromethorphan and quinidine (DM/Q) for pseudobulbar affect have all been used in MS patients. Unfortunately, the neuropsychiatric symptoms do not seem to respond as well as neurological symptoms to high-dose steroid treatment, even with concomitant psychotropic therapy [2]. This questions whether psychiatric symptoms are directly or indirectly related to MS course. Case reports in children also suggest long-term learning difficulties after a psychotic presentation of MS.

## Clinical Pearls

1. Though relatively rare, MS can present with psychiatric symptoms in the absence of neurological signs and should be considered in the differential diagnosis of patients presenting with acute-onset or atypical psychiatric symptoms.
2. Because the spectrum of presentation is so broad, a high index of suspicion for organic etiologies of new-onset psychiatric symptoms is required. Hyperacute onset, lack of prodrome, atypical features, poor response to treatment, and "soft" neurological symptoms are signs of potential organic etiology.

3. In the early stages of evaluation, the differential diagnosis must be kept broad including rheumatologic conditions, autoimmune encephalitis (particularly anti-NMDA encephalitis), inborn errors of metabolism, and other conditions as well as demyelination.
4. Management of MS patients with comorbid psychiatric diagnoses is complex and best approached with a multidisciplinary team. Steroids are not contraindicated but should be used cautiously in these patients. Both non-pharmacological and pharmacological treatment strategies have been used in these patients. Unfortunately, the psychiatric manifestations appear more resistant to treatment than the physical symptoms.

# References

1. Haussleiter IS, Brüne M, Juckel G. Psychopathology in multiple sclerosis: diagnosis, prevalence and treatment. Ther Adv Neurol Disord. 2009;2(1):13–29.
2. Fermo SL, Barone R, Patti F, Laisa P, Cavellaro TL, Nicoletti A, Zappia M. Outcome of psychiatric symptoms presenting at onset of multiple sclerosis: a retrospective study. Mult Scler. 2010;16(6):742–8.
3. Sullivan MJL, Weinshenker B, Mikail S, Edgley K. Depression before and after diagnosis of multiple sclerosis. Mult Scler. 1995;1(2):104–8.
4. Zarei M, Chandran S, Compston A, Hodges J. Cognitive presentation of multiple sclerosis: evidence for a cortical variant. J Neurol Neurosurg Psychiatry. 2003;74(7):872–7.
5. Vincent A, Buckley C, Schott JM, Baker I, Dewar BK, Detert N, Clover L, Parkinson A, Bien CG, Omer S, Lang B, Rossor MN, Palace J. Potassium channel antibody-associated encephalopathy: a potentially immunotherapy-responsive form of limbic encephalitis. Brain. 2004;127(3):701–12.
6. Drozdowicz LB, Bostwick JM. Psychiatric adverse effects of pediatric corticosteroid use. Mayo Clin Proc. 2014;89(6):817–34.
7. Minden SL, Feinstein A, Kalb RC, Miller D, Patten SB, Bever C, Schiffer RB, Gronseth GS, Narayanaswami P. Evidenced-based guideline: assessment and management of psychiatric disorders in individuals with MS. Neurology. 2014;82(2):174–81.

# Chapter 4
# Multiple Sclerosis in the Extremely Young

Y. Daisy Tang and Vikram V. Bhise

## Case Presentation

A 3-year-old girl with no significant past medical history developed URI symptoms and ongoing daily fever followed by ataxia and drowsiness 3 weeks later. On physical examination, the child was somnolent but responsive. She had a right-sided preferential gaze and self-correctable right-sided neck flexion. Extraocular movements were intact. Her examination also showed bilateral non-sustained ankle clonus and right-sided leaning with a steppage gait. Her father had a history of Hashimoto's hypothyroidism.

Serum WBC count was 23,300/μL with a normal differential. Lumbar puncture showed 88 WBCs with 63% neutrophils, 0 RBCs, 41 mg/dL protein, and 47 mg/dL glucose. Four unique oligoclonal bands were present in the CSF. Brain MRI demonstrated multifocal patchy areas of T2 hyperintensity, some of which enhanced, in the subcortical white matter, brainstem, left thalamus, hypothalamus, bilateral cerebellar peduncles, and bilateral cerebellar white matter (Fig. 4.1a and b). Spinal cord imaging was normal.

She was treated with 2 g/kg IVIG divided over 5 days for presumed acute disseminated encephalomyelitis (ADEM) with mild improvement in her symptoms. The patient was discharged to an inpatient subacute rehabilitation facility with improvement to mild residual unsteadiness, dysmetria, and intermittent left eye deviation on discharge. Six weeks after initial presentation, she was readmitted for

Y.D. Tang, M.D.
Advocare, Sinatra and Peng Pediatrics, West Orange, NJ, USA
e-mail: ydaisytang@gmail.com

V.V. Bhise, M.D. (✉)
Pediatrics, Neurology, Rutgers – Robert Wood Johnson Medical School, Child Health Institute, 89 French Street, Suite 2200, New Brunswick, NJ 08901, USA

Division of Child Neurology, Department of Pediatrics, New Brunswick, NJ, USA
e-mail: bhisevi@rwjms.rutgers.edu

© Springer International Publishing AG 2017
E. Waubant, T.E. Lotze (eds.), *Pediatric Demyelinating Diseases of the Central Nervous System and Their Mimics*, DOI 10.1007/978-3-319-61407-6_4

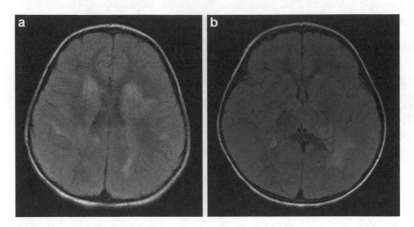

**Fig. 4.1** Initial T2 FLAIR imaging shows multifocal white matter lesions, at times appearing confluent

the reappearance of ataxia. The patient was treated with a 5-day course of IV methylprednisolone 20 mg/kg daily with significant improvement in her symptoms and discharged on an 8-week course of oral prednisone taper. The day after her last dose of prednisone, symptoms of unsteadiness recurred prompting hospital admission again. She was treated with a single dose of IVIG 2 g/kg followed by another 5-day course of IV methylprednisolone 20 mg/kg daily with full clinical recovery on the 4th hospital day. At each admission her brain imaging revealed new or larger hyperintense T2 and gadolinium-enhancing lesions with resolution of old lesions, including new lesions in the splenium of the corpus callosum (Fig. 4.2a and b) and cervical spinal cord spanning five vertebral lengths.

Serum NMO IgG was negative twice; and repeat CSF testing demonstrated 2 oligoclonal bands and 9 WBCs with 66% lymphocytes. Three months after her last episode, she again developed ataxia and was admitted for treatment. MRI showed new hyperintense T2 lesions including bilateral thalamic lesions and a new callosal-enhancing lesion. The patient was diagnosed with relapsing-remitting multiple sclerosis and started on glatiramer acetate 20 mg daily injections and given two additional monthly pulses of IV methylprednisolone 20 mg/kg daily for 3 days. Eight weeks after the initiation of glatiramer acetate, the child has an additional relapse characterized by ataxia followed 6 days later by development of a sixth cranial nerve palsy. She developed new asymptomatic subcortical white matter lesions after 5 months on glatiramer acetate but thereafter remained symptom-free with a normal neurological examination and stable brain and spinal neuroimaging at 9, 12, and 19 months on therapy.

## Clinical Questions

1. What are the features differentiating MS from NMO and ADEM at this age?

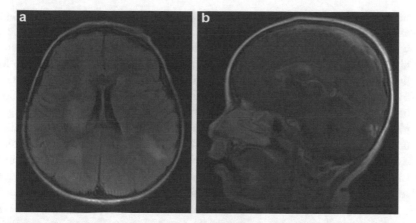

**Fig. 4.2** Repeat imaging from the second hospital admission again shows multifocal white matter lesions but in a different distribution (i.e., some lesions have disappeared, while new lesions are seen). Imaging on the right done 3 months later demonstrates an enhancing lesion in the corpus callosum

2. What is unique about MS in prepubertal children?
3. How frequently do young children with MS experience relapses?
4. What are the expected outcomes for pediatric-onset MS?
5. What is the treatment for relapsing-remitting MS in young children?

## Diagnostic Discussion

1. ADEM is typically a monophasic event but can be indistinguishable from the first manifestation of multiple sclerosis, especially in young children [1]. Patients with ADEM have varied neurological clinical manifestations, including, by definition, changes in mental status and multifocal clinical findings. Multifocal lesions are present on neuroimaging involving both gray and white matter in the supratentorial and infratentorial regions, which most often entirely resolve over time. The basal ganglia, thalami, and spinal cord are also frequently involved. Symptoms may fluctuate within 3 months of symptom onset as part of the initial event. Nevertheless, at least 10% of children with ADEM experience a "multiphasic" episode with new or recurrent symptoms that include encephalopathy 3 or more months after the initial episode. However, as in this case, it may herald a relapsing-remitting disorder such as MS, especially if encephalopathy is not present. A third episode unequivocally represents a chronic demyelinating disorder.

MS, on the other hand, is a relapsing disease in this age group distinguished by CNS lesion dissemination in both space and time [2]. The lesion pattern on MRI can be distinctive, showing juxtacortical, periventricular, infratentorial, and spinal cord involvement, as well as lesions perpendicular to the long axis of the corpus callosum ("Dawson fingers"). However, there are no specific MRI findings differentiating MS from ADEM on baseline scan. Cord lesions in MS tend to be shorter than in ADEM where the cord is more diffusely involved. CSF white cell counts typically range from 0 to 30 cells/mm$^3$, but counts can be higher. Though CSF oligoclonal bands are found in 90% of children with MS, they are not often detected in younger children initially (35%) and develop later over the course of the disease. Conversely, in children with ADEM, oligoclonal bands are transiently seen in up to 30% of patients. Further complicating the picture is the observation that 20% of children diagnosed with MS have an initial demyelinating event meeting all criteria for ADEM. It is recommended to monitor brain MRI scans during the first few years after a first demyelinating event suspect of ADEM as silent MRI changes on follow-up scans can develop that are suggestive of MS and may prompt initiation of preventative treatment.

Neuromyelitis optica (NMO) is another relapsing demyelinating disease that can also be indistinguishable from ADEM or MS at the time of first attack [3]. Typical attacks include optic neuritis, longitudinally extensive transverse myelitis, and brainstem syndromes. CSF oligoclonal band testing is often negative. The aquaporin-4 IgG antibody is highly specific for this disorder but is not present in all cases. Therefore, a seronegative presentation of NMO remains a differential diagnosis in such a patient. The distinction from MS is important as the disorder responds to a different array of therapies.

2. MS onset is rare prior to puberty, and the majority of prepubertal children have a polyfocal initial presentation, with ataxia being especially common. Unlike older MS patients, fever, seizures, and encephalopathy occur more commonly in children under 10 years of age. Impaired cognitive performance has also been documented in at least one-third of MS patients with short disease duration under the age of 17 years and may be present in as high as two-thirds of prepubertal children with MS [2]. Other features common to MS such as visual changes or sensory deficits can be notoriously difficult for both parents and physicians to detect given the limited communication skills of very young children. Boys and girls are equally represented (1:1) in this age group, unlike the female predominance (~80%) in teenagers and adults.

    Hyperintense T2 lesions on MRI in very young patients often appear not only less well defined and more widespread but may resolve on subsequent imaging in contrast with teenagers and adults with MS [4]. As such, initial MRI scans can easily be confused for a diagnosis of ADEM. CSF studies show less frequent positivity for oligoclonal bands and higher neutrophil counts in younger children with MS [5].

3. Relapse frequency is variable depending on age. Adolescent patients often have their second attack within 1 year of the initial attack, whereas younger children demonstrate longer intervals between events, possibly in part related to underdiagnosing mild relapses in that age group [2]. The median length of time between the first and second attacks is 6 years in the younger population. Recovery from relapses in younger children also appears to be better.

4. Childhood-onset relapsing-remitting MS is associated with a favorable short-term prognosis. However, these patients still have a 50% risk of transitioning to sec-

ondary progressive MS within 23 years after disease onset, compared to 10 years within disease onset in adult patients [2]. Studies suggest disease duration, greater frequency of relapses, and briefer attack intervals in early disease are linked to a higher risk of progression. While disability accumulation is slower, those with childhood-onset MS achieve disability milestones at a younger age than in adult-onset cases, which may substantially limit their activities as young adults.

5. Similar to adults and teenagers, pulsed high-dose corticosteroids (20–30mg/kg daily for 3–5 days) remain the mainstay of therapy in young children with acute demyelinating episodes [6]. Occasionally additional treatment with plasma exchange or IVIG is needed if steroid treatment is not sufficient to help with recovery. While there are no FDA-approved therapies for pediatric MS, studies in adults demonstrating reduction in relapses have led to the use of many of these drugs in children, including but not limited to glatiramer acetate and interferon beta. On rare occasions, supplementary strategies include monthly pulses of intravenous steroids or IVIG. Immunomodulatory therapy may reduce the risk of disability related to poor recovery from relapses and appears effective in early disease. While practitioners sometimes opt for the newer oral and IV MS therapies for adolescents, treatments such as fingolimod, natalizumab, teriflunomide, and dimethyl fumarate for the very young MS age group have not yet been evaluated for safety and are not advised for first-line use.

## Clinical Pearls

1. ADEM and NMO are the main differential diagnoses of pediatric multiple sclerosis. The signs and symptoms of the initial event of childhood-onset MS may mimic those characteristic of ADEM or NMO. In these patients, time will aid in establishing the diagnosis. MRI findings can be critical to help distinguish between the diseases—multiple T2-bright lesions in specified brain regions and spinal cord in MS versus large, globular, asymmetric lesions seen in ADEM versus lesions centered on the optic nerve, spinal cord, and periaqueductal brainstem in NMO. However, in young children with MS and NMO, brain lesions are often large and poorly circumscribed making the distinction difficult. Oligoclonal bands unique to the CSF, though known to occur in patients with ADEM and NMO, further raise the suspicion for a diagnosis of MS, although they can be missing at first in very young children.

2. Ataxia, fever, seizures, and encephalopathy occur more frequently in children with MS compared to adults. Cognitive morbidity is a significant concern in these young patients as they are actively developing multiple skills at this point in their lives. Younger children demonstrate longer intervals between attacks compared to adolescents, but relapses can be underdiagnosed in younger patients. Those with pediatric-onset relapsing-remitting MS have a good short-term prognosis overall compared to adults with the disease but reach disability milestones at an earlier age than their adult counterparts.

3. Standard treatment for acute demyelination in young children involves pulsed high-dose glucocorticosteroids as in adults. There are no FDA-approved medications for pediatric MS; however, glatiramer acetate and interferon beta are frequently used in children based on overall safety profile and observational studies with these drugs in children. On occasion, additional treatment may be considered including monthly pulses of IV steroids or IVIg. Experience with newer oral and IV therapies in very young children with MS is limited; thus, these are not currently advised for first-line treatment in this age category.

# References

1. Krupp LB, Tardieu M, Amato MP, Banwell B, Chitnis T, Dale RC, et al. International Pediatric Multiple Sclerosis Study Group criteria for pediatric multiple sclerosis and immune-mediated central nervous system demyelinating disorders: revisions to the 2007 definitions. Multiple sclerosis. 2013;19(10):1261–7.
2. Banwell B, Ghezzi A, Bar-Or A, Mikaeloff Y, Tardieu M. Multiple sclerosis in children: clinical diagnosis, therapeutic strategies, and future directions. Lancet Neurol. 2007;6(10):887–902.
3. Alper G. Acute disseminated encephalomyelitis. J Child Neurol. 2012;27(11):1408–25.
4. Chabas D, Castillo-Trivino T, Mowry EM, Strober JB, Glenn OA, Waubant E. Vanishing MS T2-bright lesions before puberty: a distinct MRI phenotype? Neurology. 2008;71(14):1090–3.
5. Chabas D, Ness J, Belman A, Yeh EA, Kuntz N, Gorman MP, et al. Younger children with MS have a distinct CSF inflammatory profile at disease onset. Neurology. 2010;74(5):399–405.
6. Yeh EA, Weinstock-Guttman B. The management of pediatric multiple sclerosis. J Child Neurol. 2012;27(11):1384–93.

# Chapter 5
# Breakthrough Disease in Pediatric MS

Yulia Y. Orlova, Robert I. Thompson-Stone, and Vikram V. Bhise

## Case Presentation

**Case 1** The patient is a 12-year-old girl with a history of relapsing-remitting multiple sclerosis diagnosed at 8 years of age. She initially presented with distal right leg weakness and had neurologic findings consistent with a central lesion. A brain MRI scan showed multiple, bilateral T2 hyperintense foci in the periventricular white matter and juxtacortical region (see Fig. 5.1a) with a symptomatic gadolinium-enhancing lesion. No disease-modifying therapy was initiated at that time, and she made a full recovery.

Six months later, she developed a new right-sided hemiparesis and was found to have several new gadolinium-enhancing lesions (see Fig. 5.1b) on repeat MRI. She was diagnosed with relapsing-remitting multiple sclerosis after the work-up excluded other possible causes. She initiated daily subcutaneous glatiramer acetate 20 mg but 3 months later experienced new left facial weakness and diplopia.

Her MRI scan at the time of the relapse showed three new supratentorial lesions along with a new contrast-enhancing brain stem lesion (see Fig. 5.1c). Although

Y.Y. Orlova, M.D.
University of Florida College of Medicine, McKnight Brain Institute,
Neurology Department, 1149 Newell Drive, Rm L3-100, Gainesville, FL 32611, USA
e-mail: Yulia.Orlova@neurology.ufl.edu

R.I. Thompson-Stone, M.D.
University of Rochester Medical Center, 601 Elmwood Ave., Box 631, Rochester,
NY 14642, USA
e-mail: robert_stone@urmc.rochester.edu

V.V. Bhise, M.D. (✉)
Pediatrics, Neurology, Rutgers – Robert Wood Johnson Medical School, Child Health
Institute, 89 French Street, Suite 2200, New Brunswick, NJ 08901, USA

Division of Child Neurology, Department of Pediatrics, New Brunswick, NJ, USA
e-mail: bhisevi@rwjms.rutgers.edu

© Springer International Publishing AG 2017
E. Waubant, T.E. Lotze (eds.), *Pediatric Demyelinating Diseases of the Central
Nervous System and Their Mimics*, DOI 10.1007/978-3-319-61407-6_5

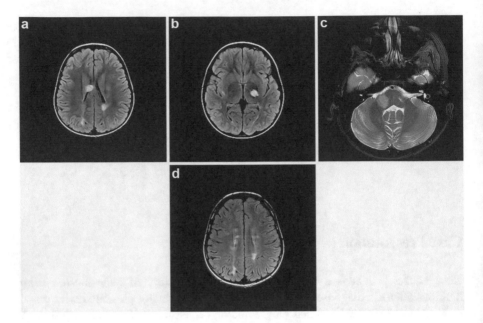

**Fig. 5.1** (**a**) Axial, FLAIR MR image demonstrating intracallosal, periventricular, and juxtacortical T2 hyperintense lesions at the time of initial presentation. (**b**) Axial, FLAIR MR image demonstrating a new T2 hyperintense lesion spanning the left lateral thalamus, and posterior limb of the internal capsule. (**c**) Axial, T2-weighted MR image demonstrating a new brain stem T2 hyperintense lesion in the region of the right lateral pontomedullary junction and middle cerebellar peduncle. (**d**) Axial, FLAIR MR image demonstrating accumulation of typical, discrete periventricular predominant T2 hyperintense lesions

treatment with glatiramer acetate had been too short to consider breakthrough on this medication, she was switched to subcutaneous interferon beta-1a three times weekly and titrated up to a dose of 44 μg per injection. Despite good compliance with treatment, she had another relapse about 1 year after starting interferon therapy that consisted of facial myokymia with hemifacial contracture. There were several new lesions on repeat brain MRI.

At the time of that relapse, a switch to a second-line disease-modifying therapy was discussed due to breakthrough disease on interferon. Drugs discussed included cyclophosphamide and natalizumab, but the parents wished to continue on interferon therapy. Monthly intravenous immunoglobulin (IVIg) infusions were added to interferon therapy. At the time of IVIg initiation, her EDSS was 3.0 (mild gaze-evoked nystagmus, right-sided hemiparesis, and right upper extremity dysmetria). She remained stable for 1 year but then developed a left homonymous hemianopia. There were new lesions on subsequent follow-up MRI scans (see Fig. 5.1d). In consideration of alternative therapies to include natalizumab, she was found to be positive for serum JC virus antibodies. The patient's parents declined natalizumab; therefore, fingolimod 0.5 mg p.o. once daily was started. At the time of this writing, she has been on that treatment for 6 months without side effect. The patient has had a single relapse 4 weeks after initiating therapy that consisted of 1 week of vertigo and ataxia but has since been relapse-free.

**Case 2** A 13-year-old boy initially presented with right-sided hemiparesis and joint pain after a near-fall while riding his bike. Acute injuries were ruled out. The brain MRI revealed multiple bilateral periventricular, subcortical, juxtacortical, infratentorial, and callosal white matter lesions, many of which were enhancing (see Fig. 5.2a, b), thus meeting 2010 McDonald criteria for relapsing-remitting MS. There were also numerous T1 hypointense lesions ("black holes") on imaging, along with one cervico-medullary junction T2-bright lesion and a non-enhancing lesion at the level of T10–11. CSF testing detected 9 unique oligoclonal bands and an elevated IgG index at 0.9 (normal ≤0.84). Testing for MS mimics was negative. He was treated with a 5-day course of 1000 mg IV methylprednisolone, followed by a 2-day course of IVIg totaling 2 g/kg and improved. He was subsequently started on subcutaneous interferon beta-1a 44 μg three times weekly. His neurological examination returned to normal within 2 months.

The patient tolerated interferon well for 5 months, though he missed the third month of his treatment. Two months after the initial presentation, he had an episode of leg weakness that resolved within a few hours (that did not meet criteria for an MS exacerbation). Approximately 1 month later, he developed right-sided hemisensory loss that lasted for 1 week. He was seen after resolution of his symptoms, and his neurological examination was normal; however, his follow-up brain MRI had dramatically worsened with multiple new infratentorial lesions, including right midbrain and left pontine (see Fig. 5.2c, d), as well as multiple new gadolinium-enhancing foci bilaterally.

The patient was switched to natalizumab after the confirmation of negative JC virus antibody status. He tolerated monthly infusions of natalizumab 300 mg well. Ten months after the initial infusion, his follow-up brain MRI revealed a significant decrease in the size of multiple demyelinating lesions with no new enhancing foci (see Fig. 5.2e, f). There have been no further relapses during 19 months of ongoing therapy.

## Clinical Questions

1. What is the definition of active disease?
2. What is considered inadequate treatment response or breakthrough disease, i.e., what are the criteria for switching therapy?
3. How should the clinician best manage inadequate treatment response?
4. How long does it take for MS drugs to take effect, and thus how long should one wait to switch therapy in the setting of breakthrough disease?
5. Is there a role for IVIg and plasma exchange in breakthrough disease?
6. What would be the options for treatment in Case 1 after the episode of left homonymous hemianopia?

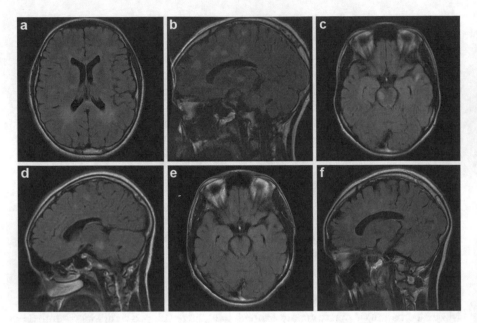

**Fig. 5.2** Axial (**a**) and sagittal (**b**) T2 FLAIR image depicts multiple subcortical and periventricular lesions at initial presentation. Three months later, multiple new lesions are present, including a new large lesion in the right midbrain identified on axial (**c**) and sagittal (**d**) FLAIR sequences. Follow-up brain MRI 10 months after the initial infusion of natalizumab shows a significant decrease in infratentorial T2 hyperintense lesions (**e** and **f**)

## Diagnostic Discussion

1. The MS Phenotype Group in 2013 updated the concept of disease activity in order to provide temporal information about the ongoing disease process that may impact the prognosis and therapeutic decisions [1].

    Activity is determined by clinical or MRI findings. Clinical activity implies the presence of recurrent relapses, which are defined as acute or subacute episodes of new or increased neurological dysfunction lasting for at least 24 h that are followed by complete or partial recovery in the absence of fever or infection. In addition, disease activity can manifest as an increase in disability. MRI activity is defined as the presence of contrast-enhancing T1 foci or new or unequivocally enlarging T2 hyperintense lesions. Debate still remains over what is the optimal time frame for assessing disease activity, but a 6–12-month interval is considered reasonable. Some clinical manifestations can be very subtle, especially in cognitive and visual domains, and require close monitoring for detection.

    Assessment and interpretation of other MRI parameters to measure tissue damage, such as black hole evolution and brain volume loss, are still not standardized. Additional measures such as optical coherence tomography (OCT), body fluid biomarkers, and newer MRI metrics have yet to be validated as outcomes of disease activity.

2. There is no consensus on the definition of breakthrough disease. The terms inadequate treatment response and partial therapeutic effectiveness are used interchangeably to express treatment failure, although the treatment may be biologically active while not meaningfully shutting down inflammatory processes. The International Pediatric MS Study Group proposed a working definition for inadequate treatment response in pediatric MS patients on full-dose therapy for a minimum of 6 months with full adherence [2]. To meet the definition, at least one of the following needs to be present: an increase or lack of reduction in relapse rate, new T2 or contrast-enhancing T1 lesions on a new MRI compared to a baseline MRI obtained shortly after treatment initiation, or two or more clinical relapses within a 12-month period or less. Additional features that may be considered when defining inadequate treatment response include poor recovery from a relapse, accumulation of disability, and rapid cognitive decline [3]. The mechanism of action, pharmacokinetics, and pharmacodynamics of the specific agent should be taken into account when considering switching therapy as most agents are not fully effective immediately. Poor adherence to therapy and discontinuation of medication due to side effects are both risk factors for developing breakthrough disease activity.

3. The management of breakthrough disease in the pediatric population is often extrapolated from studies done in the adult population. However, there is no consensus on the definition of breakthrough disease and no clear guidelines on management of breakthrough MS, even in adults with the disease. None of the available disease-modifying therapies have been approved for pediatric MS use, and data regarding their possible long-term effects on normal physiological development are lacking. Physical development, cognitive maturation, and pubertal changes are significant concerns for potential disruption unique to the pediatric population. Moreover, long-term effects on the developing immune system in children remain entirely unknown.

Several options are present for switching therapies in refractory or breakthrough MS (Table 5.1): change between first-line (injectable) therapies (i.e., interferon beta or glatiramer acetate), switch to second-line and/or third-line therapy, or add-on monthly pulses of high-dose steroids or IVIg [4]. In the first scenario, patients can move from one drug category (i.e., interferon or glatiramer acetate) to the other [5]. In addition, patients on low-dose interferon (weekly IM injections) may be advanced to high-dose interferon (three times a week or every other day subcutaneous injections). It is critical to screen patients with breakthrough disease for nonadherence. In patients with evidence of aggressive disease, rapid escalation or initiating treatment up front with a second-line agent may be reasonable strategies.

Second-line disease-modifying therapies include natalizumab, rituximab, fingolimod, teriflunomide, and dimethyl fumarate. Natalizumab has shown a strong reduction in clinical and MRI measures of disease activity in randomized controlled trials, and several small cohorts document its safe use in children with MS although with limited follow-up duration. No cases of progressive multifocal leukoencephalopathy (PML) have been reported in this age group to date,

**Table 5.1** Disease-modifying therapies approved for adults and used in pediatric multiple sclerosis

| Agent | Dosage/route | Side effects | Warning |
|---|---|---|---|
| First-line therapies | | | |
| Interferon beta-1a | 22 μg or 44 μg via subcutaneous injection three times weekly | Flu-like symptoms, transient transaminase elevation, bone marrow suppression, abnormal thyroid function, local injection site reaction | |
| Interferon beta-1a | 30 μg via intramuscular injection once weekly | | |
| Interferon beta-1b | 0.25 mg via subcutaneous injection every other day | | |
| Peginterferon beta-1a | 125 μg via subcutaneous injection every 14 days | | |
| Glatiramer acetate | 20 mg daily or 40 mg three times per week via subcutaneous injection | Injection site reaction, lipoatrophy, rash, panic attack-like with dyspnea or chest pain | |
| Second-line therapies | | | |
| Natalizumab | 300 mg or 3–6 mg/kg intravenously every 4 weeks | Hypersensitivity reaction, headache, elevated white blood cell count, anemia, PML, transaminase elevation, herpes encephalitis, and meningitis | Higher risk for PML in patients with JC virus antibody-positive status, prior immunosuppressant treatment, and/or greater than 2 years of therapy |
| Rituximab | 500–750 mg/m$^2$ intravenously, maximum 1000 mg, administered as 2 doses 2 weeks apart, or 375 mg/m$^2$, maximum 500 mg, 4 doses 1 week apart | Infusion reaction, fulminant reactivation of hepatitis B, PML in previously immunosuppressed patients | Avoid patients with a history of hepatitis B, active TB in pregnancy |

(continued)

**Table 5.1**  (continued)

| Agent | Dosage/route | Side effects | Warning |
|---|---|---|---|
| Fingolimod | 0.5 mg oral capsules PO daily | Bradycardia and/or atrioventricular conduction block after first dose, infection including rare PML and *Cryptococcus*, macular edema, decreased pulmonary function, serum transaminase elevation, hypertension, lymphopenia | First dose observation required, unexpected deaths in patients with prior history of heart or vascular disease, or combination with drugs increasing QT |
| Teriflunomide | 7 mg or 14 mg tablets PO daily | Infection, hepatotoxicity, potential teratogenicity, skin reaction, elevation of blood pressure, peripheral neuropathy, acute renal failure, interstitial lung disease, Stevens-Johnson syndrome | Requires cholestyramine or activated charcoal washout for accelerated elimination |
| Dimethyl fumarate | 240 mg PO twice daily | Flushing, abdominal pain, diarrhea, nausea, pruritus, rash, erythema, lymphopenia, rare opportunistic infections (PML) | |
| Third-line therapies | | | |
| Mitoxantrone | 12 mg/m$^2$ intravenously every 3 months; maximum cumulative dose: 140 mg/m$^2$ | Temporary blue discoloration of sclera and urine, nausea, alopecia, menstrual disorders including amenorrhea and infertility, infections, cardiac toxicity, severe local tissue damage with extravasation, acute myelogenous leukemia, myelosuppression | Lifelong risk for cardiomyopathy and leukemia, requires yearly quantitative LVEF evaluation even following discontinuation |

(continued)

**Table 5.1** (continued)

| Agent | Dosage/route | Side effects | Warning |
|---|---|---|---|
| Cyclophosphamide | 600–1000 mg/ m² intravenously, administered monthly with the minimum dose required to decrease white blood cell counts at day 10–12 to less than 3000/mm³ | Nausea, vomiting, increased susceptibility to infection, alopecia, amenorrhea, infertility, hemorrhagic cystitis | Caution in patients desiring future pregnancy, long-term risk of bladder and hematologic malignancies |

*PML* progressive multifocal leukoencephalopathy

although the numbers of children treated with this agent are small. While children are less likely to be positive for JC virus, they should still be tested for JC virus exposure prior to initiation of natalizumab and every 6–12 months thereafter. Data on the use of rituximab in pediatric MS is also limited [6]. There is also a concern for PML with this agent but much less so than with natalizumab. In addition, an increased risk of infections exists. While optimal dosing of rituximab is unclear for pediatric MS, it is extrapolated from regimens currently used for pediatric rheumatologic and oncologic diseases as well as the regimen used in adult MS.

There is limited data in children on the safety and tolerability of the recently FDA-approved oral medications (fingolimod, teriflunomide, and dimethyl fumarate), which are first-line therapies in adult patients. Despite the lack of data, the use of these agents is increasing for adolescents with MS especially for fingolimod and dimethyl fumarate. Nevertheless, the oral agents still tend to be avoided in prepubescent children due to their unknown long-term safety. International multicenter randomized trials are currently underway in the pediatric population for all three oral agents approved for adult MS.

Third-line therapy includes medications with high toxicity (mitoxantrone and cyclophosphamide). Treatment with mitoxantrone is no longer recommended for use in the pediatric population due to its lifelong cardiomyopathy and leukemia risk, save for exceptional cases. Cyclophosphamide may be considered when other treatments have failed; however, serious side effects include severe infections, amenorrhea, sterility, bladder cancer, and secondary malignancies.

Repeat brain imaging is recommended within months of switching to a new disease-modifying therapy to use as new baseline for future reference.

Finally, combination therapy with pulse corticosteroids or IVIg can be used for short-term management, though evidence to support its benefit is lacking.

4. Currently there are no validated biomarkers available to predict the treatment response at the time of initiation of MS drugs; However, clinical and radiological criteria are used to assess therapeutic effect on disease activity. Clinical criteria

to switch therapy remain somewhat arbitrary. It has been proposed that any relapse on therapy, especially during the first 5 years of the disease should raise the question about poor therapeutic response and may warrant a switch in therapy, though each therapy must be considered individually.

Studies show that natalizumab reduces disease activity on MRI criteria by 1 month after the first infusion with continued benefit as long as treatment continues [7]. The effect on annualized relapse rate can similarly be seen as early as 3 months from the beginning of therapy.

The use of clinical and MRI parameters in predicting further disease activity in adults treated with interferon beta is well published, and a measurable effect should be expected by 3 months with high-dose interferon beta.

Several studies showed that maximum efficacy of glatiramer acetate could be delayed up to 6 months. There is a more significant decrease in T2 lesion volume for patients treated with interferon beta during the first year but not during years 2 and 3, compared to those treated with glatiramer acetate. Thus, the presence of new T2 lesions alone within the first few months in a patient treated with glatiramer acetate is not necessarily a reliable prognostic factor for poor response to treatment.

5. Several case reports suggest a possible benefit for IVIg and plasma exchange in pediatric MS for symptomatic treatment of an acute demyelinating event if corticosteroid therapy is contraindicated or ineffective. In a patient with a fulminant relapse, 3–7 every other day sessions of plasma exchange can be considered. IVIg is also sometimes used as an add-on therapy (e.g., 1 g/kg every 3–4 weeks) for patients with frequent exacerbations, but its benefit is unclear. There have been no controlled trials of IVIg use in pediatric MS, although small trials in adult MS have indicated that IVIg may marginally decrease disease activity on MRI while there is no evidence of decreased relapse frequency.

6. Several options can be considered in a patient who shows accumulation of disability, high MRI activity, and continued exacerbations despite well-conducted first-line therapy [8]. In Case 1, treatment could be escalated to second-line therapy because of failure of at least one first-line therapy despite good compliance. Natalizumab is an interesting option due to its relatively prompt efficacy. The presence of JC virus antibody in this patient with aggressive disease is a relative contraindication for natalizumab due to the risk of PML that begins after 1 year of therapy. If natalizumab is initiated despite positive JC virus antibody status, discussions with the patient and family about potential risks and benefits should occur regularly.

Alternatively, oral therapies may also be considered. Like with several other disease-modifying therapies, oral agents can lead to distinct alterations in immunosurveillance. The use of fingolimod has been associated with a higher rate of varicella zoster infection in the adult population (including systemic infections) and several cases of herpes encephalitis. At least two cases of PML have also occurred in a patient with no prior treatment with natalizumab, and several cases of *Cryptococcus* infections have been reported. Fingolimod also causes temporary bradycardia following first-dose administration most of which are asymptomatic; several cases of unexpected death have been reported in adults with cardiac comorbidities or taking medications that can alter QT conduction. Additional side effects include skin cancer, macular edema, and liver toxicity. There is no information available on its use in pediatrics. Teriflunomide, an active metabolite of the rheumatoid arthritis drug leflunomide, is also a once-daily medication with adverse effects including elevated liver enzymes, alopecia, skin rashes, peripheral neuropathy, and hypertension. A major safety concern is teratogenicity particularly due to its prolonged half-life. Dimethyl fumarate is a twice-daily oral medication with a good safety record and side effects limited to flushing, gastrointestinal discomfort mostly during the first 2 months of therapy, and lymphopenia. Several cases of PML have occurred in the setting of prolonged lymphopenia but at a much lower rate than for natalizumab. Until results from clinical trials in pediatric MS become available, new therapies approved for adult MS must be used cautiously as second-line therapies.

## Clinical Pearls

- Clinical disease activity implies the presence of recurrent relapses that are followed by complete or partial recovery in the absence of fever or infection. MRI activity is defined as the presence of contrast-enhancing T1 lesions or new or unequivocally enlarging T2 hyperintense lesions.
- Before switching therapy due to inadequate treatment response, patients on first-line therapies should be treated with full doses for at least 6 months with good adherence to therapy. However, in the setting of a particularly fulminant early disease course, this may not always be possible.
- There is no consensus on criteria for inadequate treatment response. Proposed criteria include two or more clinical relapses within a 12-month period, one or more severe relapses per year, sustained increase in disability over 6 months, or new interim MRI activity in the form of new or enlarging T2 lesions or new T1 contrast-enhancing lesions.
- There are several options in managing breakthrough MS: switch between first-line therapies (interferon beta or glatiramer acetate) or advance to second-line therapies.
- Most of the studies of safety and tolerability for MS therapies are done in adults and should be extrapolated to the pediatric population with caution.

# References

1. Lublin FD, Reingold SC, Cohen JA, Cutter GR, Sørensen PS, Thompson AJ, et al. Defining the clinical course of multiple sclerosis: the 2013 revisions. Neurology. 2014;83(3):278–86.
2. Chitnis T, Tenembaum S, Banwell B, Krupp L, Pohl D, Rostasy K, et al. Consensus statement: evaluation of new and existing therapeutics for pediatric multiple sclerosis. Mult Scler. 2012;18(1):116–27.
3. Coyle PK. Switching therapies in multiple sclerosis. CNS Drugs. 2013;27(4):239–47.
4. Yeh EA, Waubant E, Krupp LB, Ness J, Chitnis T, Kuntz N, et al. Multiple sclerosis therapies in pediatric patients with refractory multiple sclerosis. Arch Neurol. 2011;68(4):437–44.
5. Banwell B, Bar-Or A, Giovannoni G, Dale RC, Tardieu M. Therapies for multiple sclerosis: considerations in the pediatric patient. Nat Rev Neurol. 2011;7(2):109–22.
6. Beres SJ, Graves J, Waubant E. Rituximab use in pediatric central demyelinating disease. Pediatr Neurol. 2014;51(1):114–8.
7. Kappos L, O'Connor PW, Polman CH, Vermersch P, Wiendl H, Pace A, et al. Clinical effects of natalizumab on multiple sclerosis appear early in treatment course. J Neurol. 2013;260(5):1388–95.
8. Wingerchuk DM, Carter JL. Multiple sclerosis: current and emerging disease-modifying therapies and treatment strategies. Mayo Clin Proc. 2014;89(2):225–40.

# Chapter 6
# Neuromyelitis Optica Spectrum Disorder with Neuropsychiatric Presentation

Timothy E. Lotze and Elizabeth A. McQuade

## Case Presentation

An 11-year-old previously healthy girl presented with complaints of acute onset of diplopia and right exotropia on examination. The family history was notable for an estranged father with a reported diagnosis of multiple sclerosis and a maternal great aunt with schizophrenia. A gadolinium-enhanced brain MRI showed bilateral but asymmetric longitudinally extensive hyperintense T2 lesions extending from the deep gray nuclei to the periaqueductal regions and cerebral peduncles (Figs. 6.1, 6.2, and 6.3). Additional lesions were seen in the periventricular regions and mesial temporal lobes as well as the frontal gray matter. There was no gadolinium enhancement of the lesions. MRI of the cervical spine was normal. CSF studies showed 9 WBC (2% neutrophils, 95% lymphocytes, 3% monocytes), 0 RBC, normal protein 24 mg/dL, normal glucose 76 mg/dL (serum 147 mg/dL), IgG index 0.54, (0.3–0.7 normal range), and no oligoclonal bands. The findings were thought to be consistent with an acquired demyelinating disease, and she received a 5-day course of methylprednisolone 1000 mg IV. During this treatment, she developed auditory and visual hallucinations along with expressive aphasia. These resolved with completion of intravenous corticosteroid therapy. It was unclear as to whether her mental status changes were a side effect of her steroid treatment or part of her clinical syndrome. She was diagnosed at that time with acute disseminated encephalomyelitis.

T.E. Lotze, M.D. (✉) • E.A. McQuade, M.D.
Division of Neurology and Developmental Neuroscience, Department of Pediatrics,
Baylor College of Medicine, Texas Children's Hospital, 6701 Fannon CC 1250,
Houston, TX 77030, USA
e-mail: tlotze@bcm.edu; eamcquad@texaschildrens.org

© Springer International Publishing AG 2017
E. Waubant, T.E. Lotze (eds.), *Pediatric Demyelinating Diseases of the Central Nervous System and Their Mimics*, DOI 10.1007/978-3-319-61407-6_6

**Fig. 6.1** T2 flair
hyperintensity in the right
midbrain involving the
cerebral peduncles and
periaqueductal gray
regions (onset)

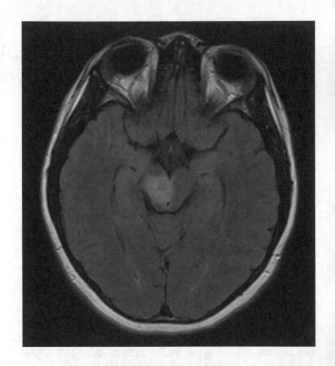

**Fig. 6.2** T2 flair
hyperintensity extending
rostrally in the right
midbrain (onset)

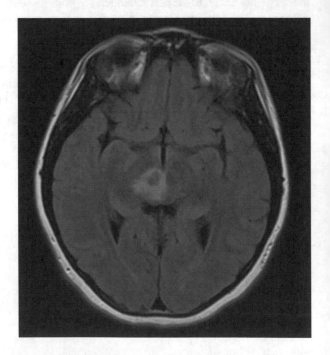

**Fig. 6.3** T2 flair
hyperintensity involving
the right thalamus (onset)

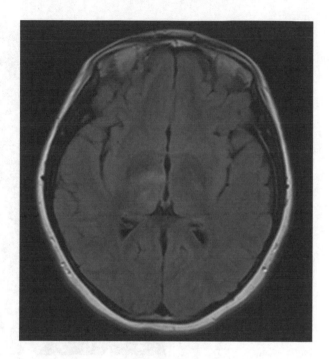

Within 2 months, she returned with paresthesia in the right arm and leg. A repeat brain MRI demonstrated improvement in the brainstem lesion but interval development of a hyperintense T2 lesion in the left caudate nucleus, bilateral basal ganglia, left thalamus, and left external capsule (Figs. 6.4, 6.5, and 6.6). She was again treated with high-dose methylprednisolone for 5 days but had coincidental recurrence of hallucinations, paranoia, hyper-religiosity, and selective mutism that persisted after discontinuation of her steroid treatment. She was additionally treated with IVIG 2 gm/kg divided over 5 days. While her sensory complaints improved, her paranoia and abnormal behaviors persisted. In consideration of her initial presenting diagnosis of ADEM, this second event was considered to be a protracted course of the initial attack, and disease-modifying therapy was not initiated.

Six months later, she returned with new persistent headaches, nausea, right arm and leg paresthesia and weakness, diplopia, dysarthria, dysphagia, ataxia, and enuresis. She continued to have psychiatric disturbances described as "night terrors," insomnia, visual hallucinations, fearfulness, anxiety, emotional lability, poor school performance, and paranoid mistrust of her family. She developed aggressive behaviors and pseudo-seizures characterized by "fainting and unresponsiveness." Repeat contrast-enhanced brain MRI showed a new T2-hyperintense gadolinium-enhancing lesion in the right middle cerebellar peduncle and continued presence of the prior mentioned lesions (Fig. 6.7). MRI of the entire spine was again normal. Labs including ANA, SSA/B, antiphospholipid antibodies, hepatic function tests, thyroid function studies, serum AQP-4 Ab, and angiotensin converting enzyme level were all negative or normal. Steroids were avoided secondary to concerns for wors-

**Fig. 6.4** Slight
improvement of the T2
hyperintensity of the right
midbrain (2 months)

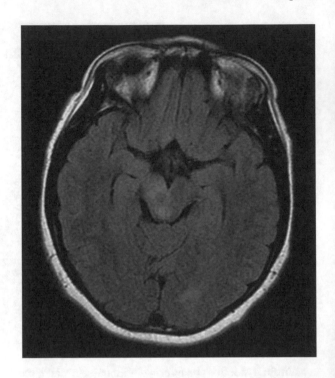

**Fig. 6.5** Slight
improvement of T2
hyperintensity in deep
midbrain structures (2
months)

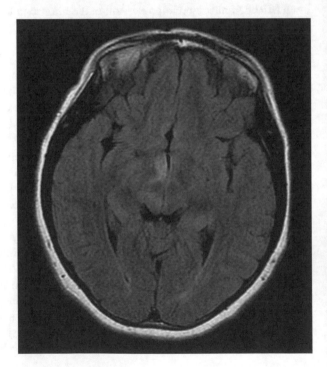

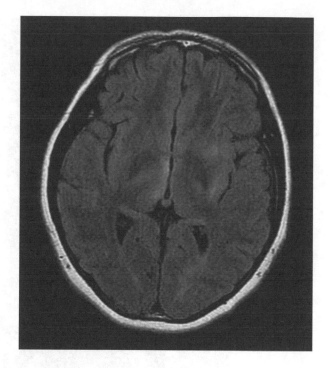

**Fig. 6.6** Interval development of a hyperintense T2 lesion in the left caudate nucleus, bilateral basal ganglia, left thalamus, and left external capsule (2 months)

ening her psychiatric symptoms, and she received IVIG 2 gm/kg over 5 days. She was also started on risperidone with some improvement in her behaviors.

The clinical findings were not thought to be typical of multiple sclerosis; however, she did not meet prior 2007 diagnostic criteria for NMO. Therefore, treatment for possible multiple sclerosis was initiated with glatiramer acetate. Interferons were specifically avoided secondary to concerns of exacerbating her psychiatric disease. Despite this treatment, she continued to have interval attacks of psychiatric symptoms over the next 5 years with psychosis and mood disturbances to include an attempted suicide for which she required inpatient psychiatric hospitalization. These symptoms responded to treatment with olanzapine and valproic acid.

In addition to these psychiatric concerns, she had repeated neurological attacks of ataxia, diplopia, and decreased expressive speech. Interval MRIs showed waxing and waning of her lesions (Figs. 6.8, 6.9, 6.10, 6.11, 6.12, 6.13, and 6.14). Repeated tests for serum and CSF AQP-4 Ab were negative. Repeat CSF was notable only for elevated IgG index of 0.8 with no oligoclonal bands. Secondary to her atypical course, additional investigations for inborn errors of metabolism, Wilson's disease, and a chromosomal microarray for genetic disorders were performed with negative results. Along with ongoing glatiramer acetate, she was started on pulse monthly IVIG 1 gm/kg/dose and mycophenolate mofetil 1000 mg twice daily.

Over the next year, her MRI brain lesions remained inactive. However, she continued to require intermittent inpatient psychiatric care. She additionally developed

**Fig. 6.7** New
T2-hyperintense
gadolinium-enhancing
lesion in the right middle
cerebellar peduncle (6
months)

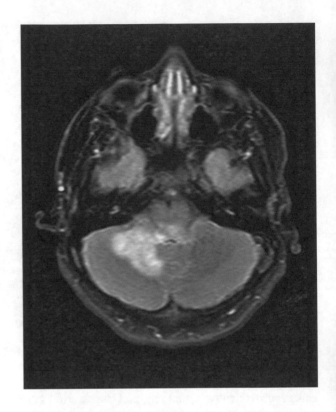

**Fig. 6.8** T2 flair
hyperintensity involving
the cerebral peduncles and
occipital horns of the
lateral ventricles (9
months)

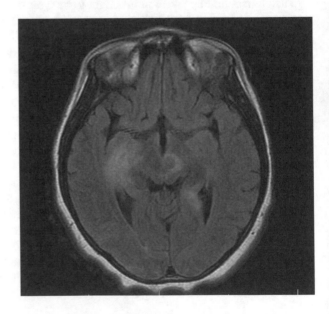

**Fig. 6.9** T2 flair hyperintensity involving the right thalamus, right posterior limb of the internal capsule, and periventricular area of the left occipital horn (9 months)

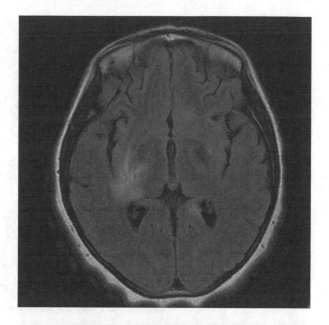

**Fig. 6.10** T2 flair hyperintensities surrounding the periventricular areas (9 months)

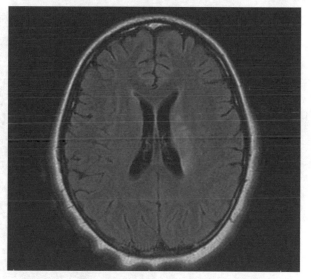

comorbid central hypothyroidism and diabetes mellitus which were thought to be related to her antipsychotics.

Five years after her initial presentation, she developed right arm and leg weakness in association with a tumefactive lesion in the left hemispheric white matter. Repeat serum studies at that time demonstrated a positive AQP-4 Ab titer. CSF studies were not performed. She was then diagnosed with NMO. Glatiramer acetate was discontinued, and she began treatment with rituximab 1000 mg/dose for two

**Fig. 6.11** T2 flair hyperintensities in periventricular areas as well as involving the corpus callosum (9 months)

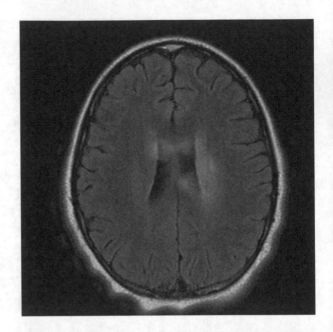

**Fig. 6.12** T2 flair hyperintensities of the pons and medulla (9 months)

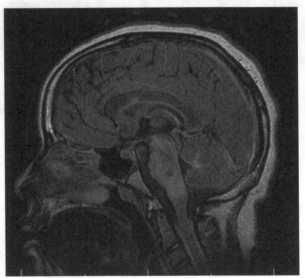

initial doses followed by booster dosing of 1000 mg every 6 months. In the interval of 2 years of follow-up, she had no further clinical attacks. She did require ongoing psychiatric treatment but no longer had active psychosis or agitated behaviors. She was able to complete her high school education with accommodations.

**Fig. 6.13** T2 flair
hyperintensities of the
thalami and right internal
capsule (35 months)

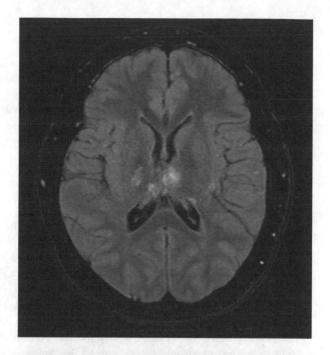

**Fig. 6.14** Right-sided T2
flair hyperintensity (35
months)

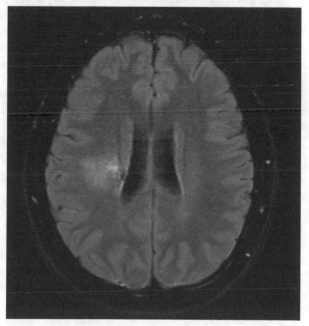

## Clinical Questions

1. What neuropsychiatric problems and neurocognitive effects are seen in NMO?
2. What is the utility of AQP-4 Ab serum tests, and how often does one covert to seropositive?
3. What are the acute and long-term treatments in NMO with psychiatric complications in pediatrics?

## Diagnostic Discussion

1. The prevalence of psychiatric comorbidities has not been well defined for NMO. The underlying mechanism by which aquaporin-4 antibody-mediated disease might produce neuropsychiatric sequelae is unclear, and the long-term outcome for such patients is unknown. Interestingly, AQP4 antibodies have been discovered in some cases of anti-NMDA receptor (NMDAR) encephalitis—a disease where psychiatric comorbidities are common. Titulaer et al. described an association between anti-NMDAR encephalitis and NMO. Among a cohort of 12 patients with anti-NMDAR encephalitis plus clinical or MRI features of demyelinating syndrome that occurred sequentially in time, five cases were proven to be NMO. Of the four patients who were AQP-4 Ab positive, all were first diagnosed with NMO and 11–80 months later had an episode of anti-NMDAR encephalitis. The fifth patient was seronegative for AQP-4 Ab and first developed anti-NMDAR encephalitis followed by an NMO episode 1 month later. In another cohort of 11 patients, anti-NMDAR encephalitis plus clinical or MRI features of demyelination occurred simultaneously. Of these, five patients were found to have NMO. All five were positive for AQP4 and NMDAR antibodies. Although three had typical NMO symptoms, two of these patients were actually asymptomatic for NMO; however, both had abnormal brain MRIs [1]. The occurrence of psychiatric disease in a patient with NMO should prompt the clinician to test for NMDAR antibodies, as this might further explain the presenting clinical syndrome.

   Although there are no clear conclusive differences in neurocognitive effects between MS and NMO, studies have shown that both disorders affect cognitive function. The exact prevalence of neurocognitive deficits in NMO is unknown. Similar to MS, NMO has been associated with problems in executive function, long- and short-term memory, as well as speed of information. Abnormal performance in verbal fluency and attention deficits have also been reported. It seems possible that these changes might also influence one's quality of life and susceptibility to depression; however, there has not been a consensus on this assumption. On the contrary, comorbid factors such as fatigue and depression may have primary causative roles in cognitive impairment.

There is no clear correlation between imaging findings and neuropsychiatric and cognitive disease manifestations of NMO. McKeon et al. published a study of 88 seropositive children with NMO that found 68% had abnormalities detected on brain MRI. This study also observed that 45–55% of children with NMO have symptoms that may correlate with brain involvement to include behavioral changes [2]. In other studies, diencephalic and corpus callosum lesions have been reported in association with behavioral changes and abnormal cognition, as well as motor dysfunction [3]. A study by Blanc comparing 28 patients with NMO to 28 healthy controls found that NMO patients had global and focal brain atrophy of white matter (sparing gray matter). Of these patients, 15 had cognitive dysfunction, which was correlated to the amount of global and focal white matter atrophy [4]. However, NMO patients without obvious brain involvement on MRI have also been found to have cognitive abnormalities. A study done by He et al. showed that memory problems, attention deficits, and decreased information processing speed are worse both during and after acute relapse of NMO even without MRI-detected brain involvement [5]. Possible explanations for this include the ubiquitous expression of AQP4 in the brain and microscopic effects of antibody-mediated attacks and cytokines released during these. In support of this consideration are the results of histopathological study of cortex biopsies in six NMO patients where there was evidence for neuronal loss in layers II, III, and IV along with meningeal inflammation [6].

Thus, as with MS, the burden of cognitive disease in patients with NMO may not correlate with imaging findings or the level of other functional disabilities found on clinical presentation. In addition, NMO has been known to co-occur with other inflammatory autoimmune CNS diseases such as systemic lupus erythematosus, antiphospholipid antibody syndrome, and Sjogren syndrome. Independent of NMO, these disorders have been associated with neurocognitive deficits that might further impact patient outcomes in this area [7].

2. Our patient was tested for AQP-4 Ab early in her disease course. However, her initial serum test was negative. She seroconverted to a positive antibody result in her serum years later during a subsequent exacerbation. A recent multicenter comparison of the current commercial assays showed that the ELISA detection method had a sensitivity of 60%, while a cell-based assay (CBA) methodology had a sensitivity of 68%, and both had 100% specificity. Used together, the CBA and ELISA tests had a sensitivity of 72% [8]. Thus, even the most sensitive assays will not pick up all cases of NMO on initial analysis, and this may provide an explanation for our patient's initial false negative report. If NMO spectrum disorder is considered a strong possibility, yet serum antibody testing is negative, CSF analysis for the presence of APQ4 antibodies might improve the diagnostic yield. Seroconversion from positive to negative titers has been previously described in case reports; however, the frequency of this is not currently known. A retrospective analysis in children showed that out of seven patients with AQP-4 Ab seropositivity, one was initially seronegative but converted to seropositive during a later relapse. This patient also showed return to seronegative status after

immunosuppressant therapy. Jarius et al. described a retrospective analysis of the AQP-4 Ab in eight adult patients and the relationship of this antibody to disease activity. In this analysis, AQP-4 Ab titers were higher during disease relapse and lower when disease was in remission. This analysis also showed that the AQP-4 Ab decline corresponded with immunosuppressant treatment. However, in three patients continuing on immunosuppressant therapy, a rise in AQ4B-Ab levels was not followed by clinical relapse [9]. Further studies are needed to better determine how tracking antibody status in NMO spectrum disorder might help to guide long-term treatment decisions.

3. There is no specific treatment regimen for NMO with psychiatric disturbances in children. In fact, some treatment for NMO may exacerbate mental illness. Acute exacerbations of pediatric NMO are typically treated with IV methylprednisolone. Agitation, excitation, and sleep disturbances are frequent adverse drug effects reported in steroid use [10]. Both our patient and other retrospective case reports indicate worsening of psychiatric symptoms with exposure to steroids.

In a review of the literature, Drozdowicz et al. reported that in adults, there is a trend toward euphoria and hypomania as the more common adverse events occurring early in the treatment course, whereas depression is more common in prolonged courses. However, some case studies documented events late in therapy or even after it had been stopped, ranging from mild mood swings to frank psychosis. When psychiatric symptoms improve with initiation of treatment such as rituximab, then a causal relationship between NMO and psychiatric changes is suggested. The relationship is not as clear when psychiatric symptoms continue despite stable neurologic disease. In adults, the psychiatric side effects of steroids had a dose-responsive effect although this has not been well studied in children [10]. If there is concern for worsening of psychiatric symptoms during steroid treatment, the therapy should be reduced or stopped. Plasmapheresis and sometimes IVIG are considered as an alternate for acute disease exacerbation. Rituximab may provide the best option for long-term disease management in these patients and, in some studies, has shown overall superiority over azathioprine and mycophenolate mofetil in relapse prevention [11]. The effects of acute and chronic regimens on underlying neuropsychiatric disorders in NMO are unknown, and further investigations are needed to monitor psychiatric disease in association with relapse, treatment, and over time.

## Clinical Pearls

1. Psychiatric symptoms have been described in both adults and pediatrics with NMO. Such patients should be investigated for comorbid disorders to include anti-NMDAR encephalitis, sending a metabolic panel, as well as testing for various autoimmune conditions, such as lupus erythematosus.

2. Used together, the CBA and ELISA tests have a 72% sensitivity for detecting NMO. In seronegative patients with high suspicion for NMO, repeat testing is

important, as seroconversion can occur and further clarify the diagnosis. Testing of CSF can also be helpful in some cases.

3. There is no tailored treatment for psychiatric comorbidities of pediatric NMO. Steroids may exacerbate psychiatric symptoms in which case plasmapheresis or in some cases IVIG should be considered as a better treatment option. Rituximab may be optimal for long-term treatment of these patients. Other agents include mycophenolate mofetil and azathioprine.

# References

1. Titulaer M, Hoftbreger R, Iizuka T, Leypoldt F, McCracken L, Cellucci T, et al. Overlapping demyelinating syndromes and anti-N-methyl-D-aspartate receptor encephalitis. Ann Neurol. 2014;75(3):411–28.
2. McKeon A, Lennon V, Lotze T, Tenenbaum S, Ness J, Rensel M, et al. CNS aquaporin-4 autoimmunity in children. Neurology. 2008;71(2):93–100.
3. Kim H, Paul F, Lana-Peixoto M, Tenembaum S, Asgari N, Palace J, et al. MRI characteristics of neuromyelitis optica spectrum disorder: an international update. Neurology. 2015;84(11):1165–73.
4. Blanc F, Noblet V, Jung B, Rousseau F, Renard F, Bourre B, et al. White matter atrophy and cognitive dysfunctions in neuromyelitis optica. PLoS One. 2012;7(4):e33878.
5. He D, Chen X, Zhao D, Zhou H. Cognitive function, depression, fatigue, and activities of daily living in patients with neuromyelitis optica after acute relapse. Int J Neurosci. 2011;121(12):677–83.
6. Saji E, Arakawa M, Yanagawa K, Toyoshima Y, Yokoseki A, Okamoto K, et al. Cognitive impairment and cortical degeneration in neuromyelitis optica. Ann Neurol. 2013;73(1):65–76.
7. Blanc F, Zephir H, Lebrun C, Labauge P, Castelnovo G, Fleury M, et al. Cognitive functions in neuromyelitis optica. Arch Neurol. 2008;65(1):84–8.
8. Waters P, McKeon A, Leite M, Rajasekharan S, Lennon V, Villalobos A, et al. Serologic diagnosis of NMO: a multicenter comparison of aquaporin-4-IgG assays. Neurology. 2012;78(9):665–71.
9. Jarius S, Aboul-Enein F, Waters P, Kuenz B, Hauser A, Berger T, et al. Antibody to aquaporin-4 in the long-term course of neuromyelitis optica. Brain. 2008;131(11):3072–80.
10. Drozdowicz L, Bostwick J. Psychiatric adverse effects of pediatric corticosteroid use. Mayo Clin Proc. 2014;89(6):817–34.
11. Kessler R, Mealy M, Levy M. Treatment of neuromyelitis optica spectrum disorder: acute, preventive, and symptomatic. Curr Treat Options Neurol. 2015;18(1):2.

# Chapter 7
# Pediatric Tumefactive Demyelination

Michael A. Lopez and Timothy E. Lotze

## Case Summary

A previously healthy right-handed 14-year-old boy presented with 1 month of cognitive impairment and behavioral changes. A week prior to symptom onset, he was diagnosed and treated for presumed streptococcal pharyngitis. Subsequently, he was noted to have progressive short-term memory impairment, word finding difficulty, dysfluency, and misjudging spatial relationships. He additionally began to complain of bilateral retro-orbital pain and pressure, vomiting, gait instability, and staring episodes and was occasionally disoriented to place. His blood counts, electrolytes, and liver function tests were unremarkable.

At presentation to the hospital, a gadolinium-enhanced MRI brain was performed and demonstrated multiple bihemispheric T2 hyperintense tumefactive lesions with incomplete rings of enhancement (see Fig. 7.1). A gadolinium-enhanced MRI spine revealed no evidence of spinal cord involvement. Cerebrospinal fluid analysis revealed WBC 0, RBC 36, protein 31 mg/dL, and glucose 72 mg/dL. There were no oligoclonal bands. The IgG index was normal. A broad infectious evaluation was negative including parasitic, bacterial, and fungal cultures/immunoassays from both blood and CSF. Initial diagnostic considerations included neoplasm or intracranial infection. Therefore, the patient underwent a biopsy of a left temporal lesion which

M.A. Lopez, M.D., Ph.D.
Developmental Neuroscience and Department of Pediatrics, Baylor College of Medicine,
Texas Children's Hospital, 6701 Fannon CC 1250, Houston, TX 77030, USA
e-mail: michaell@bcm.edu

T.E. Lotze, M.D. (✉)
Division of Neurology and Developmental Neuroscience, Department of Pediatrics,
Baylor College of Medicine, Texas Children's Hospital, 6701 Fannon CC 1250,
Houston, TX 77030, USA
e-mail: tlotze@bcm.edu

© Springer International Publishing AG 2017
E. Waubant, T.E. Lotze (eds.), *Pediatric Demyelinating Diseases of the Central Nervous System and Their Mimics*, DOI 10.1007/978-3-319-61407-6_7

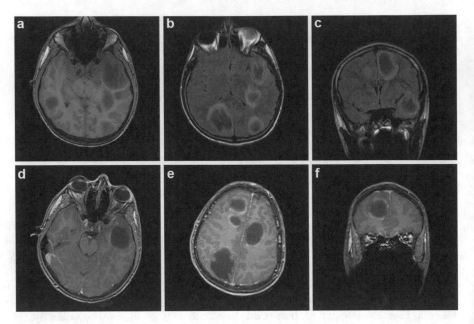

**Fig. 7.1** (**a**) T1-weighted non-contrast axial image demonstrating large hypointense lesions in the juxtacortical and deep white matter. (**b** and **c**) T2-FLAIR sequences demonstrating a peripheral rim of T2 hyperintensity with minimal mass effect. (**d–f**) T1 gadolinium-enhanced sequences demonstrating "broken rims" of enhancement around several of the lesions

revealed no infectious or neoplastic etiologies. The pathological report demonstrated microscopic fragments of unremarkable brain tissue in a background of blood, occasional inflammatory cells, and occasional clusters of macrophages. Myelin stains were not performed.

He was diagnosed with tumefactive demyelinating disease and started treatment with intravenous methylprednisolone 1 g daily for 5 days. He did not have any significant response to methylprednisolone and went on to receive a total of six plasma exchanges over 10 days. After completing plasma exchange, he was able to return home with an oral steroid taper and outpatient rehabilitation. At the time of discharge, his neurological status had improved with normal orientation, strength, tone, coordination, and sensation. However, he continued to have ongoing speech impairment including problems in comprehension, naming, and repetition. He was able to give three-word phrases, but his fluency was reduced. He also continued to have gait instability and visual-spatial impairment. Three months after his presentation, his motor and language impairments had completely resolved. However, he complained of persistent neurocognitive difficulties to include perseverative thoughts and actions, short-term memory difficulties, attention problems, and anxiety.

# Clinical Questions

1. What historical, examination, and ancillary diagnostic study findings help to distinguish tumefactive demyelination from other diagnostic considerations?
2. What are the radiographic studies that help to differentiate tumefactive demyelination from other brain lesions?
3. When should we recommend brain biopsy?
4. Are there specific acute treatments for tumefactive demyelination?
5. What is known about the prognosis including recurrence risk and neurological outcome in patients with tumefactive demyelination?

# Diagnostic Discussion

1. In the largest study ($N = 168$) of patients with biopsy-proven tumefactive demyelinating lesions (TDL), the majority (61%) presented as a first-time neurological event [1]. The remaining patients either had a previous diagnosis of multiple sclerosis (MS) or a history of another antedated neurological event consistent with demyelination. Patients with TDL can present with hemispheric or posterior fossa involvement including cognitive, motor, sensory, or cerebellar changes [1]. In our case, the patient presented with short-term memory impairment, difficulty with expressive speech, and imbalance. This progressed to include evidence of increased intracranial pressure as manifested by headache and vomiting, which is commonly seen in children with TDL.

   Cerebral abscess and brain tumors are two TDL mimics that should be in the differential diagnosis. Clinical features that would be suggestive of CNS infection include fever, toxic appearance, or an immunocompromised patient. Other findings, such as altered mental status, headache, focal deficits, and seizures might be shared between TDL and TDL mimics [2]. Infectious risk factors could include an immunocompromised host, travel to high-risk areas, and exposures to pathogens with a predilection for central nervous system (CNS) invasion. Specific pathogens might include parasites (*Angiostrongylus cantonensis*, *Toxoplasma gondii*), bacteria (*Bartonella*, *Borrelia burgdorferi*, *Mycobacterium tuberculosis*, and *Treponema pallidum*), and viruses (cytomegalovirus, human immunodeficiency virus, and JC virus). In an at risk patient, one might additionally consider fungal pathogens, i.e., *Aspergillus*, *Candida*, and *Cryptococcus*.

   Neurosarcoidosis is a systemic disease that can lead to multifocal CNS lesions with enhancement and increased T2 signal. It is most prevalent in African Americans and women. If suspected, a systemic evaluation for uveitis, erythema nodosum, pulmonary infiltrates, or hilar adenopathy should be done. CSF might show increased mononuclear pleocytosis with elevated IgG index and the presence of oligoclonal bands as with TDL. Serum may show elevated angiotensin-converting enzyme.

Brain tumor, lymphoma, and cerebral metastasis can produce multifocal lesions with edema and mass effect. In children, a solitary brain lesion is more suspicious for neoplasia and represents a more difficult diagnostic challenge. In contrast, children with TDL tend to have more than one lesion. Brain tumors that can mimic TDLs include astrocytomas (either high or low grade), oligodendrogliomas, and CNS lymphomas. Primary CNS lymphoma is rare in children. Systemic lymphoma maybe more readily recognized by a chronic time course, systemic symptoms (fever, night sweats, weight loss), and examination finding such as diffuse lymphadenopathy. It is important that steroids are withheld during an evaluation for CNS lymphoma because steroids may alter MRI and pathologic findings thus complicating the diagnosis. A careful evaluation for systemic malignancy could include a chest x-ray, CT chest, abdomen, and pelvis, and CT-PET. An ophthalmological examination is also important to evaluate for ocular involvement that can co-occur with primary CNS lymphoma or sarcoid. In this case, the patient had an illness time course of 1 month, without systemic malignant symptoms, or evidence of lymphadenopathy.

A lumbar puncture to analyze CSF is critical to evaluate tumor-like CNS lesions unless there are clinical signs of a life-threatening cerebral herniation. The CSF profile in demyelinating disease may reveal elevated white blood count, positive oligoclonal bands, or an elevated IgG index. The protein should be normal, gram stain and cultures should be negative and cytology without neoplastic cells.

2. Differentiating tumefactive demyelinating lesions from a brain tumor or cerebral abscess can be challenging. Radiographically, TDLs appear as large lesions (>2 cm) with perilesional edema without or with mass effect that is usually milder than with brain tumors.

CT is often the first emergent imaging study performed. Hypodense lesions on CT are characteristics of demyelination or infection and would be atypical for a high-grade tumor, which are more often hyperdense. Pyogenic abscesses are solitary in 50% of cases but can also be multifocal [2]. They are usually located at the gray-white junction encountered along arterial distributions and can have perilesional edema.

Contrast-enhanced MRI is important to further clarify the diagnosis. Lesion location can help to better refine differential diagnostic considerations. Multifocal lesions in typical locations for demyelination, such as juxtacortical, infratentorial, corpus callosum, periventricular, and deep white matter regions are consistent with TDL. Most common CNS tumors of childhood are solitary and more likely to occur in the posterior fossa. It is also especially important to evaluate the optic nerve and spinal cord as lesions in these locations would be supportive of demyelination.

Well-circumscribed borders are commonly seen in cases of tumefactive demyelination [3] as well as multifocal abscesses, CNS lymphoma, and other tumors. Other useful MRI signal characteristics of TDL include isointense to markedly hypointense signal on T1-weighted sequences, a hypointense rim on T2-weighted studies, and increased diffusion coefficient within the lesion. The presence of diffusion restriction at the rim of the lesion on diffusion-weighted imaging is variable with studies reporting this finding in 50–70% [4]. In contrast, cerebral abscesses and high-grade tumors tend to show diffusion restriction throughout the lesion.

The MRI enhancement pattern following contrast administration is particularly useful for evaluating TDL. Demyelinating lesions can have a variety of enhancement patterns. The classic pattern associated with MS is a "broken ring" or incomplete ring of peripheral enhancement with the opening oriented toward the cortex. Abscesses tend to have a solid smooth rind of enhancement with orientation toward the ventricles. Tumors can have heterogeneous or homogenous enhancement that involves the whole lesion, rather than just the borders.

MR spectroscopy can sometimes be beneficial in distinguishing a high-grade malignancy from demyelination. The former tends to show an inversion of the choline/creatine peaks, representing increased cell turnover and metabolic demands. On MR spectroscopy, tumefactive demyelination may show increased choline to $N$-acetyl-aspartate ratio similar to that seen in neoplasia. However, unlike neoplasia, the ratio in tumefactive demyelination tends to decrease with time as opposed to remaining stable as would be expected in neoplasia. Therefore, serial MR spectroscopy may be more informative than a single imaging series.

3. Brain biopsy may be avoided in patients where demyelination is likely such as:

   (a) Patients with a history of prior neurologic event(s) that resolved or a known demyelinating condition (CIS, MS)
   (b) Multifocal lesions in typical locations for demyelination including juxtacortical, infratentorial, corpus callosum, periventricular, and deep white matter regions
   (c) A classic demyelinating pattern such as an incomplete ring of enhancement open toward the cortex
   (d) The absence of any infectious risk factors with a CSF profile consistent with demyelination

   While these features can be helpful, it may be necessary to obtain a brain biopsy to rule out neoplasia, infection, or sarcoid, especially in the case of isolated lesions. If possible, the biopsy should be performed before steroid treatment. Once steroids are deemed safe, an empiric trial may reveal a rapid clinical improvement that in combination with serial imaging can provide further evidence of a demyelinating process rather than abscess or tumor.

4. First-line symptomatic treatment for TDL is high-dose corticosteroids, such as methylprednisolone 30 mg/kg/dose (maximum 1000 mg) daily for up to 5 days. Plasma exchange can be considered as a second-line therapy if corticosteroids are ineffective within weeks of treatment. Pediatric patients with a solitary lesion are the most challenging to diagnose, and a biopsy might be indicated if CSF is unrevealing [5, 6].

5. As TDLs are rare, there is limited and conflicting data regarding prognosis, especially in pediatric populations. It has been reported that patients with a single isolated tumefactive lesion have a lower risk of progression to definite multiple

sclerosis. However, in a large group of 85 patients with their first demyelinating event of biopsy-proven tumefactive demyelination, 70% went on to develop definite or probable multiple sclerosis within 4 years [1]. Half of the patients had multifocal and half monofocal lesions on presentations. In this same cohort, four of the seven patients that were under the age of 18 years developed MS. A more recent study [7] showed 18 of 31 (58.1%) children with TDL progressed to MS over a median period of 3.3 months. Our patient met 2010 McDonald criteria for MS as MRI lesions were disseminated in space (involving subcortical and periventricular areas) and in time (as several silent lesions enhanced after injection of contrast). As such, the risk of relapse is substantial, and the patient could benefit from early initiation of disease-modifying therapy.

## Clinical Pearls

1. In patients where brain tumor and cerebral abscess are in the differential, it is important to also consider TDL.
2. There is variability of radiographic features in patients with TDL. However, features suggestive of TDL include ring-enhancing lesions on MRI, locations typical for demyelination, and milder mass effect/edema than seen in tumors/abscess. The use of other imaging modalities such as MR spectroscopy can help further characterize changes suggestive of the etiology. Serial imaging may be necessary to ensure no evidence of an alternate diagnosis.
3. The prognosis of patients with TDL is uncertain. The majority of patients develop MS relapses during follow-up.

## References

1. Lucchinetti CF, et al. Clinical and radiographic spectrum of pathologically confirmed tumefactive multiple sclerosis. Brain. 2008;131(Pt 7):1759–75.
2. Luthra G, et al. Comparative evaluation of fungal, tubercular, and pyogenic brain abscesses with conventional and diffusion MR imaging and proton MR spectroscopy. AJNR Am J Neuroradiol. 2007;28(7):1332–8.
3. Altintas A, et al. Clinical and radiological characteristics of tumefactive demyelinating lesions: follow-up study. Mult Scler. 2012;18(10):1448–53.
4. Yao J, et al. Clinical and radiological characteristics of 17 Chinese patients with pathology confirmed tumefactive demyelinating diseases: follow-up study. J Neurol Sci. 2015;348(1–2):153–9.
5. Hardy TA, Chataway J. Tumefactive demyelination: an approach to diagnosis and management. J Neurol Neurosurg Psychiatry. 2013;84(9):1047–53.
6. Morin MP, et al. Solitary tumefactive demyelinating lesions in children. J Child Neurol. 2011;26(8):995–9.
7. Yiu EM, et al. Clinical and magnetic resonance imaging (MRI) distinctions between tumefactive demyelination and brain tumors in children. J Child Neurol. 2014;29(5):654–65.

# Chapter 8
# Radiologically Isolated Syndrome

Katherine DeStefano and Naila Makhani

## Case Presentation

A 16-year-old girl with a past medical history of asthma was taken to the hospital after she developed acute-onset chest tightness, shortness of breath, brief visual changes, and slowed speech while running at school. She was running 250 m sprints at an outdoor track practice when she had sudden onset of chest tightness and shortness of breath. When leaning over to catch her breath, she noted her vision "blacked out" in both eyes for 10 s before returning entirely to normal. In addition, she briefly felt light-headed and nauseous. Her symptoms improved immediately upon sitting down. She denied having any symptoms of headache, numbness, weakness, or altered consciousness. However, she was noted by teachers to have "slow speech," which was not otherwise characterized (i.e., no slurred speech, facial weakness, or word-finding difficulties) for roughly 1 h. She was born full term after an uncomplicated pregnancy and denied any previous history of transient neurologic symptoms including numbness, weakness, paresthesia, vision alteration, bowel or bladder symptoms, or Lhermitte's symptom. She had a normal neurological examination. Initial evaluation was performed with a non-contrast CT scan of the head, which demonstrated frontally predominant white matter hypodensities. A subsequent brain MRI revealed numerous (>9) T2 white matter hyperintense lesions without enhancement including periventricular (>3), juxtacortical, and subcortical lesions. A cervical spine MRI with and without contrast was normal, and a lumbar puncture revealed

K. DeStefano, M.D., M.S. (✉)
Department of Neurology, Yale University School of Medicine,
333 Cedar Street, New Haven, CT 06510, USA
e-mail: katherine.destefano@yale.edu

N. Makhani, M.D., M.P.H.
Yale University School of Medicine, Yale New Haven Hospital,
333 Cedar Street, LMP 3088, New Haven, CT 06510, USA
e-mail: naila.makhani@yale.edu

© Springer International Publishing AG 2017
E. Waubant, T.E. Lotze (eds.), *Pediatric Demyelinating Diseases of the Central Nervous System and Their Mimics*, DOI 10.1007/978-3-319-61407-6_8

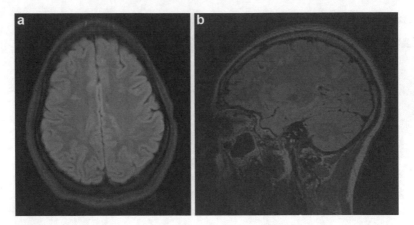

**Fig. 8.1** (**a** and **b**) Brain MRI showing ovoid T2 hyperintense lesions

two white cells and protein of 18 mg/dL. A serologic workup including vitamin B12, ANA, dsDNA, rheumatoid factor, anti-SSA and anti-SSB, NMO IgG, and HIV was unremarkable. She was discharged home with a diagnosis of syncope related to exercise-induced asthma. She was subsequently seen in follow-up as an outpatient where she was found to be clinically stable without any further episodes of neurologic symptoms and a normal neurological examination (Fig. 8.1a, b).

## Clinical Questions

1. What is the definition of the radiologically isolated syndrome (RIS)?
2. What tests should be done to rule out other causes of white matter lesions?
3. Does RIS increase the risk of developing clinically isolated syndrome (CIS) or multiple sclerosis (MS)?
4. What are the best predictive factors for developing CIS or MS?
5. How should patients with RIS be followed over time?

## Diagnostic Discussion

1. Even before the era of MRIs, postmortem autopsy studies revealed the presence of clinically silent demyelinating lesions in asymptomatic individuals [1]. With the advent of MRIs, increased use of imaging, and advances in imaging techniques has come an increase in the detection of incidental MRI findings in the central nervous system (CNS). While some lesions are nonspecific, many are highly suggestive of demyelination given their morphology and location within brain parenchyma (e.g., ovoid, well-circumscribed, periventricular, juxtacortical,

infratentorial). In 2009, Okuda and colleagues introduced the term radiologically isolated syndrome (RIS) to describe patients without any clinical symptoms of MS with MRI abnormalities highly suggestive of demyelinating disease [2]. Proposed diagnostic MRI criteria for RIS included T2 lesions that are (1) ovoid, well-circumscribed, and homogeneous foci with or without involvement of the corpus callosum; (2) >3 mm and fulfill at least three of four Barkhof Criteria for dissemination in space (DIS)[1]; (3) not consistent with a vascular pattern; and (4) not explained by another disease process.

2. Crucial to the diagnosis of RIS is ruling out other medical conditions that could explain the observed MRI brain lesions. This is typically done by blood test analysis including, but not limited to CBC (to look for signs of infection), Lyme disease titers (particularly in endemic areas), antinuclear antibody, double-stranded DNA antibodies, anti-SSA and anti-SSB antibodies, rheumatoid factor, vitamin B12, homocysteine and methylmalonic acid, antiphospholipid antibody screen, thyroid function tests, and HIV testing. Cerebrospinal fluid (CSF) analysis and visual evoked potential (VEP) testing may also be helpful to exclude other diagnoses (particularly CNS infection) and to look for signs of subclinical demyelination, respectively.

3. Several adult cohorts have shown that RIS increases the risk that a patient will go on to develop a first clinical attack consistent with a diagnosis of either clinically isolated syndrome (CIS) or MS [2, 3]. Given that RIS is a relatively new entity, there is limited natural history data in adults and no longitudinal studies in the pediatric population. The approach to children with RIS must therefore be extrapolated from the limited adult data. Several adult studies have shown that individuals with RIS have a roughly 30% risk of being diagnosed with CIS or MS after 5 years [2, 3]. In a 2009 study with a cohort of 44 patients (> 16 years of age) with RIS, 10 of the 30 patients who had follow-up developed CIS or MS (by 2005 McDonald criteria) after a median of 5.4 years [2]. After a median of 2.7 years of follow-up, radiologic progression (consisting of new T2 lesions, enhancing lesions, or enlarging lesions) occurred in 59% of patients. While the majority of adult RIS patients who progress clinically do so with an acute clinical event, a smaller percentage have an initial event that goes on to fulfill criteria for primary progressive MS.

4. Once patients with RIS are identified, it would be ideal to be able to determine which patients are most likely to progress to CIS or MS. Okuda et al. have shown that in adults with RIS, asymptomatic spinal cord lesions were associated with a substantial increase in the odds of developing a clinical demyelinating event or primary progressive MS (odds ratio 75.3 with 95% confidence interval 16.1–350.0 and $p < 0.0001$, 84.0% positive predictive value, sensitivity 87.5%, and specificity 91.5%) [4]. These findings were independent of brain T2 lesion load or the

---

[1] Barkhof Criteria for DIS: (1) at least nine T2 hyperintense lesions or one gadolinium-enhancing lesion, (2) at least three periventricular lesions, (3) at least one infratentorial lesion, (4) at least one juxtacortical lesion [6].

presence of enhancement. Thus, patients with asymptomatic lesions in both the brain and the spinal cord carry a higher risk of clinical progression than those patients with brain lesions alone. Additionally, there was a relationship between age at RIS presentation and subsequent risk of CIS or PPMS; for every 10-year increase in age, the odds of a later clinical attack were reduced (OR 0.38 [0.15–0.97]; $p = 0.043$) [4]. In analyzing the 5-year risk of developing an initial clinical event, Okuda et al. found that 34% of patients with RIS experienced a clinical event consistent with a demyelinating event and that the presence of lesions in the spinal cord, age < 37, and male sex were the most important predictors of clinical symptom onset [5]. Given the association with higher risk of clinical progression, spinal imaging should be considered for prognostic purposes in patients with RIS.

5. Although there are no official consensus guidelines for how to follow patients with RIS, two basic approaches are frequently employed: (a) wait expectantly for a clinical attack and (b) actively follow with imaging. While some clinicians will observe closely for a first clinical attack, many others choose to follow patients with serial MRIs to determine whether patients are accruing new lesions over time. Some clinicians will follow patients with annual MRIs. The frequency of neuroimaging can further be tailored based on the presence or absence of known predictive factors for clinical progression. Given the debate about the necessity of treating patients with RIS and lack of clinical trials with disease modifying therapies (DMTs), it is difficult to make generalized statements about standardized care of RIS patients. While studies have shown the use of a DMT in adults with a clinically isolated syndrome (CIS) will delay progression to MS, to date we have no such studies for RIS as clinical trials are still ongoing in adults RIS patients. There currently are no FDA-approved drugs for RIS, and in general, the use of a DMT is not routinely recommended outside of clinical trials. This is in large part because some RIS patients will never develop a clinical event (even with long-term follow-up) and the use of DMTs is not without risk of adverse events or side effects. Future studies are necessary to better determine not only the long-term prognosis of RIS in children but also the role of DMTs, if any, in altering the natural history of RIS in both adults and children.

## Clinical Pearls

1. In any suspected case of RIS, first rule out other possible causes of CNS lesions.
2. Roughly 30% of adult RIS patients will develop a first clinical attack or meet diagnostic criteria for MS within 5 years. The natural history of pediatric RIS remains unknown.
3. Given the predictive value of asymptomatic spinal cord lesions in adult RIS patients, it is suggested that cervical and thoracic cord imaging is obtained in children with RIS.

4. More research is necessary, in both adult and pediatric populations, to better ascertain the prevalence of RIS, the natural history of RIS, and how to best monitor and possibly treat patients with RIS.

# References

1. Engell T. A clinical patho-anatomical study of clinically silent multiple sclerosis. Acta Neurol Scand. 1989;79(5):428–30.
2. Okuda DT, Mowry EM, Beheshtian A, Waubant E, Baranzini SE, Goodin DS, Hauser SL, Pelletier D. Incidental MRI anomalies suggestive of multiple sclerosis: the radiologically isolated syndrome. Neurology. 2009;72(14):800–5.
3. Lebrun C, Bensa C, Debouverie M, Wiertlevski S, Brassat D, et al. Association between clinical conversion to multiple sclerosis in radiologically isolated syndrome and magnetic resonance imaging, cerebrospinal fluid, and visual evoked potential. Arch Neurol. 2009;66(7):841–6.
4. Okuda DT, Mowry EM, Cree BAC, Crabtree EC, Goodin DS, Waubant E, Pelletier D. Asymptomatic spinal cord lesions predict disease progression in radiologically isolated syndrome. Neurology. 2011;76(8):686–92.
5. Okuda DT, Siva A, Kantarci O, Inglese M, Katz I, et al. Radiologically isolated syndrome: 5-year risk for an initial clinical event. PLoS One. 2014;9(3):e90509.
6. Barkhof F, Filippi M, Miller DH, et al. Comparison of MRI criteria at first presentation to predict conversion to clinically definite multiple sclerosis. Brain. 1997;120(11):2059–69.

# Chapter 9
# Anti-glutamic Acid Decarboxylase Limbic Encephalitis

Robert Rudock, Jason Helis, and Soe S. Mar

## Case Presentation

A 6-year-old African American boy, diagnosed 6 months prior with type I diabetes, presented with simple partial seizures of his right hand. His seizures rapidly progressed over several days to epilepsia partialis continua, involving the right face, arm, and leg. An EEG showed epileptiform discharges and slowing of the left hemisphere. Two weeks after the initial seizure, he became obtunded and aphasic. The seizures were refractory to multiple antiseizure medications and corticosteroids. He was intubated and placed on a continuous midazolam infusion on day 17 of illness.

Serum evaluations for herpes simplex virus, mycoplasma, varicella zoster virus, cytomegalovirus, Epstein-Barr virus, and human herpesvirus 6 were negative. Thyroid function studies, serum ammonia, serum lactate, anti-DNA antibodies, rheumatoid factor, lupus anticoagulant, pro-time, partial thromboplastin time, protein C, protein S, and antithrombin III were all normal. Cerebral spinal fluid studies that included evaluation for herpes simplex virus, cryptococcal antigen, fungal, as well as viral and bacterial cultures were also normal. His serum anti-GAD65 titer was 3484 U/ml (positive >4.0 U/ml) at the time of his diagnosis of diabetes, but islet

R. Rudock, M.D. M.B.A.
Division of Pediatric and Developmental Neurology, Department of Neurology,
Washington University in St. Louis School of Medicine, 660 S. Euclid Ave,
Campus Box 8111, St. Louis, MO 63110-1094, USA
e-mail: rjrudock@wustl.edu

J. Helis, M.D. M.S.
Maine Medical Partners Neurology, 49 Spring Street, Scarborough, ME 04074, USA
e-mail: helisj@neuro.wustl.edu

S.S. Mar, M.D. (✉)
Department of Neurology, Washington University School of Medicine, St. Louis, MO, USA
e-mail: mars@wustl.edu

© Springer International Publishing AG 2017
E. Waubant, T.E. Lotze (eds.), *Pediatric Demyelinating Diseases of the Central Nervous System and Their Mimics*, DOI 10.1007/978-3-319-61407-6_9

**Fig. 9.1** MRI (FLAIR sequences) 6 days after presentation: this image shows hyperintense lesion of the cerebellum. The child was still conscious at this time

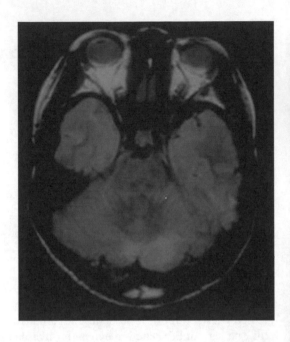

cell antibodies were negative. At the time of development of epilepsia partialis continua, his serum anti-GAD65 titers were 19,610 U/ml (positive >1.0 U/ml). Cerebral spinal fluid anti-GAD 65 titers were 3325 U/ml. He also had positive serum anti-islet cell antibodies at 10,240 Juvenile Diabetes Foundation Units (reference range: negative).

An MRI of the brain was obtained at the time of initial presentation and was normal. Repeat MRI taken 6 days after presentation showed a hyperintense lesion in the cerebellum (FLAIR sequence) (see Fig. 9.1). Another MRI performed 26 days after presentation showed lesions located in the left frontal and occipital cortex (FLAIR sequence) (see Fig. 9.2).

Treatment consisted of high-dose IV steroids (2 mg/kg/day), intravenous immunoglobulin, and plasmapheresis. After an initial 5-day course of daily plasmapheresis, his anti-GAD 65 antibodies fell to 4491 U/ml. His aphasia improved and he became seizure-free. Repeat cycles of plasmapheresis were continued and their timing spaced out over the next several months. He improved clinically to his baseline mental status 3 months after initiation of plasmapheresis. His serum anti-GAD65 antibodies stabilized between 5000 and 6000 U/ml.

## Clinical Questions

1. What is a paraneoplastic syndrome?
2. When should anti-GAD encephalitis be considered in a differential diagnosis?

**Fig. 9.2**  26 days after presentation: this MRI shows additional lesions in the left frontoparietal cortex as well as the left occipital cortex

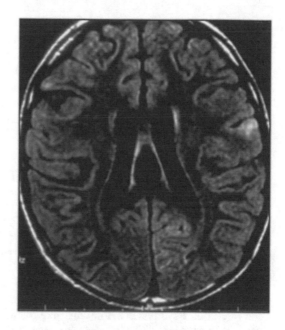

3. What other conditions are associated with positive GAD65 antibodies?
4. What are the most effective treatment options for patients with anti-GAD encephalitis?
5. What are the long-term outcomes for patients with established encephalitis related to elevated GAD65 antibodies?

## Diagnostic Discussion

### *What Is a Paraneoplastic Syndrome?*

Paraneoplastic syndromes represent a discreet group of illnesses caused by the indirect effects of malignancy. The unique symptoms of a particular syndrome are theorized to be the result of immunologic cross-reactivity between tumor antigens and specific sites along the neuroaxis [1].

These central nervous system antibody-associated syndromes tend to be separated into two general categories [2]. The first category, classic paraneoplastic disorders, produces antibodies that target intracellular neuronal antigens and is nearly always accompanied with an underlying cancer. While especially rare in children, several adult-onset paraneoplastic antibodies have been described, including anti-Hu, anti-Ma, and anti-Ri. Conversely, the nonclassic or autoimmune disorders, such as anti-GAD encephalitis and anti-NMDA receptor encephalitis, target intracellular synaptic proteins or antigens on the cell surface of neurons, respectively, and affect both the adult and pediatric populations; they are only sometimes associated with malignancy. Anti-NMDA receptor encephalitis, for example, nicely illustrates this variability in tumor association, which interestingly appears to be related to age. In women older than 18 years of age with positive anti-NMDA receptor antibodies, nearly 45% will have an associated ovarian teratoma. In girls less than 14 years old, however, fewer than 9% will have a teratoma identified [2].

## When Should Anti-GAD Encephalitis Be Considered in a Differential Diagnosis?

Anti-glutamic acid decarboxylase antibody-associated limbic encephalitis (AGADE) typically presents with psychiatric changes, subacute memory loss, and seizures. Any previously healthy child or teenager who suddenly presents with these symptoms should be evaluated for anti-GAD encephalitis once more common encephalitic causes (i.e., HSV encephalitis, anti-NMDA, and other infections) have been ruled out. Psychiatric symptoms may include depression, mood disturbance, visual hallucinations, and/or anxiety; memory difficulties, sleep disturbance, apraxia, and ataxia may also occur [3]. Seizures may appear clinically and electro-graphically focal or generalized, resulting in patients often being given an initial diagnosis of new-onset temporal lobe epilepsy before anti-GAD encephalitis is considered. The frequency of status epilepticus and epilepsia partialis continua in these children with elevated GAD antibodies is not well described. Associated seizures, however, are extremely difficult to treat and are often refractory to multiple antiepileptic medications.

While an initial brain MRI may appear normal, thus reinforcing a diagnosis of idiopathic epilepsy, imaging may in fact take up to several years to show T2 hyperintensity changes, most commonly in the temporal lobes and hippocampus. MRI changes are not exclusive to the temporal lobes and may also be seen in other cortices as well as the cerebellum [3]. Temporal lobe involvement may initially be misinterpreted as possible HSV encephalitis during the initial workup. Cerebrospinal fluid analysis, like with other forms of limbic encephalitis, may reveal elevated protein, a lymphocytic predominant pleocytosis, and/or oligoclonal bands [1].

## What Other Conditions Are Associated with Positive GAD65 Antibodies?

Glutamic acid decarboxylase (GAD) is an intracellular enzyme, which acts to convert glutamate into GABA. There are currently two known GAD isoforms: 65 and 67 kDa [4]. GAD is found in large quantities in the dentate gyrus of the hippocampus and in CA1 [5], as well as beta cells in the pancreas. While AGADE has just recently begun to be described in the pediatric literature, in adults positive GAD65 antibodies are well known to be associated with stiff person syndrome, cerebellar ataxia, paraneoplastic conditions, and diabetes mellitus [3, 6]. The pathologic mechanism in adults and children is theorized to be similar, mainly that antibodies interfere or prevent the production of GABA through enzymatic inhibition of GAD [7].

Anti-GAD encephalitis patients may also have endocrinologic disorders such as common variable immunodeficiency or type I diabetes mellitus [3]. Moreover, the clinical significance of elevated GAD antibodies in the setting of neurologic disease is not currently fully understood. Given that approximately 60% of patients with DM 1 have elevated GAD antibodies at baseline, such antibodies may not be as useful of a marker for neurologic disease, but may instead, as some researchers have suggested, simply represent a nonspecific autoimmune finding [8]. Nevertheless, this overlap may still be a result of subtle antigenic differences between GAD antibodies associated with neurologic sequela and those associated with diabetes [9]. Therefore, if anti-GAD antibodies are found in a patient with symptoms consistent with limbic encephalitis, further testing for GABA-A and GABA-B antibodies may help to guide treatment. GABA-A positive patients are less likely to have an underlying paraneoplastic syndrome but tend to have a more severe encephalitic presentation and are at least partially responsive to treatments [10]. Concurrent GABA-B positivity, while more rare, is strongly associated with neoplasms, especially small cell lung cancer (SCLC) in adults [11]. Therefore, thorough evaluation for an underlying malignancy is suggested in any patient with limbic encephalitis and elevated GAD65 antibodies.

## What Are the Most Effective Treatment Options for Patients with Anti-GAD65 Encephalitis?

Initial treatment for anti-GAD encephalitis in children may include high-dose IV steroids, IVIG, and/or plasmapheresis. Mild symptoms at presentation, in the setting of positive antibodies, may prompt the health care provider to recommend treatment options such as steroids or IVIG. If the disease presentation is more severe, however, a treatment approach that more quickly removes the offending antibodies, such as plasmapheresis, may be warranted. Mycophenolate mofetil, cyclophosphamide, and rituximab have also been tried both to halt disease progression and maintain disease remission, albeit with inconsistent results. Of these three immune-modulating drugs, rituximab may have the greatest benefit, according to several case reports [3, 12]. Trending anti-GAD antibody titers may also provide a clinical utility, as there have been accounts of a proportional relationship between titers and seizure control, at least in adults [13].

# What Are the Long-Term Outcomes for Patients with Established Encephalitis Related to Elevated GAD65 Antibodies?

Long-term clinical outcome data is extremely limited, but according to a recent study by Haberlandt et al., three out of four pediatric patients with elevated anti-GAD antibody-associated limbic encephalitis had persistent symptoms at greater than 2.5 years following treatment initiation; only one patient made a complete recovery [14]. Furthermore, it is currently unknown whether or not patients may require lifelong immune-modulatory treatments. Nevertheless, response to treatment tends to be less effective in antibody-mediated encephalitides that target intracellular antigens, over those that target antigens on the cell surface [1], presumably because of current treatment options ability to reach the intended target.

## Clinical Pearls

1. The clinical significance of elevated GAD65 antibodies in children with limbic encephalitis-like symptoms is not fully understood, and pediatric cases are just beginning to be described in the literature; therefore, pediatric AGADE may be an underdiagnosed disease.
2. GAD65 antibodies should be checked in any patient who presents with subacute to chronic onset of difficult to treat seizures of unknown cause with psychiatric symptoms after more common diseases are ruled out.
3. Rituximab may offer the best treatment response but should only be entertained after treatment options with fewer side effects, such as IV steroids, IVIG, and plasmapheresis, have been tried.
4. Clinical outcome data is still being collected, but current evidence suggests that pediatric patients with anti-GAD65 antibody-associated limbic encephalitis tend to require long-term treatment and have persistent symptoms.

## References

1. Mustafa K, Yasmin K. Paraneoplastic syndromes affecting the nervous system. In: Swaiman KF, Ashwal S, Ferriero DM, editors. Pediatric neurology: principles & practice, vol. 4th ed. Philadelphia: Mosby; 2007.
2. Dalmau J, Rosenfeld MR. Autoimmune encephalitis update. Neuro-Oncology. 2014;16(6):771–8.
3. Mishra N, Rodan LH, Nita DA, Gresa-Arribas N, Kobayashi J, Benseler SM. Anti-glutamic acid decarboxylase antibody associated limbic encephalitis in a child: expanding the spectrum of pediatric inflammatory brain diseases. J Child Neurol. 2014;29(5):677–83.

4. Manto MU, Laute MA, Aguera M, Rogemond V, Pandolfo M, Honnorat J. Effects of anti-glutamic acid decarboxylase antibodies associated with neurological diseases. Ann Neurol. 2007;61(6):544–51.
5. Sloviter RS, Dichter MA, Rachinsky TL, Dean E, Goodman JH, Sollas AL, et al. Basal expression and induction of glutamate decarboxylase and GABA in excitatory granule cells of the rat and monkey hippocampal dentate gyrus. J Comp Neurol. 1996;373(4):593–618.
6. Saiz A, Blanco Y, Sabater L, Gonzalez F, Bataller L, Casamitjana R, et al. Spectrum of neurological syndromes associated with glutamic acid decarboxylase antibodies: diagnostic clues for this association. Brain. 2008;131(10):2553–63.
7. Christgau S, Aanstoot HJ, Schierbeck H, Begley K, Tullin S, Hejnaes K, et al. Membrane anchoring of the autoantigen GAD65 to microvesicles in pancreatic beta-cells by palmitoylation in the NH2-terminal domain. J Cell Biol. 1992;118(2):309–20.
8. Vincent A, Dale RC. Autoimmune channelopathies and other antibody-associated neurological disorders. In: Dale RC, Vincent A, editors. Inflammatory and autoimmune disorders of the nervous system in children. London: Mac Keith Press; 2010. xvi, 504 p., 8 p. of plates p.
9. Vianello M, Keir G, Giometto B, Betterle C, Tavolato B, Thompson EJ. Antigenic differences between neurological and diabetic patients with anti-glutamic acid decarboxylase antibodies. Eur J Neurol. 2005;12(4):294–9.
10. Petit-Pedrol M, Armangue T, Peng X, Bataller L, Cellucci T, Davis R, et al. Encephalitis with refractory seizures, status epilepticus, and antibodies to the GABAA receptor: a case series, characterisation of the antigen, and analysis of the effects of antibodies. Lancet Neurol. 2014;13(3):276–86.
11. Boronat A, Sabater L, Saiz A, Dalmau J, Graus F. GABA(B) receptor antibodies in limbic encephalitis and anti-GAD-associated neurologic disorders. Neurology. 2011;76(9):795–800.
12. Korff CM, Parvex P, Cimasoni L, Wilhelm-Bals A, Hampe CS, Schwitzgebel VM, et al. Encephalitis associated with glutamic acid decarboxylase autoantibodies in a child: a treatable condition? Arch Neurol. 2011;68(8):1065–8.
13. Kanter IC, Huttner HB, Staykov D, Biermann T, Struffert T, Kerling F, et al. Cyclophosphamide for anti-GAD antibody-positive refractory status epilepticus. Epilepsia. 2008;49(5):914.
14. Haberlandt E, Bast T, Ebner A, Holthausen H, Kluger G, Kravljanac R, et al. Limbic encephalitis in children and adolescents. Arch Dis Child. 2011;96(2):186–91.

# Chapter 10
# Anti-NMDA Receptor Antibody Encephalitis

Tristan T. Sands, Katherine Kedzierski, and Naila Makhani

## Case Presentation

Case 1  A 14-year-old girl presented with seizures and altered mental status 1 week after an upper respiratory tract infection. During the 3 days prior to admission, her family had noted confusion, behavioral changes, and bizarre language. A brief episode of unresponsiveness and cyanosis led the family to seek care in the emergency department where she had an observed generalized seizure treated with lorazepam. On initial evaluation, she was febrile and tachycardic. She was lethargic and mumbling incoherent phrases but had an otherwise non-focal neurological examination. She was loaded with intravenous fosphenytoin and empirically started on antibiotics and acyclovir. Cerebral spinal fluid (CSF) analysis revealed 24 white blood cells per microliter (92% lymphocytes) with normal protein and glucose. Bacterial cultures and CSF viral studies (VZV, HSV1/2, EBV, CMV, and enterovirus) were negative. Brain MRI showed a subtle T2 signal abnormality along the right medial temporal lobe and subtle enhancement along the inferior anterior temporal pole. Over the next several days, she became progressively encephalopathic and developed respiratory instability requiring intubation, tem-

T.T. Sands, M.D., Ph.D. (✉)
Division of Child Neurology, Columbia University Herbert and Florence
Irving Medical Center, 180 Fort Washington Avenue, Harkness Pavilion 5,
New York, NY, 10032, USA
e-mail: tts27@cumc.columbia.edu

K. Kedzierski, M.D.
Waterbury Neurology, 1625 Straits Turnpike, Suite 307, Middlebury, CT 06762, USA
e-mail: kasiaked@gmail.com

N. Makhani, M.D., M.P.H.
Yale University School of Medicine, Yale New Haven Hospital,
333 Cedar Street, LMP 3088, New Haven, CT 06510, USA
e-mail: naila.makhani@yale.edu

© Springer International Publishing AG 2017
E. Waubant, T.E. Lotze (eds.), *Pediatric Demyelinating Diseases of the Central
Nervous System and Their Mimics*, DOI 10.1007/978-3-319-61407-6_10

perature dysregulation, and hypertensive crises requiring transfer to intensive care. She subsequently developed dystonic limb movements and orofacial dyskinesias. EEG showed frontally predominant generalized rhythmic delta with shifting laterality and generalized periodic discharges with excess delta/theta in the awake state without normal sleep architecture, suggestive of moderate diffuse or multifocal cerebral dysfunction and cortical hyperexcitability. Anti-NMDA receptor antibody testing returned positive at a titer of 1:320 in CSF and 1:2560 in serum. Pelvic CT revealed a calcified left ovarian mass, which was resected and confirmed to be an ovarian teratoma on pathology. She was treated with 5 days of IV corticosteroids, plasmapheresis (five exchanges in 10 days), intravenous immunoglobulin (2 g/kg over 5 days), and rituximab (500 mg/m$^2$ on days 1 and 14). There was minimal initial clinical improvement, and she was started on monthly pulse cyclophosphamide (800 mg/m$^2$), which was continued for 12 months. Follow-up EEG demonstrated "extreme delta brush" (Fig. 10.1a). Rituximab was readministered after 8 months following CD19 count reconstitution. Eighteen months after first presentation, she is ambulating, has recovered her speech, and is independent in her activities of daily living.

**Case 2** A 13-year-old girl with a history of truncus arteriosus repaired in infancy presented with 3 weeks of episodic right limb stiffening. Four weeks prior, she had complained of profound fatigue requiring modification of her physical education program. One week later, she fell and lost consciousness after her right leg stiffened while walking. The episode was accompanied by right leg weakness and numbness. She was admitted with concern for her cardiac history, but an echocardiogram and EKG were stable. Brain MRI was normal. EEG captured an episode of involuntary right leg shaking without electrographic correlate, and she was diagnosed with non-epileptic seizures. Over the next 2 weeks, she developed multiple episodes per day of recurrent right leg stiffening and shaking. She was started on levetiracetam empirically without benefit. She returned to the emergency department with hourly episodes of right limb stiffening over 12 h and was treated with anticonvulsants for presumed status epilepticus. Repeat EEG was normal apart from excessive beta activity deemed likely secondary to benzodiazepines. She was monitored with EEG over several days, and a slow (~1 Hz) and irregular tremor at the right ankle was recorded without electrographic change. After 60 h of unremarkable EEG recording, the patient developed sudden onset of focal status epilepticus with seizures characterized clinically by tonic posturing of the right arm and/or leg and electrographically by an alpha frequency recruiting rhythm maximal at P3 (Fig. 10.1b). A repeat brain MRI revealed enhancement over the left parietal convexity (Fig. 10.1c). CSF analysis revealed ten leukocytes with a lymphocytic predominance. Her anti-NMDA receptor antibody testing returned negative in serum, but positive in CSF. Pelvic imaging did not detect any ovarian masses. She was treated with a 5-day pulse IV steroid course at her local hospital.

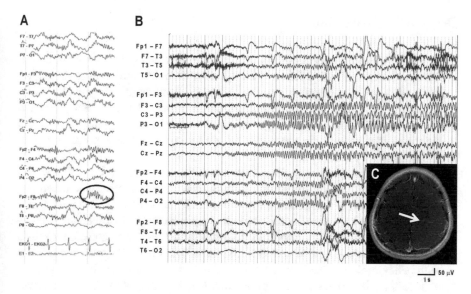

**Fig. 10.1** Electroencephalographic features of patients with NMDA encephalitis. (**a**) Interictal EEG from the first case. Extreme delta brush (*circled*), characterized by beta frequency waveforms superimposed on a delta wave. (**b**) Focal seizure recorded in the second case. Ictal onset is comprised of rhythmic, sharply contoured 11 Hz activity, maximal at the left central-parietal leads. Clinically the seizure was characterized by dystonic posturing of the right upper and lower extremities. (**c**) MRI of the brain from the same patient, showing subtle gyral pattern of contrast enhancement in perirolandic cortex, corresponding to the ictal focus. (**b, c**) Reprinted from Sands TT, Nash K, Tong S, Sullivan J. Focal seizures in children with anti-NMDA receptor antibody encephalitis. Epilepsy Res; 2015; 112:31–6, with permission from Elsevier

## Clinical Questions

1. What are the clinical and ancillary diagnostic features of anti-NMDA receptor encephalitis?
2. What is the spectrum of imaging features seen in anti-NMDA receptor encephalitis?
3. What acquired demyelinating diseases may occur in patients with anti-NMDA receptor encephalitis?
4. What is the pathogenesis of anti-NMDA receptor encephalitis?
5. What treatment regimens are used for anti-NMDA receptor encephalitis?
6. What determines prognosis in anti-NMDA receptor encephalitis?
7. Given these two different clinical presentations of anti-NMDA receptor encephalitis, when should the diagnosis be considered?
8. What is the role of serum versus CSF antibody titers?
9. Can patients with anti-NMDA receptor encephalitis relapse?

# Diagnostic Discussion

1. Anti-NMDA receptor encephalitis is an increasingly recognized cause of noninfectious encephalitis in children. It surpassed enteroviral infection as the underlying etiology in cases referred to the California Encephalitis Project [1]. While there is a predilection for young women, children under 18 years of age account for nearly 40% of patients [2]. Approximately 40% of patients under 12 years old are males, but females are more affected with increasing age, representing over 80% of cases by adulthood.

   Anti-NMDA receptor encephalitis is typically characterized by behavioral changes, sleep, memory and speech disturbances, seizures, movement disorders, autonomic dysregulation, and progressive deterioration of mental status. A history of a viral-like prodrome can be elicited from about 70% of patients. Herpes simplex encephalitis is a precursor to anti-NMDA receptor encephalitis in a small subset of patients. Whereas >75% of patients over 18 years old present with behavioral, cognitive, or memory changes, nearly 50% of children present with either seizures or a movement disorder [2]. A variety of hyperkinetic movement disorders, typically multiple, occur in children with anti-NMDA receptor encephalitis [3]. Orofacial dyskinesias are common. Myorhythmia, an unusual slow coarse irregular tremor, was observed in one of the patients described above. Autonomic instability, with frequent autonomic crises, is often characterized by blood pressure lability, heart rate changes, temperature dysregulation, and central hypoventilation, may require intensive care unit management, and is a particular source of morbidity and mortality.

   CSF analysis often reveals a lymphocytic pleocytosis, but it may also be normal. Elevations in protein, opening pressure, and IgG index and unique CSF oligoclonal bands have all been described. Infectious etiologies may be difficult to distinguish clinically early in the disease course [1]. EEG is abnormal in over 90% of patients (typically diffusely slow, disorganized, and with lack of normal sleep architecture), although it can be normal early in the disease course. About 33% of patients, will develop a distinctive "extreme delta brush" pattern (Fig. 10.1a), which may correlate with more severe disease [4]. Generalized rhythmic delta is another described interictal pattern. Seizures are often focal and electrographically have an ictal onset characterized by rhythmic alpha frequency activity (Fig. 10.1b) [5].

2. At disease onset, 35% of patient show nonspecific radiological findings, rising to 50% over the course of the disease. A spectrum of abnormalities may be seen with brain MRI including cortical and subcortical T2 hyperintensities and leptomeningeal enhancement, thought to reflect myelin disruption and subtle compromise of the blood-brain barrier (Fig. 10.2). Such findings can mimic demyelinating disease or infection, creating diagnostic challenges. In a subgroup of patients, MRI demonstrates frank comorbid demyelinating disease.

3. In a cohort of 691 patients with anti-NMDA receptor encephalitis, clinical and/or radiological findings of demyelination were found in 23 (3.3%) [6].

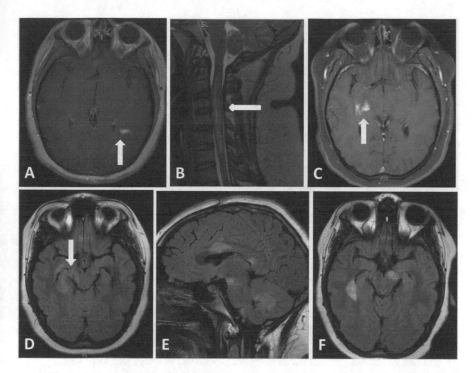

**Fig. 10.2** Spectrum of imaging findings observed in anti-NMDAR encephalitis. (**a**) Initial contrast-enhancing lesion; (**b**) longitudinally extensive transverse myelitis; (**c**) continued development of contrast-enhancing lesions; (**d**) retrochiasmatic optic neuritis; (**e**, **f**) continued accumulation of T2/FLAIR hyperintense lesion burden

Importantly, 11 of these patients manifested the first signs and symptoms of demyelination concurrently with an acute presentation of NMDA encephalitis without other discrete episodes of clinical demyelinating syndromes. These patients were more likely to have infratentorial or spinal cord involvement and 5/12 harbored antibodies to aquaporin-4 (AQP4). Of the 12 remaining patients who presented with symptoms of demyelinating disease before or after their episode of NMDA receptor encephalitis, 4 had AQP4 antibodies and another patient was diagnosed with neuromyelitis optica without AQP4 antibodies. All aquaporin-4 positive patients had onset of a clinical demyelinating syndrome prior to onset of NMDAR encephalitis. Anti-MOG antibodies are also common in these patients, though the significance of this finding is unclear. Clinical features of demyelination in those with anti-NMDAR encephalitis may include attacks of optic neuritis and transverse myelitis (consistent with clinical NMO), brainstem syndromes, and multifocal neurological symptoms/signs with or without fever and encephalopathy (ADEM-like). Recognition of the co-occurrence of demyelinating disease and NMDA receptor encephalitis is crucial, as management and prognosis differ for each condition (discussed below).

4. The NMDA receptor is a ligand-gated, calcium permeable, ion channel that functions as a coincident detector, opening in response to glutamate only in the setting of depolarization. It plays a critical role in long-term potentiation, the cellular basis for learning and memory. In anti-NMDA receptor encephalitis, intrathecally synthesized IgG antibodies bind to an extracellular hinge on the N-terminus of the GluN1 subunit. The result is receptor cross-linking and internalization with functional loss of NMDA receptor-mediated currents akin to the effects of pharmacologic receptor blockade by agents such as ketamine and phencyclidine [6]. This is in contrast to the complement-mediated mechanism of toxicity triggered by the AQP4 antibodies in NMO that results in marked tissue cavitation and necrosis observed on histopathology [7]. These pathological differences likely account for the relative treatment responsiveness and lower morbidity of NMDA receptor encephalitis in comparison to NMO.
Ovarian teratomas are identified in 46% of young women with anti-NMDA receptor encephalaitis, but this association is age-dependent with teratomas identified in only 6% of girls <12 years [2]. Ovarian teratomas contain neural tissue expressing the NMDA receptor and are thought to play a role in exposing the antigenic target to the immune system. Other tumors are rare and mainly reported in adults, but isolated cases of neuroblastoma and ovarian cystadenofibroma have been reported in pediatric patients. Patients with NMDAR encephalitis and comorbid demyelinating disease appear to have lower rates of ovarian teratoma, consistent with a general increased predisposition to autoimmunity [6].

5. Retrospective studies have demonstrated that first-line immunotherapy, consisting of a combination of pulse glucocorticoid infusions, plasmapheresis, intravenous immunoglobulin, and oopherectomy for teratoma, is associated with improved modified Rankin Scale (mRS) scores at 24-month follow-up. Good outcome, defined as a mRS of 0–2, is seen in 97% of patients receiving first-line therapy as compared with 71% of patients not receiving immunomodulatory treatment [2]. In the approximately 50% of patients who demonstrate no response within 4 weeks, second-line therapy with rituximab (375 mg/m$^2$ weekly for 4 weeks or 500 mg/m$^2$ on day 1 and 14) and/or cyclophosphamide (750–800 mg/m$^2$ monthly) is associated with improved mRS at 24 months with 78% of patients receiving second-line therapy achieving scores of 0–2 as compared to 55% of those receiving no further immunotherapy [2]. Supportive care and symptom management are also critical. Importantly, while patients with NMDAR encephalitis and concurrent demyelinating disease often respond to first-line immunotherapy for the period of encephalitis, episodes of clinical demyelination in these patients often require more aggressive second-line therapies and result in greater neurological deficits [6].

6. In one series of 577 patients with NMDAR encephalitis, 81% overall had a good outcome (mRS 0–2) at 24 months [2]. Favorable prognosis is associated with lower disease severity within 4 weeks of onset, defined by maximum mRS, no intensive care admission, and early treatment. In a multivariable analysis, second-line immunotherapy was also associated with increased likelihood of good outcome. Deficits in memory, attention, and executive function may persist.

Children often require an individualized educational plan on returning to school. Comorbid demyelinating disease carries a higher risk of residual neurological sequelae.

7. Anti-NMDA receptor encephalitis should be considered in severe cases of encephalitis, but also in children presenting subacutely with new unexplained movement disorders especially when accompanied by behavioral change, systemic symptoms, frank seizures, and progressive encephalopathy. Inpatient EEG monitoring may be helpful to characterize such movements, to exclude or confirm seizures, and to identify other distinctive features such as extreme delta brush that can be helpful in suggesting a diagnosis of anti-NMDA receptor encephalitis [5]. Anti-NMDA receptor encephalitis should also be considered in patients with atypical presentations of demyelinating disease, including prominent psychiatric symptoms, dyskinesias or autonomic dysfunction, or ADEM-like initial phenotypes.

8. At the time of diagnosis, IgG antibodies to the GluN1 NMDA receptor subunit are detectable in the CSF of 100% of reported patients, but remain absent in the serum in 13% of patients. CSF titers correlate more closely than serum titers with disease severity, outcomes, and relapses [8]. Moreover, approximately 10% of the healthy general population has nonspecific serum antibodies to a component of the NMDA receptor, which are not distinguished in routine testing. Therefore, CSF analysis is indispensible in diagnosis and management.

9. Up to 25% of patients with anti-NMDA receptor encephalitis experience a relapsing course [2]. Relapse is less likely for patients in whom an ovarian teratoma is identified and removed and for patients without ovarian teratomas who receive second-line therapies. Of note, while CSF titers generally decrease over time in response to immunotherapy therapy, they may persist even when patient clinically recover [9]. A baseline CSF titer once a patient has improved can be useful to have as a baseline if there is a subsequent question of relapse as CSF titers have been reported to rise at the time of acute symptom exacerbations.

## Clinical Pearls

1. Anti-NMDA receptor encephalitis presents with a characteristic constellation of behavioral change, memory/cognitive disturbance, seizures, and movement disorders, but there is individual variability in disease severity at presentation and progression.

2. When clinical symptoms are suggestive, the diagnosis of anti-NMDA receptor encephalitis is confirmed by detection of CSF anti-NMDA receptor antibodies, which are highly specific.

3. MRI findings may mimic demyelinating disease or infection and create diagnostic challenges for providers.

4. Recognition of comorbid demyelinating disease and NMDA receptor encephalitis is critical, as it profoundly affects treatment and outcome.

5. Prognosis is favorable in the majority of children, but recovery may be protracted. Prognosis is improved by prompt initiation of immunotherapy and tumor removal. In patients with both NMDA receptor encephalitis and demyelinating disease, response to therapy is lower and residual deficits are more significant.

# References

1. Gable MS, Sheriff H, Dalmau J, Tilley DH, Glaser CA. The frequency of autoimmune $N$-methyl-D-aspartate receptor encephalitis surpasses that of individual viral etiologies in young individuals enrolled in the California Encephalitis Project. Clin Infect Dis. 2012;54(7):899–904.
2. Titulaer MJ, McCracken L, Gabilondo I, Armangue T, Glaser C, Iizuka T, Honig LS, Benseler SM, Kawachi I, Martinez-Hernandez E, et al. Treatment and prognostic factors for long-term outcome in patients with anti-NMDA receptor encephalitis: an observational cohort study. Lancet Neurol. 2013;12(2):157–65.
3. Baizabal-Carvallo JF, Stocco A, Muscal E, Jankovic J. The spectrum of movement disorders in children with anti-NMDA receptor encephalitis. Mov Disord. 2013;28(4):543–7.
4. Schmitt SE, Pargeon K, Frechette ES, Hirsch LJ, Dalmau J, Friedman D. Extreme delta brush: a unique EEG pattern in adults with anti-NMDA receptor encephalitis. Neurology. 2012;79(11):1094–100.
5. Sands TT, Nash K, Tong S, Sullivan J. Focal seizures in children with anti-NMDA receptor antibody encephalitis. Epilepsy Res. 2015;112:31–6.
6. Titulaer MJ, Hoftberger R, Iizuka T, Leypoldt F, McCracken L, Cellucci T, Benson LA, Shu H, Irioka T, Hirano M, et al. Overlapping demyelinating syndromes and anti-$N$-methyl-D-aspartate receptor encephalitis. Ann Neurol. 2014;75(3):411–28.
7. Lucchinetti CF, Mandler RN, McGavern D, Bruck W, Gleich G, Ransohoff RM, Trebst C, Weinshenker B, Wingerchuk D, Parisi JE, Lassmann H. A role for humoral mechanisms in the pathogenesis of Devic's neuromyelitis optica. Brain. 2002;125(Pt 7):1450–61.
8. Moscato EH, Peng X, Jain A, Parsons TD, Dalmau J, Balice-Gordon RJ. Acute mechanisms underlying antibody effects in anti-$N$-methyl-D-aspartate receptor encephalitis. Ann Neurol. 2014;76(1):108–19.
9. Gresa-Arribas N, Titulaer MJ, Torrents A, Aguilar E, McCracken L, Leypoldt F, Gleichman AJ, Balice-Gordon R, Rosenfeld MR, Lynch D, et al. Antibody titres at diagnosis and during follow-up of anti-NMDA receptor encephalitis: a retrospective study. Lancet Neurol. 2014;13(2):167–77.

# Chapter 11
# Pediatric Central Nervous System Vasculitis

Jennifer P. Rubin

## Case Presentation

A 6-year-old right-handed female initially presented with several weeks of frontal headaches and intermittent fevers (38.4–39.5 °C). Her symptoms progressed to include fatigue, mental status changes, and an inability to walk unassisted due to her mental status and truncal ataxia. She was admitted 20 days into her illness, and her exam demonstrated encephalopathy characterized by moaning in bed with no intelligible words being spoken but able to follow simple commands. She would not fix or follow on vision examination although formal ophthalmologic exam was normal. While there was no appreciable focal weakness or sensory deficits, she was hyperreflexic in all limbs and had sustained clonus in her ankles bilaterally with an extensor plantar response.

Brain MRI with and without contrast demonstrated numerous areas of asymmetric patchy, ill-defined T2/FLAIR hyperintense lesions primarily subcortical in location, throughout both cerebral hemispheres, as well as T2 hyperintense lesions in the thalami, brainstem, and cerebellum (Fig. 11.1). There were not dedicated orbital sequences, but the optic nerves appeared normal. There was no associated gadolinium enhancement or restricted diffusion. Brain MRA and spine MRI were normal.

Laboratory evaluation revealed an elevated white blood cell count (20,000/μL with neutrophilic predominance), sedimentation rate (62 mm/h), and C-reactive protein (2.8 mg/dL), with negative antinuclear and antiphospholipid antibodies. Additional studies included CSF analysis, which demonstrated two white blood cells, elevated protein (73 mg/dL), and normal glucose. Serum and CSF infectious studies were negative, including viral and bacterial studies, HIV negative. Continuous EEG monitoring obtained on admission demonstrated a severe diffuse

J.P. Rubin, M.D. (✉)
Ann and Robert H. Lurie Children's Hospital of Chicago,
225 East Chicago Avenue, Box 51, Chicago, IL 60611-2605, USA
e-mail: jerubin@luriechildrens.org

© Springer International Publishing AG 2017                                    83
E. Waubant, T.E. Lotze (eds.), *Pediatric Demyelinating Diseases of the Central Nervous System and Their Mimics*, DOI 10.1007/978-3-319-61407-6_11

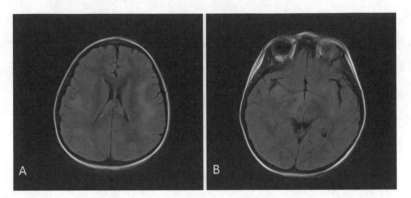

**Fig. 11.1** Numerous asymmetric patchy subcortical T2/FLAIR hyperintense lesions throughout both cerebral hemispheres (**a**), as well as the thalami, brainstem, and cerebellum (**b**)

slow wave abnormality, maximal over the left temporal region, and a prolonged nonconvulsive seizure originating in the right frontotemporal area with EEG improvement after rectal diazepam and fosphenytoin.

Given her encephalopathy and multifocal CNS abnormalities, the initial diagnosis of acute demyelinating encephalomyelitis (ADEM) was made. She was treated with IV methylprednisolone 30 mg/kg/dose intravenously for 5 days followed by an oral steroid taper for 2 weeks.

Prior to completing her oral prednisone taper, her headache recurred but was now associated with right eye pain and blurred vision suggestive of right optic neuritis. Her ophthalmologic exam demonstrated an afferent pupillary defect (APD) in her right eye and visual acuity of only light perception on that side. She had normal vision in the left eye. Brain MRI with attention to the orbits demonstrated new involvement of the right optic nerve characterized by increased T2 signal intensity and patchy enhancement of the right optic nerve. The previously noted lesions were otherwise unchanged in their appearance. Her sedimentation rate remained elevated (45 mm/h). CSF analysis revealed a slight pleocytosis of seven cells (81% lymphocytes, 18% monocytes with normal cytology) with normal protein, glucose, and lactate. IgG index and oligoclonal band studies were negative, and opening pressure was not measured. CSF and serum neuromyelitis optica (NMO) aquaporin-4 IgG antibodies were negative.

The event was considered to be a continuation of her initial presentation with a protracted course, given the close temporal association between the two presentations. She was again treated with high-dose intravenous methylprednisolone and discharged home with a slow prednisone taper over the next 4 months.

Nine months later, when she had been off of steroids for 5 months, she presented with pain on movement of the left eye associated with blurred vision. She did not have associated headache or encephalopathy. Ophthalmological examination revealed best-corrected visual acuity of 20/100 in the left eye with color desaturation and disc edema, consistent with left optic neuritis. Her right eye was normal. MRI of the brain and orbits with and without contrast demonstrated new enhancing

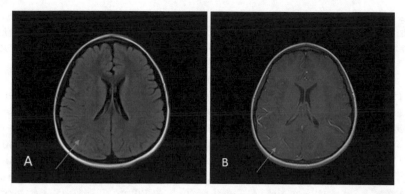

**Fig. 11.2** New T2/FLAIR hyperintensity in the right parietal lobe (*arrow A*) with enhancement on T1 post-contrast imaging (*arrow B*)

**Fig. 11.3** Post-contrast T1 sequences demonstrate bilateral optic nerve enhancement, which was new on the left

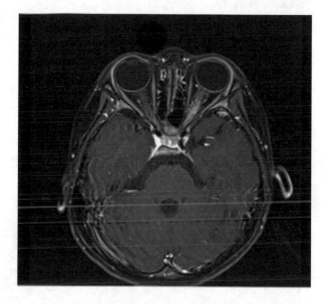

lesions in the right parietal lobe (Fig. 11.2), persistence of the prior right optic nerve enhancement, and new left optic nerve enhancement (Fig. 11.3). CSF profile was significant for pleocytosis with 30 cells (54% lymphocytes, 37% monocytes) with normal protein, glucose, and IgG index. CSF NMO aquaporin-4 IgG antibody and OCB were negative.

Given recurrent symptoms of steroids and prior headaches and multifocal lesions, the main concern was CNS vasculitis. Conventional cerebral angiography was normal, which does not exclude the possibility of small vessel vasculitis, so a brain biopsy was pursued. A biopsy was performed of an enhancing right parietal lobe lesion. This demonstrated multiple foci of perivascular inflammatory infiltration with damage to the vessel wall seen as a discontinuous smooth muscle layer fenestrated by lymphocytes

(Fig. 11.4). These findings were most consistent with primary CNS angiitis, as the child did not have any symptoms of a systemic autoimmune disease. Her sedimentation rate was normal, and lupus anticoagulant, antinuclear antibody, double-stranded DNA, anti-Ro/SS, anti-La/SSB, and neuromyelitis optica antibodies were negative. She did not have skin rashes, joint swelling, anemia, or renal involvement.

She was treated with cyclophosphamide infusions (500 mg/m$^2$) once monthly, for a total of six infusions, and prednisone 2 mg/kg/day which was transitioned to mycophenolate mofetil (MMF) 600 mg/m$^2$ divided twice daily.

Over the subsequent 18 months, she was appeared to have complete remission of her CNS vasculitis, with an essentially normal MRI brain, aside from gliosis of the prior biopsy site noted. She was weaned off of MMF after 18 months of therapy. However, 9 months later, she presented again with left optic neuritis characterized by blurred vision and optic nerve enhancement on MRI. She was restarted on steroids and mycophenolate mofetil, which was continued for an indefinite treatment course at that time.

In continued follow-up for the past 2 years on therapy, she has had a normal examination and no evidence for new disease on her brain MRI. While she is in a regular classroom and meeting grade-level expectations, she does require tutoring in mathematics.

## Clinical Questions

1. What clinical features provide clues for a diagnosis of CNS angiitis versus multiple sclerosis (MS) in children?

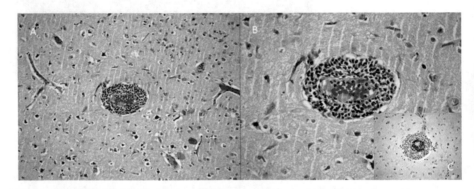

**Fig. 11.4** Sections from the parietal lobe at ×20 magnification (**a**) show the cerebral cortex with numerous neurons and associated oligodendroglial cells. In the center, there is a dense perivascular inflammatory infiltrate mainly composed of lymphocytes and plasma cells. The lymphocyte population consisted of a mixture of CD3-positive T cells and CD20-positive B cells (not shown). At ×40 magnification (**b**), the composite images show lymphocytes pushing up on the endothelial basement membrane. The smooth muscle actin (SMA) immunostain in the bottom right (**c**) shows damage to the vessel consisting of a discontinuous smooth muscle layer fenestrated by lymphocytes

2. How do paraclinical data, including MRI and CSF analysis, support the diagnosis?
3. What additional diagnostic evaluation should be performed?
4. When should secondary CNS angiitis be suspected?
5. What is the typical treatment and prognosis for pediatric CNS angiitis?


# Diagnostic Discussion

1. Childhood primary angiitis of the central nervous system (cPACNS) is a rare inflammatory brain disease which targets the vasculature of the central nervous system to include the brain and/or the spinal cord. The historical incidence is unknown due to the small number of cases reported, but the condition has been increasingly recognized. The disease is characterized by newly acquired neurologic deficits with angiographic and/or histological evidence of CNS vasculitis in the absence of an associated systemic vasculitic condition. Two forms of the disease have been described to involve either small vessels or large-medium vessels.

   Constitutional symptoms of small vessel cPACNS include fever and chronic fatigue in 50% of children. Other clinical clues include new cognitive deficits, such as a decline in school performance, and headaches. Seizures are a fairly common (80%) clinical symptom at diagnosis and occur more frequently in children compared to adults. In contrast, fever and headaches are uncommon presenting symptoms in children with MS, although they may have seizures.

   Children with large or medium vessel vasculitis less often have the constitutional symptoms of small vessel disease but do have headaches, seizures, cognitive declines, and neuropsychiatric manifestations of their disease. In addition, they can present with transient ischemic events, with focal neurologic symptoms initially waxing and waning, followed by acute strokes. The middle cerebral artery is most commonly affected.

   Optic neuropathy and myelopathy have been rarely reported to occur in patients with PACNS, thus mimicking an inflammatory demyelinating disease such as multiple sclerosis (MS). However, CNS angiitis has not been reported to co-occur with MS in either children or adults, and it does not respond to adult MS disease-modifying therapies.

2. Previously healthy children presenting with new neurologic deficits require prompt evaluation for inflammatory, infectious, and prothrombotic conditions. Inflammatory markers including ESR, CRP, and leukocyte count may be elevated in children with cPACNS, but, by definition, identification of an underlying systemic inflammatory disease is consistent with a secondary CNS vasculitis.

   Brain MRI with and without contrast is the imaging modality of choice to detect inflammatory lesions. Lesions are best viewed on T2/FLAIR sequences. In small vessel CNS vasculitis, the dynamic, evanescent lesions are highly variable in location, but are most commonly found in the subcortical white matter and cortical gray matter versus the typical white matter and corpus callosal lesions in multiple sclerosis. Lesions may enhance after injection of gadolinium, although contrast enhancement is present in less than 50% of children with active angiitis at diagnosis. The lesions may demonstrate restricted diffusion. Children with acute disseminated encephalomyelitis (ADEM) more commonly have large, multiple asymmetric subcortical, and white matter lesions, as well as involving the gray matter of the thalami and basal ganglia; lesions confined to the corpus callosum are rare.

CSF analysis typically demonstrates mild to moderately increased CSF protein and/or cell count with a mild to moderate CSF lymphocytosis. Oligoclonal banding may be present. Negative inflammatory markers and normal CSF do not exclude the possibility of CNS vasculitis even before steroid therapy.

3. Children with small vessel vasculitis typically have normal conventional angiography and MRA findings. However, in cases of medium and large vessel vasculitis, angiography may demonstrate proximal vessel stenosis, vessel tortuosity, or beading. Since the differential diagnosis of CNS vasculitis includes infection, demyelinating conditions, and other systemic inflammatory diseases, if angiography negative, brain biopsy is recommended prior to initiating long-term treatment. Lesional biopsies ideally should include leptomeninges, cortex, and white matter of enhancing lesions. The majority of biopsies in cPACNS demonstrate lymphocytic, nongranulomatous lesions, as well as vessel wall invasion with intramural infiltration of lymphocytes. The presence of viral inclusions, microglial nodules, or significant loss of myelin suggests a different diagnosis.

4. CNS vasculitis may also develop in the context of a systemic infections or autoimmune conditions. Infections are the most urgent concern; therefore, a comprehensive infectious evaluation is mandatory (Table 11.1). Secondary CNS vasculitis may occur in children with underlying systemic rheumatologic disease, including systemic lupus erythematosus and polyarteritis nodosa. Serum markers of systemic diseases should be thoroughly assessed (Table 11.1).

5. Children with small vessel cPACNS require several years of immunosuppressive therapy. In one open-label cohort study, children were given induction therapy with seven pulses of 500–700 mg/m$^2$ intravenous cyclophosphamide every 4 weeks and started on prednisone 2 mg/kg daily (maximum 60 mg daily) with a small weaning of the dose occurring every 4 weeks. The patients then received maintenance therapy with either mycophenolate mofetil (MMF) 800–1200 mg/m$^2$/day (maximum 2000 mg daily) or azathioprine 2–3 mg/kg/day (maximum 150 mg daily).

Remission can be defined as absence of disease activity via history and examination and no new active disease on neuroimaging. One outcome study noted at 24 months of follow-up that 70% of patients had a good outcome characterized by a normal neurological examination or only mild, non-impairing deficits. Twenty percent of patients can experience a relapse after discontinuation of treatment.

**Table 11.1** Laboratory workup for suspected childhood inflammatory brain diseases

| Markers of inflammation/disease activity |
| --- |
| Erythrocyte sedimentation rate |
| C-reactive protein |
| Complete blood count |
| Immunoglobulin G |
| Complement C3 |
| von Willebrand factor antigen |
| **Autoantibodies** |
| Antinuclear antibodies |
| Extractable nuclear antigens (ENA) if ANA positive |
| Double-stranded DNA antibodies |
| Rheumatoid factor |
| Antineutrophil cytoplasmic antibodies (cANCA, pANCA) |
| Anticardiolipin antibodies |
| **Prothrombotic workup** |
| Protein C |
| Protein S |
| Activated protein C |
| Anti-thrombin III |
| Fibrinogen |
| Plasminogen |
| Homocysteine |
| Factor V Leiden gene mutation |
| MTHFR gene mutation |
| Prothrombin gene mutation |
| Lupus anticoagulant |
| **Cerebrospinal fluid analysis** |
| Opening pressure |
| Cell count |
| Protein |
| Glucose |
| Cytology |
| Oligoclonal IgG |
| Lactate |
| Amino acids |
| **CNS antibodies (in serum and CSF)** |
| Suspected neuromyelitis optica: |
| • Aquaporin-4 antibodies |
| Suspected NMDA-R encephalitis: |
| • NMDA receptor NR1/NR2 heteromer antibodies |
| Suspected immune-mediated limbic encephalitis: |
| • Voltage-gated potassium channels (VGKC) antibodies |
| • Glutamic acid decarboxylase (GAD) antibodies |
| • GABA(B1) or GABA(B2) receptor antibodies |

From Benseler S, Pohl D. Childhood central nervous system vasculitis. Handb Clin Neurol. 2013;112:1065–78. With permission from Elsevier

Most relapses will occur shortly after treatment is stopped, but some patients have been reported to have a relapse more than 12 months after discontinuation of therapy.

Treatment of large and medium vessel central nervous system vasculitis typically includes a combination of immunosuppressive therapy and antithrombotic therapy. Larger studies are necessary to establish more evidence-based treatment protocols.

## Clinical Pearls

1. Childhood primary CNS vasculitis is an inflammatory brain disease characterized by newly acquired neurologic deficits and angiographic and/or histological evidence of CNS vasculitis, in the absence of an associated systemic condition.
2. In contrast to multiple sclerosis, children with cPACNS may have headaches and fevers. Brain MRI demonstrates evanescent lesions most commonly found in the subcortical white matter and cortical gray matter versus the typical white matter and corpus callosal lesions in multiple sclerosis.
3. Although laboratory data and neuroimaging may provide diagnostic clues, conventional angiography and/or brain biopsy are necessary to confirm diagnosis.
4. Secondary causes of CNS vasculitis, including infections and systemic autoimmune disease, should be reasonably excluded.
5. Long-term treatment of small vessel cPACNS consists of immunosuppressive therapy with induction therapy for 6 months followed by maintenance therapy for at least 18 months.

## Further Reading

1. Benseler S, Pohl D. Childhood central nervous system vasculitis. Handb Clin Neurol. 2013;112:1065–78.
2. Hutchinson C, Elbers J, Halliday W, Branson H, Laughlin S, Armstrong D, Hawkins C, Westmacott R, Benseler SM. Treatment of small vessel primary CNS vasculitis in children: an open-label cohort study. Lancet Neurol. 2010;9(11):1078–84.
3. Lanthier S, Lortie A, Michaud J, Laxer R, Jay V, deVeber G. Isolated angiitis of the CNS in children. Neurology. 2001;56(7):837–42.
4. Twilt M, Benseler S. CNS vasculitis in children. Mult Scler Relat Disord. 2012;2:162–71.

# Chapter 12
# Neuroinflammatory Disease in Association with Morphea (Localized Scleroderma)

E. Ann Yeh and Bianca Weinstock-Guttman

## Case

A 13-year-old girl of South Asian descent presented with a history of seizures since 7 years of age. The seizures were initially characterized by left-sided clonic shaking and drooling lasting under 5 min. After 1 year, the seizures evolved to left-sided nonrhythmic shaking accompanied by drooling and followed by confusion, left-sided weakness for 5–10 min, and postictal sleep lasting 1–2 h. Multiple anticonvulsants, including valproic acid, benzodiazepines, carbamazepine, and phenytoin had been tried without adequate seizure control. At presentation, her anticonvulsant regimen included oxcarbazepine (450 mg PO BID), levetiracetam (1750 mg PO BID), and lamotrigine (200 mg PO BID). However, her seizures continued to occur up to four times per month.

Her physical examination was remarkable for eczema over the right arm and a depressed area over the right forehead noted by the family to have been present since she was 5 years old (Fig. 12.1). Neurological examination, including mental status, cranial nerve, and motor, sensory, cerebellar, and gait examination, was within normal limits.

Throughout the course of her epilepsy, multiple EEGs, including long-term video EEGs were performed. At the time of her first seizure, an EEG with sleep was within normal limits; 2 years later, a long-term video EEG was performed and was also within normal limits. Due to persistence of her seizures, a repeat video EEG

E.A. Yeh, M.D. (✉)
Department of Pediatrics, Division of Neurology, The Hospital for Sick Children, University of Toronto, 555 University Avenue, Toronto, ON, Canada, M5G 1X8
e-mail: ann.yeh@sickkids.ca

B. Weinstock-Guttman, M.D.
Department of Neurology, State University of New York at Buffalo, 100 High Street, Buffalo, NY 14203, USA
e-mail: Bweinstock-guttman@kaleidahealth.org

© Springer International Publishing AG 2017
E. Waubant, T.E. Lotze (eds.), *Pediatric Demyelinating Diseases of the Central Nervous System and Their Mimics*, DOI 10.1007/978-3-319-61407-6_12

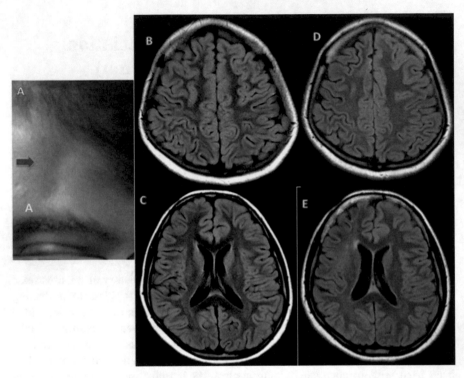

**Fig. 12.1** (**a**) Skin lesion of the right forehead. (**b** and **c**) Axial FLAIR images at presentation. Evidence for the skin lesion can be seen in the subcutaneous fat in the right frontal area. (**d** and **e**) Progression of the frontal lesion 5 years later, with evidence for frontal atrophy and hyperintensity at the frontal horn of the right lateral ventricle. Note the prominent abnormality in the frontal subcutaneous fat corresponding with the skin lesion

monitoring was performed 5 years after her initial presentation and showed focal slowing over the right frontal and parietal regions. Epileptiform discharges were also seen bifrontally and over the right central region.

While an MRI brain without contrast was normal at the time of her first seizures, a subsequent MRI done 5 years later showed right medial frontal T2 hyperintensities with interval volume loss and increased T2 hyperintensity in the insular cortex (Fig. 12.1).

A brain biopsy was performed at that time of the frontal abnormality but was nondiagnostic, only identifying areas of gliosis. A repeat biopsy done 2 years later showed cortical thinning with more extensive gliosis and neuronal loss. In addition, there were many perivascular CD3 positive T-cells, but few B-cells were seen.

Rheumatologic workup was negative apart from mildly elevated ESR (23), CRP (3.5), and a persistent positive ANA (1:640). A diagnosis of chronic, focal autoimmune encephalitis associated with morphea was made. Therapy was initiated to include monthly pulse cyclophosphamide (750–1000 mg/m$^2$ for 6 months) along with monthly pulse steroids (methylprednisolone 1 g IV monthly) followed by a slow oral steroid wean for 6 months. The patient experienced stabilization of the MRI abnormalities and of seizures after 6 months of therapy with cyclophosphamide.

## Clinical Questions

1. What key feature of the history and physical examination suggests that an underlying inflammatory etiology might be considered in this child's case?
2. How will repeat brain MRI help in the event that localized scleroderma is noted on physical examination in a child with focal seizures?
3. What additional workup might be helpful if a facial lesion such as that noted above is found in a child with chronic, focal seizures?
4. How does information from pathologic studies of LS help us to derive a treatment plan?
5. What is known about the anticipated clinical course in children with focal neuroinflammation associated with linear sclerosis?

## Diagnostic Discussion

1. In this particular case, the child was noted to have a skin lesion on the forehead. The picture in Fig. 12.1 depicts a skin lesion highly suggestive for morphea or localized scleroderma (LS). LS occurs in approximately 1–3/100,000 children and consists of localized fibrosis of the skin, usually limited to the skin and subcutaneous tissue, without underlying organ involvement [1]. LS is a process whereby inflammation is followed by fibrosis and vascular injury characterized by inflammatory infiltrates, vascular intimal thickening, stenosis, and superimposed thrombotic events. Twenty-five percent of children with LS have extra-dermatologic manifestations, the most common of which are articular, ocular, and neurologic. Linear sclerosis is the most common subtype and may also be referred to as "en coup de sabre" and, when leading to facial hemiatrophy, Parry-Romberg syndrome. It occurs in about half of children, and while lesions may occur anywhere, lesions of the head and face are common (25%) [2], with neurologic complications occurring in 17% of children with head/face lesions [3]. In this case, careful physical examination revealing the skin abnormality together with the history of intractable seizures may lead to suspicion of an underlying inflammatory etiology affecting the central nervous system.

    No large-scale longitudinal studies evaluating progression of neurologic manifestations in children with LS have been performed. The most common brain MRI features include white matter lesions (25.5%), an abnormal gyral pattern (13.2%), and cerebral atrophy (10%). One small retrospective study ($n = 9$) and one case report suggest that progression of MRI lesions, either in the form of progressive growth of T2 hyperintense lesions or progressive atrophy, may occur in some cases over the course of years [4, 5]. In this patient's case, progressive atrophy and increase in size of hyperintense lesions developed slowly over the course of 5 years. Thus, serial MRI scans may be useful for following and identifying disease progression and response to treatment.

2. While no single serum biomarker is associated with LS, one-fifth of children with linear sclerosis have elevated ESR, and almost half of children with linear sclerosis have elevated ANA (42% of LS). Eosinophilia, elevated serum IgG, rheumatoid factor (RF), and anti-dsDNA have been reported in this cohort as well. Given the high rate of positivity of these markers, especially ESR and ANA, a basic rheumatological workup, including ESR, CRP, ANA, and RF, may be useful in determining whether ongoing systemic inflammation is present. Furthermore, CSF testing may reveal the presence of oligoclonal banding, and as such, a lumbar puncture may be useful although not specific [6]. Skin biopsy can also help characterize the disease.

3. In this case, the brain biopsy showed T-cell predominance. This is in keeping with what is seen in skin biopsies of LS, which have positive staining for CD4 and CD8 T-cells, with a CD4 cell predominance. While RCTs for the treatment of neurologic manifestations of LS have not been published, case reports suggest the use of immunotherapy may halt disease progression. The use of immunotherapies such as pulse (high-dose) corticosteroids and/or cyclophosphamide for at least 6 or 12 months have been described, as have other immunotherapies such as methotrexate (1 mg/kg/week. SC), azathioprine, and mycophenolate mofetil (<1.25 m², 600 mg/m² 40–50 kg or 1.25–1.5 m², 750 mg BID; >50 kg or >1.5 mg/ m², 1000 mg BID) (therapy dosing listed where consensus guidelines for treatment of localized scleroderma in children available) [7]. Published data about therapy is limited to single case reports, and efficacy for controlling neurologic symptoms is therefore unknown. Nonetheless, knowledge of the predominant inflammatory nature of the skin and brain lesions may be used to guide the decision to initiate immunotherapy and to choose a therapy that will target T-cells.

4. While LS skin lesions may "burn out" within 3–5 years, the clinical course of the neurological manifestations is less clear. However, as noted above, progressive MRI abnormalities and seizures have been described in several case series, suggesting the possibility of intractable seizures and the potential need for early, aggressive immunotherapy to prevent disease progression [4]. Our case presented with an insidious onset and little clear evidence for progressive enlargement of lesions, but others may present with multifocal lesions with progressive encroachment in different territories (Fig. 12.2a, d). Alternatively, T2 hyperintense lesions may regress (Fig. 12.2b, e). Enhancement pattern can also be variable, with multifocal lesions (Fig. 12.2c, f). Additional neurological deficits have been reported as well as chronic headaches localizing to the area of the CNS lesions. Of note, in a review of reported cases of LS with neurologic complications, epilepsy was seen in 41%, and an abnormal EEG was found in two-thirds [6].

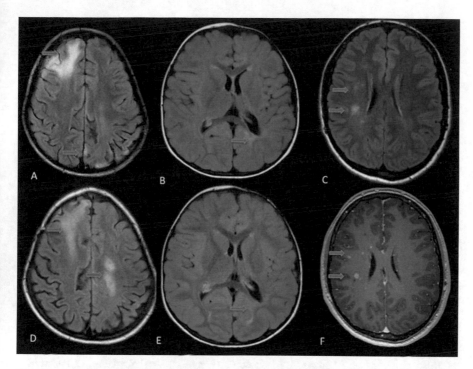

**Fig. 12.2** MRI scans from three different children demonstrating the range of MRI brain abnormalities that may exist in association with morphea. (**a** and **d**) Two MRI scans (axial T2 FLAIR images) spaced 1 year apart in a child, aged 6 years, with new onset seizures who developed intractable epilepsy. (**b** and **e**) Two MRI scans (axial T2 FLAIR images) spaced 1 year apart of a child, aged 1 year old at first scan, with a mild hemiparesis and congenital morphea. (**c**) An MRI scan (Axial T2 FLAIR) image, and (**f**) is an axial T1 image with gadolinium showing enhancement of the lesions of a 15-year-old boy with long-standing morphea and headaches

# Clinical Pearls

1. Examination of the skin and joints may yield clues as to underlying diagnosis in cases of intractable focal epilepsy.
2. Repeat neuroimaging should be performed in children with persistent and intractable focal seizures. In LS, the imaging may reveal either progressive hemiatrophy or T2 hyperintense lesions on the ipsilateral side of the skin lesion, which may enhance on T1-weighted imaging after administration of gadolinium contrast.
3. Treatment with immunosuppressants may delay progression of lesions or be associated with improvement in cases in which active inflammatory disease related to LS is suspected. However, given the rarity of the condition, no RCTs of therapy have been performed. Careful evaluation for evidence of ongoing inflammatory activity, including serum autoimmune workup, and CSF should be performed. ANA is frequently elevated in LS. While elevation of inflammatory

markers may be present in these cases, they are non-specific, and little is known about whether serial evaluation of the markers is useful for following disease activity.

4. In some cases, brain biopsy, although non-specific, may help to establish the presence of active inflammation in intractable epilepsy when MRI, serum, and CSF analyses do not provide clear evidence for active disease: this may point to targeted therapies. However, a skin biopsy may be sufficient to confirm the diagnosis of LS.

5. Brain lesions associated with LS usually appear ipsilateral and close to the facial or scalp lesion; they may change insidiously or sometimes more rapidly, over years. Therefore, comparison with images performed over the course of several years may help to establish the presence of progressive inflammation and active disease.

# References

1. Torok KS. Pediatric scleroderma: systemic or localized forms. Pediatr Clin North Am. 2012;59:381–405.
2. Zulian F, Athreya BH, Laxer R, Nelson AM, Feitosa de Oliveira SK, Punaro MG, Cuttica R, Higgins GC, Van Suijlekom-Smit LW, Moore TL, Lindsley C, Garcia-Consuegra J, Esteves Hilario MO, Lepore L, Silva CA, Machado C, Garay SM, Uziel Y, Martini G, Foeldvari I, Peserico A, Woo P, Harper J. Juvenile localized scleroderma: clinical and epidemiological features in 750 children. An international study. Rheumatology (Oxford). 2006;45:614–20.
3. Zulian F, Vallongo C, Woo P, Russo R, Ruperto N, Harper J, Espada G, Corona F, Mukamel M, Vesely R, Musiej-Nowakowska E, Chaitow J, Ros J, Apaz MT, Gerloni V, Mazur-Zielinska H, Nielsen S, Ullman S, Horneff G, Wouters C, Martini G, Cimaz R, Laxer R, Athreya BH. Localized scleroderma in childhood is not just a skin disease. Arthritis Rheum. 2005;52:2873–81.
4. Appenzeller S, Montenegro MA, Dertkigil SS, Sampaio-Barros PD, Marques-Neto JF, Samara AM, Andermann F, Cendes F. Neuroimaging findings in scleroderma en coup de sabre. Neurology. 2004;62:1585–9.
5. Grosso S, Fioravanti A, Biasi G, Conversano E, Marcolongo R, Morgese G, Balestri P. Linear scleroderma associated with progressive brain atrophy. Brain Dev. 2003;25:57–61.
6. Amaral TN, Peres FA, Lapa AT, Marques-Neto JF, Appenzeller S. Neurologic involvement in scleroderma: a systematic review. Semin Arthritis Rheum. 2013;43:335–47.
7. Li SC, Torok KS, Pope E, Dedeoglu F, Hong S, Jacobe HT, Rabinovich CE, Laxer RM, Higgins GC, Ferguson PJ, Lasky A, Baszis K, Becker M, Campillo S, Cartwright V, Cidon M, Inman CJ, Jerath R, O'Neil KM, Vora S, Zeft A, Wallace CA, Ilowite NT, Fuhlbrigge RC. Development of consensus treatment plans for juvenile localized scleroderma: a roadmap toward comparative effectiveness studies in juvenile localized scleroderma. Arthritis Care Res. 2012;64:1175–85.

# Chapter 13
# Susac's Syndrome

Adam D. Wallace and Teri L. Schreiner

## Case Presentation

A 14-year-old previously healthy girl presented to the pediatric emergency room with complaints of headache and strange behavior for the last 2 weeks. Her parents and friends had noted that she was acting "moody" and had been more withdrawn during that time. In the 2 days prior to her initial presentation, the confusion worsened. She was having difficulty concentrating in the classroom and completing simple chores at home. Her initial examination in the ER was significant for recalling only one of three words at 5 min and mild left-sided peripheral vision loss. Her past medical history and family history were unrevealing; medications included only acetaminophen for the headaches. Toxic ingestions were denied. Hospitalization ensued, and further workup included a normal complete blood count, comprehensive metabolic profile, ammonia, and inflammatory markers. Cerebrospinal fluid studies demonstrated an increased protein (152 mg/dl.), 2 RBCs, 11 WBCs (lymphocytic pleocytosis), and normal glucose. A routine EEG demonstrated mild diffuse slowing. Initial MRI demonstrated patchy T2 hyperintensities in the body and head of the corpus callosum with corresponding T1 hypointensities (Fig. 13.1). Additional T2 hyperintensities were present in the periventricular white matter (Fig. 13.2). Audiologic evaluation was normal. Dilated eye exam demonstrated evidence of branch chain retinal occlusions bilaterally. Initial treatment for a suspected diagnosis of Susac's syndrome included methylprednisolone 30 mg/kg daily for 5 days and aspirin 81 mg. This lead to rapid improvement of encephalopathy. She was sent home only to return within a week for recurrence of her confusion. She received an additional 5-day course of high-dose intravenous methylprednisolone. Discharge was followed by a prolonged oral

A.D. Wallace, M.D. (✉) • T.L. Schreiner, M.D., M.P.H.
Department of Neurology and Pediatrics, Children's Hospital Colorado, University of Colorado-Denver, 13123 E. 16th Ave., B155, Aurora, CO 80045, USA
e-mail: adwallac13@gmail.com; teri.schreiner@ucdenver.edu

© Springer International Publishing AG 2017                                                97
E. Waubant, T.E. Lotze (eds.), *Pediatric Demyelinating Diseases of the Central Nervous System and Their Mimics*, DOI 10.1007/978-3-319-61407-6_13

**Fig. 13.1** Sagittal T1 image showing typical hypointensities in the central portion of the corpus callosum. Courtesy of Justin Honce, MD

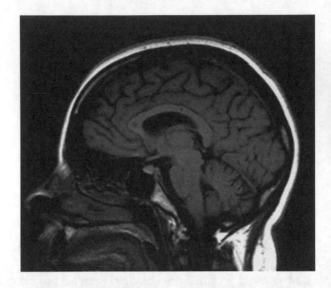

**Fig. 13.2** Axial diffusion-weighted image showing focal restricted diffusion in the posterior limb of the internal capsule and the splenium of the corpus callosum. Courtesy of Justin Honce, MD

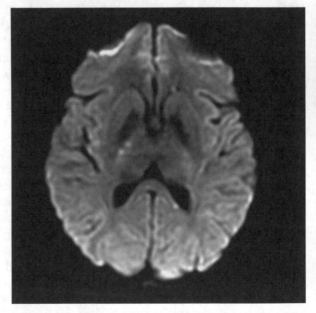

prednisone taper performed over 3 months. Follow-up audiometry demonstrated mild bilateral low-moderate frequency hearing loss, and fluorescein angiography confirmed initial findings of bilateral branch retinal artery occlusion (BRAO). Repeated attempts to wean off of oral steroids failed with recurrence of confusion. She was treated with intravenous immunoglobulin 2 mg/kg IV divided over 4 days, rituximab (375 mg/m$^2$ given at day 1 and day 14), and eventually azathioprine (initial dose of 1 mg/kg/day gradually increased to 2.5 mg/kg/day). Eighteen months following diagnosis, her disease course stabilized. Six months later, only very mild hearing loss persisted, and she was performing well in high school. Azathioprine was continued at that time.

## Clinical Questions

1. What are the characteristic clinical features of this disease?
2. What are the typical epidemiologic features of patients with Susac's syndrome?
3. Which tests are essential in the initial diagnosis and monitoring of Susac's syndrome?
4. What are the best treatment options for the underlying process, and what supportive care should also be provided?
5. What is the spectrum of clinical course and outcomes for patients with Susac's syndrome?

## Discussion

1. The syndrome of encephalopathy, branch retinal artery occlusions (BRAOs), and deafness was first reported by Dr. John O. Susac in 1979 [1]. This rare, frequently misdiagnosed, multisystem syndrome is best described as an autoimmune microangiopathic disease resulting in occlusion of the branch retinal arteries and microinfarction of the central nervous system (CNS) and cochlea. The most common presenting symptom is encephalopathy which typically has a subacute onset and varies from cognitive decline and confusion to psychiatric illness and personality changes [1, 2]. As a rule, patients with encephalopathy have corpus callosum lesions at diagnosis (discussed below) [3]. Headaches frequently precede the diagnosis [2]. BRAOs are seen bilaterally and can often be clinically silent. Symptomatic patients complain of visual field defects, blurred vision, or flashing/scintillating lights [4]. Cochlear involvement frequently starts acutely (sometimes overnight) and is manifest by low-moderate frequency hearing loss and tinnitus [4]. Unilateral involvement can be present at onset, but many evolve to include both cochleas. Additional damage to the adjacent vestibular apparatus can lead to vertigo and nystagmus [1]. Seizures occur rarely.
2. Originally described as a disease only affecting women, many cases of affected males have since been reported with the best estimate of male/female ratio of 1:3.5 [2]. Although the current largest review of Susac's cases including 304 patients found 81% of patients were between 16 and 40 years of age, pediatric cases do exist with patients as young as 2 years [2, 5]. Notably, a number of patients in the pre- and postpartum periods of pregnancy have also been reported [2].
3. Susac's syndrome is recognized as a multisystem disease; therefore, a number of studies are recommended for monitoring disease progression. Magnetic resonance

**Fig. 13.3** Axial FLAIR
image showing T2
hyperintensity adjacent to
the right lateral ventricle.
Courtesy of Justin Honce,
MD

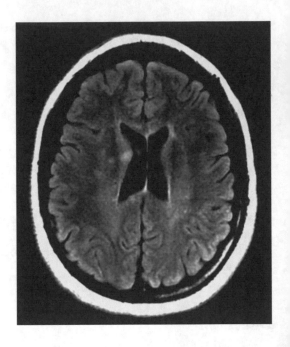

imaging (MRI), however, is essential for initial diagnosis. The hallmark finding on
MRI is involvement of the central portion of the corpus callosum with T2 hyperintense lesions sometimes referred to as "snowball" lesions [3]. These lesions eventually evolve into T1 hypointensities. These MRI findings, accompanied by any
other features of Susac's syndrome, are highly indicative of the disease. Other
changes, including subacute enhancement of callosal lesions, focal restricted diffusion of the internal capsule (Fig. 13.3), leptomeningeal enhancement, and
involvement of cerebellum, brainstem, and deep gray structures, have been
reported [2–4]. Because funduscopic examination can fail to demonstrate evidence
of subtle BRAO, fluorescein angiography is an important diagnostic tool and
should be used for disease monitoring throughout its course. This test highlights
the leakage of fluorescent material into the vessel wall indicating areas of occlusion [4]. Retinal artery wall plaques are frequently seen. These "Gass plaques" are
yellow plaques randomly located along vessel walls. These plaques are pathognomonic for the disease and may spontaneously remit [4]. Formal audiometry is the
best measure used to follow cochlear involvement. Similar to fluorescein angiography, it should be repeated during the disease course to monitor for progression.
Brainstem evoked potentials can be used in severely encephalopathic individuals.
EEG can be abnormal, most frequently with diffuse slowing, but is not considered
a necessary diagnostic tool [1, 2]. CSF studies demonstrate moderately elevated
protein and mild elevations of CSF white blood cells (WBCs), usually with a lymphocytic pleocytosis [1, 2, 4]. Oligoclonal bands are not routinely noted although
elevatedIgG synthesis can be seen [2, 4]. Cerebral angiography is not helpful.

The initial differential diagnosis of Susac's syndrome is typically broad as disease presentation can be manifest by encephalopathy alone. White matter lesions on MRI open the differential diagnosis to much more common diseases like multiple sclerosis, acute disseminated encephalomyelitis (ADEM), infectious encephalitis, neuromyelitis optica (NMO), and cerebral vasculitis. Other considerations have included stroke, malignancy, and genetic/metabolic diseases (CADASIL, MELAS, etc.) [2, 4].

4. Given the rarity of Susac's syndrome, randomized treatment trials have not been performed. The best current data is based on case reports and anecdotal evidence. Treatment generally targets an underlying autoimmune component of the disease. Although no definitive evidence of antibody-mediated disease exists in Susac's, histopathologic studies of affected tissues have demonstrated lymphocytic infiltration of the arteriolar walls and arteriolar wall thickening [2, 4]. Anti-endothelial cell antibodies (AECA) have been suggested to play a role in disease pathogenesis; yet no studies have clearly linked the two [6]. The histopathological features along with an overall favorable response to immunosuppressant therapy have made them the mainstay treatments used for both acute and maintenance therapies. Typical initial therapy includes high-dose IV methylprednisolone (10–30 mg/kg/day, max 1000 mg daily for 3–5 days). This is followed by a prolonged oral steroid taper starting at 1 mg/kg/day, max 60–80 mg/day. Weaning is dependent on continued symptom control and patient tolerance and typically occurs over 3–6 months. Rennebohm et al. recommend early initiation of intravenous immunoglobulin (IVIG) infusions, 2 mg/kg (typically divided over 2–5 days), occurring every 4 weeks for a total of six infusions [7]. Others reserve the use of IVIG for more refractory cases. More aggressive immunosuppressant therapy should be implemented when patients do not respond to initial steroid therapy or in those who have very severe presentations (profound encephalopathy). Failure to wean off of oral steroid therapy is another indication for treatment intensification. Alternative immunosuppressant medications found to be helpful include rituximab, cyclophosphamide, mycophenolate mofetil, azathioprine, and cyclosporine [7]. These options can also be considered in patients with unacceptable adverse effects from prolonged steroid therapy or progression of disease on prior therapy. Susac's syndrome shares histopathologic features with dermatomyositis, thus peaking interest in developing common treatment pathways [7].

5. The case presented here is typical of an incomplete clinical triad at initial presentation. Onset of all three characteristic features at presentation is seen in only a small minority of patients, reportedly as low as 13% [2, 4]. The complete clinical triad, however, eventually develops in the majority of patients [2]. Distinct disease types have been identified describing the timeline (monocyclic, polycyclic, and chronic continuous) and clinical features (encephalopathic and recurrent BRAO subtypes) [2, 7]. Monocyclic is characterized by less than 2 years of disease activity where polycyclic continues past 2 years with episodic worsening. Chronic continuous is a rare subtype also lasting past 2 years. Courses can be further described by their prominent clinical features [3]. As its name suggests,

the "encephalopathic subtype" is primarily characterized by encephalopathy, though hearing loss and BRAOs do eventually accompany it. Its course is typically monocyclic in nature. The presented case best fits this clinical course. The "recurrent BRAO subtype" is a less common presentation, usually less severe, typically prolonged (polycyclic or chronic continuous), and frequently occurs without significant encephalopathy [3].

The most recent evidence has demonstrated a wide spectrum of clinical outcomes. Although no formal data exists, prolonged time to treatment and an increased burden of relapses have been thought to lead to worse outcomes. Some degree of residual hearing loss and visual symptoms are present in most patients [6]. Abnormal neuropsychological outcomes were seen in over half of patients in a recent 25 patient cohort. Symptoms have ranged in severity from fatigue, mild memory deficits, and disorientation to severe cognitive dysfunction and encephalopathy.

## Clinical Pearls

1. Susac's syndrome is a multisystem disease requiring multidisciplinary care including neurologists, neuropsychologists, ophthalmologists, and audiologists.
2. Pathognomonic features of the workup include corpus callosum lesions on MRI, low-moderate frequency hearing loss, and abnormal fluorescein angiography. The key differential diagnoses are MS, ADEM, encephalitis, and vasculitis.
3. Early aggressive treatment with immunosuppressant therapy is essential to avoid poor outcomes including deafness, profound vision loss, and dementia. Treatment is frequently prolonged, especially in patients with BRAO predominant disease.
4. Although rare, Susac's syndrome is an important differential diagnosis for pediatric patients presenting with encephalopathy of unknown etiology. The clinical triad does not need to be present for its diagnosis; therefore, awareness of the diagnostic possibility should prompt screening with MRI, audiogram, and funduscopic examination.

## References

1. Susac JO. Susac's syndrome: the triad of microangiopathy of the brain and retina with hearing loss in young women. Neurology. 1994;44(4):591–3.
2. Dörr J, Krautwald S, Wildemann B, Jarius S, Ringelstein M, Duning T, Aktas O, Ringelstein EB, Paul F, Kleffner I. Characteristics of Susac syndrome: a review of all reported cases. Nat Rev Neurol. 2013;9:307–16.
3. Rennebohm R, Susac JO, Egan RA, Daroff RB. Susac's syndrome—update. J Neurol Sci. 2010;299:86–91.
4. Kleffner I, Duning T, Lohmann H, Deppe M, Basel T, Promesberger J, Dörr J, Schwindt W, Ringelstein EB. A brief review of Susac syndrome. J Neurol Sci. 2012;322:35–40.

5. Prakash G, Jain S, Gupta M, Nathi T. Susac's syndrome: first from India and youngest in the world. Indian J Ophthalmol. 2013;61:772.
6. Jarius S, Kleffner I, Dörr JM, et al. Clinical, paraclinical and serological findings in Susac syndrome: an international multicenter study. J Neuroinflammation. 2014;11:46.
7. Rennebohm RM, Egan RA, Susac JO. Treatment of Susac's syndrome. Curr Treat Options Neurol. 2008;10:67–74.

# Chapter 14
# Infectious Mimics of Multiple Sclerosis

Jennifer Martelle Tu and Emmanuelle Waubant

## Illustrative Case

A previously healthy, normally developing 11-year-old boy, who recently immigrated from Michoacán, Mexico, with his family, presented for evaluation of abnormal eye movements and left-sided weakness. His symptoms began with night sweats, high fevers, and fatigue and then progressed over a few weeks to muscle weakness, gait changes, abnormal eye movements, and intermittent urinary incontinence. He initially presented to a hospital in Mexico, but his diagnosis was unclear, and his parents reported that he received no specific treatment. The family relocated to the USA shortly thereafter, and he presented to another hospital. There, he was diagnosed with presumed acute disseminated encephalomyelitis and treated with a course of oral steroids for 3 months. He initially had some improvement in all symptoms, but then his strength and eye movements worsened a few months after being weaned off of steroids. His family had relocated again, so he presented to another hospital system where he received a 10-month course of steroids for these symptoms as well as quadruple anti-TB therapy for a positive PPD (negative chest X-ray and AFB cultures) and concern that his constellation of symptoms might reflect active tuberculosis infection. His CSF at that time demonstrated a lymphocytic pleocytosis of 59 WBC/μL, low glucose of 27 mg/dL, elevated protein of 117 mg/dL, and negative cultures including TB studies. His symptoms improved,

J.M. Tu, M.D., Ph.D. (✉)
Children's National Health System, Department of Neurology, 111 Michigan Ave NW, Washington, DC 20010, USA
e-mail: Jennifer.MartelleTu@ucsf.edu

E. Waubant, M.D., Ph.D.
Clinical Neurology and Pediatrics, Regional Pediatric MS Clinic at UCSF, University of California San Francisco, 675 Nelson Rising Lane, Suite 221, San Francisco, CA 94158, USA
e-mail: Emmanuelle.waubant@ucsf.edu

© Springer International Publishing AG 2017
E. Waubant, T.E. Lotze (eds.), *Pediatric Demyelinating Diseases of the Central Nervous System and Their Mimics*, DOI 10.1007/978-3-319-61407-6_14

although his left-sided weakness and abnormal eye movements did not completely resolve. He was stable for 9 months off of steroids before developing mild swallowing difficulty. Over this time, he was also noted to have progressive, severe scoliosis. He was eventually referred to a pediatric multiple sclerosis (MS) center for further evaluation due to brain MRI abnormalities concerning for demyelinating disease.

His exam on referral was remarkable for visual acuity 20/20 OU, optic disc pallor bilaterally, left CN VI palsy and internuclear ophthalmoplegia, left pronator drift, and left foot drop with absent Achilles reflex.

MRI scans from his initial presentation as well as a follow-up MRI performed 20 months later were available for review. The initial contrast-enhanced MRI brain and spine demonstrated intramedullary foci of gadolinium enhancement throughout the spinal cord and the brainstem with extramedullary nodular enhancement along the surface of the fourth ventricle (Figs. 14.1 and 14.2). Follow-up imaging performed 20 months later demonstrated evolution of the abnormal T2 signal within the brainstem, multiple foci of intracranial subarachnoid and intraventricular enhancement, as well as volume loss and myelomalacia with T2 prolongation of the central gray matter throughout the cervical and thoracic cord (Figs. 14.3 and 14.4). His CSF at the time of referral to the MS center was remarkable for a lymphocytic pleocytosis of 69 WBC/μL (1 RBC/μL), an elevated protein of 109 mg/dL, a low glucose of 6 mg/dL, an elevated IgG index of 2.6, and greater than five oligoclonal bands specific to the CSF. His CSF bacterial and fungal cultures from this lumbar puncture were negative. Additional extensive infectious work-up included negative investigations for borreliosis, cryptococcus, cysticercosis, CMV, brucellosis, and leptospirosis. Then, over 3 years after symptom onset, a repeat lumbar puncture obtained 1 month after evaluation by the MS center yielded CSF where AFB cultures grew at 6 weeks with *Histoplasma capsulatum*, finally establishing a diagnosis. Additional work-up revealed no other systemic fungal foci. He was treated with a 6-week course of IV liposomal amphotericin and then transitioned to oral itraconazole for 1 year. A follow-up lumbar puncture obtained 6 months into his antifungal treatment course produced a sterile culture and a benign CSF profile with only 2 WBC/μL and protein of 31 mg/dL. A repeat MRI demonstrated interval resolution of the intracranial leptomeningeal enhancement; however, there was no significant change in the T2 prolongation throughout the spinal cord or in the volume loss of the spinal cord, brainstem, and cerebellum.

## Clinical Questions

1. What are common and uncommon infectious mimics of multiple sclerosis?
2. What are potential red flags on clinical presentation?
3. What are potential laboratory red flags for infectious mimics?
4. What are radiologic red flags for infectious mimics?
5. What are typical findings associated with histoplasmosis?

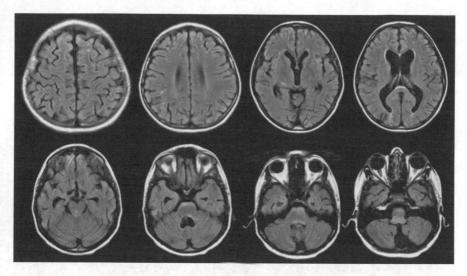

**Fig. 14.1** Axial T2 MRI demonstrating intramedullary foci of T2 prolongation through the brainstem

## Diagnostic Discussion

1. MS in the pediatric population is rare; however, it is estimated that up to 5% of MS patients experience childhood onset [1]. While diagnostic criteria were initially developed from the adult population, the most recent revisions of the McDonald criteria are now recognized as the standard method to diagnose MS in the pediatric population [2, 3]. As with adults, the exclusion of other diseases is a mainstay in diagnosing MS in pediatric patients.

   Infectious diseases can have a similar presentation to MS with regard to neurologic symptoms and radiologic findings, but atypical clinical and paraclinical "red flags" should point away from a diagnosis of MS [4, 5]. There are several infectious etiologies that can have significant overlap with MS and should be considered based on clinical and paraclinical findings [6, 7]. These can include neuroborreliosis, neurosyphilis, progressive multifocal leukoencephalopathy (PML), HIV, HTLV-1, and toxoplasmosis. Table 14.1 provides a more complete list of infectious mimics of MS and features of the patient history that might be suggestive. In the above patient, the history alone of recent immigration from Michoacán could raise concern for borreliosis, cysticercosis, brucellosis, tuberculosis, histoplasmosis, and leptospirosis.

2. The patient in our case presented with symptoms consistent with ADEM; however, each of his subsequent attacks was a nearly identical, stereotypical event. This is unusual in MS, where dissemination in space of lesions is a part of the diagnostic criteria. The initial presentation for pediatric MS patients is more often monosymptomatic with rapid onset (i.e., within hours or days) of clinical syndromes such as optic neuritis, isolated brainstem dysfunction, or isolated long-tract dysfunction [1]. However, approximately 15–20% of pediatric MS

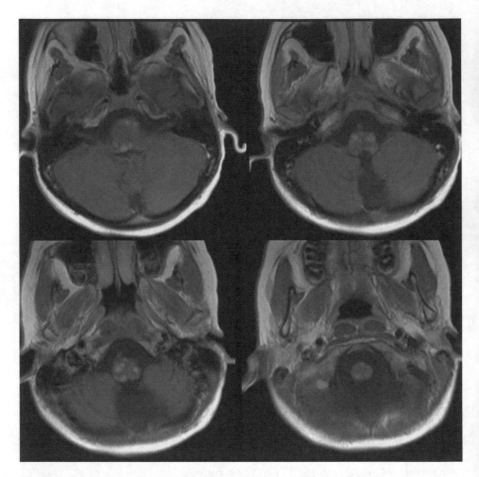

**Fig. 14.2** Axial T1 post-contrast MRI demonstrating intramedullary foci of enhancement through the brainstem with nodular enhancement along the surface of the fourth ventricle

patients have an initial presentation that is difficult to distinguish from acute disseminated encephalomyelitis (ADEM) and can include manifestations of encephalitis such as impaired level of consciousness, seizures, behavior abnormalities, vomiting, and fever [1–3]. In such cases, patients should be evaluated for alternate etiologies and followed closely. A diagnosis of MS should be delayed until there is a second non-encephalopathic event, 3 or more months after symptom onset, associated with new MRI lesions [3]. Chronic progression of neurologic deficits is very unlikely in pediatric patients with ADEM or MS. ADEM tends to be an acute monophasic event with rare relapses, whereas pediatric MS is almost exclusively a relapsing-remitting disease with less than 1% of patients having a primary progressive MS diagnosis. The following should also be considered atypical clinical findings in pediatric acquired demyelinating syndromes and prompt exploration of alternative diagnoses: extrapyramidal features, hypothalamic symptoms, hearing loss, purely progressive

**Fig. 14.3** Axial T2 MRI demonstrating volume loss and myelomalacia with T2 prolongation of the central gray matter throughout the cervical and thoracic cord

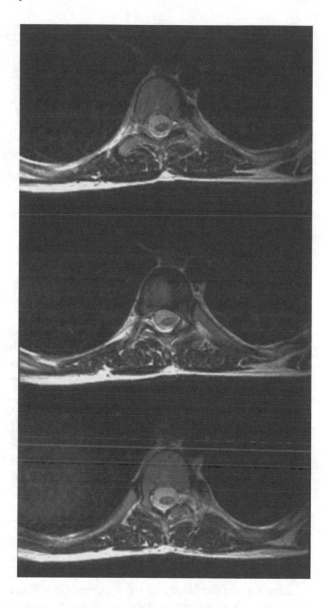

ataxia, purely pyramidal motor findings, peripheral nervous system involvement, isolated cranial neuropathies, polyradiculopathy, evidence of organ involvement suggestive of systemic disease, or constitutional symptoms, such as the night sweats and high fevers that occurred in the presented case [2, 4, 5].

3. In pediatric patients with multiple sclerosis, CSF analysis demonstrates oligoclonal bands in greater than 90% of patients, and there is a lymphocytic predominance with typically fewer than 50 WBC/μL [5]. Typically, the CSF in patients with MS demonstrates normal protein and glucose, and an elevated protein or low glucose should raise concern for an infectious or neoplastic process [8]. The CSF

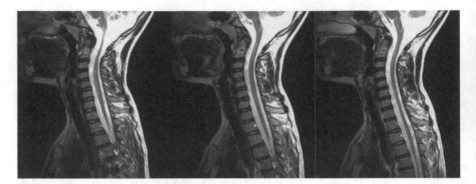

**Fig. 14.4** Sagittal T2 MRI demonstrating volume loss and myelomalacia with T2 prolongation of the central gray matter throughout the cervical and thoracic cord

analysis of the patient in our case revealed a cell count greater than 50 WBC/μL and a significantly elevated protein, both of which should have prompted evaluation for an alternative diagnosis.

4. The above illustrative case also demonstrates a few of the radiologic red flags. When evaluating imaging findings in patients suspected of having MS, specific categories to consider in the analysis include the enhancement pattern, evidence of bleeding or infarct, lesion distribution, presence of selective atrophy, and pattern of T2 hyperintensity [5]. With regard to infectious MS mimics in particular, imaging red flags include the following: meningeal enhancement; complete ring enhancement; venous sinus thrombosis; T2 hyperintensities involving the basal ganglia, thalamus, or hypothalamus; presence of hydrocephalus; lesions in the anterior temporal or inferior frontal lobes; lesions with mass effect; simultaneous enhancement of all lesions; or calcifications on CT imaging [5, 9]. In the above case, MR imaging was remarkable for meningeal and intraventricular enhancement, long segment cord involvement, and atrophy with myelomalacia. There was no demonstration of the classically described ovoid periventricular or juxtacortical lesions. Cytomegalovirus has a predilection for establishing latency in ependymal, germinal matrix, and capillary endothelium cells and thus may mimic MS with periventricular distribution of lesions. It is more often encountered in immunocompromised individuals. CMV is an outlier compared to other infections and opportunistic diseases, where callosal or periventricular lesions are rare and ventriculitis can be common [7]. Please see Table 14.2 for specific radiologic findings that may help to identify an infectious etiology.

5. Histoplasmosis meningitis is not well described in the immunocompetent pediatric population. There is one recent case report describing primary, chronic histoplasmosis meningitis in a previously healthy child where the presumed mechanism of infection was inhalation of a large inoculum while cleaning a chicken coop [10]. Histoplasmosis is more typically seen as a disseminated disease in healthy patients or as an opportunistic CNS infection in HIV or otherwise immunocompromised patients. CNS histoplasmosis, both primary and secondary, is uncommon but may present with headaches, confusion, or hydrocephalus [10].

**Table 14.1**  Important history supporting diagnosis

| Infectious mimic | Important features of patient history |
|---|---|
| Angiostrongylus cantonensis (eosinophilic meningitis) | Found mainly in Southeast Asia. Can be acquired by eating raw or undercooked snails or slugs infected with the parasite or eating raw contaminated produce |
| Bartonella hensellae (Cat scratch) | Cat exposure with scratch or bite. May have had rash or swollen lymph nodes |
| Borrelia burgdorferi (Lyme disease) | Travel to areas where Ixodes ticks (deer tick) are endemic including south and north eastern USA, along the Gulf coast, and around the Great Lakes (Lake Michigan and Lake Superior), but some species also found along Pacific coast and throughout Utah. May have history of erythema chronicum migrans |
| Brucella spp. (Brucellosis) | This entity is not common in the US but has been seen in California and Texas. The patient may have history of exposure to sheep, goats, cattle, deer, elk, or pigs, or may have a history of consuming unpasteurized, raw dairy products |
| Hepatitis C virus | Sexual contact, IVDU, vertical transmission |
| HHV-6 | Most humans exposed to HHV6 during infancy and childhood (roseola). Reactivation can be seen post transplant or in an immune compromised host |
| Histoplasma capsulatum (Histoplasmosis) | Travel to the Ohio valley, cave spelunking, AIDS or other immunosuppression, exposure to bat guano or bird droppings |
| HIV/AIDS | Sexual contact, MSM, IVDU |
| HTLV-1 | Suggested transmission is through breastfeeding or sexual contact. Can produce progressive spastic paraparesis when the spinal cord is involved. Patients infected with HTLV-1 are at risk for other opportunistic infections likely due to viral tropism |
| JC virus (Progressive Multifocal Leukoencephalopathy, PML) | JC virus is very common in the general population. PML typically occurs from JC virus reactivation during immune suppression or deficiency. A history of taking rituximab or natalizumab should raise suspicion |
| Leptospira spp. (Leptospirosis) | The incidence of leptospirosis correlates directly with the amount of rainfall, making it seasonal in temperate climates and year-round in tropical climates. Transmission occurs from contact with water contaminated with urine or feces from primary (rats, mice, moles) and secondary (deer, rabbits, cows, sheep, racoons, opossums, skunks) hosts |
| Listeria monocytogenes | Transmitted by the ingestion of contaminated food such as dairy or deli case items. This is the most common cause of infectious rhombencephalitis and may have trigeminal nerve involvement. |

(continued)

**Table 14.1** (continued)

| Infectious mimic | Important features of patient history |
|---|---|
| Mycobacterium tuberculosis | Chronic exposure to known contact, immigration from endemic areas, HIV infection, chronic steroid therapy, substance abuse |
| Mycoplasma spp. | May or may not have accompanying respiratory symptoms. Spread through contact with droplets |
| Prion disease (Creutzfeldt-Jakob) | Disease occurs world-wide. Symptoms of cognitive and memory deficits, mood changes, dysarthria, ataxia, dysphagia, or hallucinations should raise suspicion |
| Taenia solium metacestode (neurocysticercosis) | Found world wide, but usually restricted to areas where pigs are allowed to roam freely and eat human feces |
| Trematode helminth schistosome (schistosomiasis or bilharzia) | Travel to endemic areas including many parts of Africa, Asia, South America, the Caribbean, and the Middle East |
| Treponema pallidum (Syphilis) | Sexual contact, MSM |
| Tropheryma whipplei (Whipple's disease) | May have systemic features such as abdominal pain, malabsorption with diarrhea, low-grade fever, chronic cough, endocarditis, seronegative arthritis, uveitis, spondylodiscitis |

**Table 14.2** Important imaging features helping diagnosis

| Radiologic finding | Infectious mimic |
|---|---|
| Meningeal enhancement | Meningitis |
| Ventriculitis | Tuberculosis, cryptococcus, toxoplasmosis |
| Complete ring enhancement | Abscess |
| Venous sinus thrombosis | Menigitis |
| Hydrocephalus | Meningitis |
| Calcifications on CT | Cystercercosis, toxoplasmosis |
| Periventricular lesions | CMV |
| Centrum semiovale or other non-periventricular white matter lesions | Many infectious diseases (not limited to toxoplasmosis, neuroborreliosi, hepatitis C virus, HTLV-1, HIV) |
| Juxtacortical lesions | JC Virus |
| Brainstem lesions | Human herpes viruses such as Varicela zoster virus, enterovirus, Listeria monocytogenes |
| Middle cerebellar peduncle involvement | JC Virus |
| Atrophy of lower thoracic cord | HTLV-1 |
| Optic nerve involvement | Syphillis, Bartonella, toxocariasis, tuberculosis |

# Clinical Pearls

1. Infectious diseases are an important alternative consideration that must be ruled out in order to satisfy the "no better explanation" caveat for the diagnosis of MS.
2. The serologic work-up for infectious mimics needs not be exhaustive, but should instead be targeted based on risk factors, including travel, in the patient history, pertinent neurologic and systemic exam features, and brain and spinal cord imaging findings.
3. Careful attention to atypical clinical symptoms, such as high fevers and primary progression of deficits or specific radiologic abnormalities, such as meningeal enhancement or complete ring enhancement, will aid in the efficient and successful work-up of distinguishing acquired demyelinating diseases from alternative diagnoses.

# References

1. Renoux C, Vukusic S, Confavreux C. The natural history of multiple sclerosis with childhood onset. Clin Neurol Neurosurg. 2008;110(9):897–904.
2. Polman CH, Reingold SC, Banwell B, et al. Diagnostic criteria for multiple sclerosis: 2010 revisions to the McDonald criteria. Ann Neurol. 2011;69(2):292–302.
3. Krupp LB, Tardieu M, Amato MP, et al. International Pediatric Multiple Sclerosis Study Group criteria for pediatric multiple sclerosis and immune-mediated central nervous system demyelinating disorders: revisions to the 2007 definitions. Mult Scler. 2013;19(10):1261–7.
4. Miller DH, Weinshenker BG, Filippi M, et al. Differential diagnosis of suspected multiple sclerosis: a concensus approach. Mult Scler. 2008;14(9):1157–74.
5. Bigi S, Banwell B. Pediatric multiple sclerosis. J Child Neurol. 2012;27(11):1378–83.
6. Ratchford JN, Calabresi PA. The diagnosis of MS: white spots and red flags. Neurol. 2008;70(13):1071–2.
7. Rocha AJ, Littig IA, Tilbery CP. Central nervous system infectious diseases mimicking multiple sclerosis: recognizing distinguishable features using MRI. Arq Neuropsiquiatr. 2013;71(9B):738–46.
8. Freedman MS, Thompson EJ, Deisenhammer F, et al. Recommended standard of cerebrospinal fluid analysis in the diagnosis of multiple sclerosis: a consensus statement. Arch Neurol. 2005;62(6):865–70.
9. Charil A, Yousry TA, Rovaris M, et al. MRI and the diagnosis of multiple sclerosis: expanding the concept of "no better explanation". Lancet Neurol. 2006;5(10):841–52.
10. Schuster JE, Wushensky CA, Di Pentima MC. Chronic primary central nervous system Histoplasmosis in a healthy child with intermittent neurological manifestations. Pediatr Infect Dis J. 2013;32(7):794–6.

# Chapter 15
# Central Nervous System Lymphoma

Bittu Majmudar and Soe S. Mar

## Case Presentation

A previously healthy 11-year-old boy presented to an outside hospital with 2 days of fever, emesis, and headache. Brain MRI was normal, and CSF showed elevated protein of 155 with WBC 246 and 40% lymphocytes. He was diagnosed with presumed viral meningitis. Fever and emesis improved, but he continued to have headaches. Two months later, he presented with worsening headache and seizure involving right-sided numbness followed by loss of consciousness. Brain MRI now showed multiple enhancing supratentorial and parenchymal lesions with dural and leptomeningeal involvement, but the spine MRI was normal. Due to the risk of hydrocephalus and tentorial herniation, he was started on high-dose IV dexamethasone (5 mg every 6 h). Work-up for inflammatory and infectious etiologies was negative, including *Bartonella*, arbovirus, EBV, *Histoplasma*, *Blastomyces*, *Aspergillus*, *Cryptococcus*, *Toxoplasma*, *Mycoplasma*, HIV, HSV, immunoglobulin levels, neutrophil oxidative burst, and lymphocytic choriomeningitis antibody. A brain biopsy done after several days on steroids demonstrated only reactive changes. No definitive diagnosis could be made. IV dexamethasone resulted in subsequent improvement of lesion enhancement on MRI, and he was discharged home on a steroid taper. Over the following week, he developed worsening headache and increased seizures requiring readmission. On examination, he was somnolent with

B. Majmudar, M.D.
Department of Neurology, Washington University School of Medicine in St. Louis,
660 South Euclid Avenue, St. Louis, MO 63110, USA
e-mail: bmajmudar@wustl.edu

S.S. Mar, M.D. (✉)
Department of Neurology, Washington University School of Medicine, St. Louis, MO, USA
e-mail: mars@wustl.edu

© Springer International Publishing AG 2017
E. Waubant, T.E. Lotze (eds.), *Pediatric Demyelinating Diseases of the Central Nervous System and Their Mimics*, DOI 10.1007/978-3-319-61407-6_15

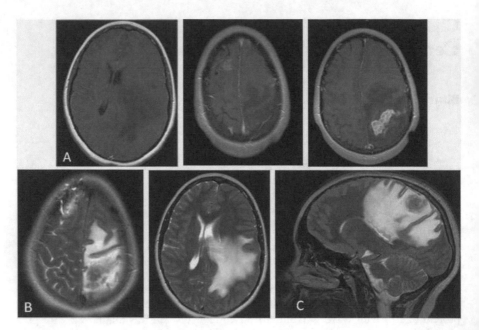

**Fig. 15.1** Axial T1 with contrast (**a**), axial T2 (**b**), and sagittal FLAIR-weighted (**c**) images of right frontal and left frontoparietal lesions with surrounding edema and mass effect

right-sided weakness and decreased sensation. Repeat brain MRI showed increased size of a left parietal enhancing lesion with T2 hyperintensity and increased edema with midline shift (Fig. 15.1). Due to the rapid progression of symptomatology and MRI findings, primary CNS lymphoma was considered. Peripheral blood smear, bone marrow analysis, chest and abdominal CT, MRI of the spine, bone scan, and repeat CSF cell, glucose, protein, and cytology were all normal. He received a second infusion of IV dexamethasone, which resulted in resolution of the right-sided weakness and improvement of the enhancing lesion on MRI. Spectroscopy centered on the brain lesion showed an elevated lipid peak, which could go along with the consideration for a demyelinating process. He was transitioned to oral steroids but deteriorated, requiring restarting of IV dexamethasone and discharge home on an IV steroid taper. The working diagnosis was tumefactive ADEM. Repeat brain MRI 1 month later continued to show improvement, and he was transitioned to oral steroids. However, 3 months later, he re-presented with headache and fever. Abdominal distension was noted, and abdominal CT at this time showed ascites with extensive lymphadenopathy. Lymph node biopsy showed Stage IV large-cell anaplastic lymphoma. Given that he previously had normal chest and abdominal CT imaging and normal bone marrow biopsy without any lymphadenopathy, the presumptive diagnosis of primary CNS lymphoma with dissemination was made. He received cytarabine, etoposide, intrathecal methotrexate, and whole-brain radiation with complete recovery and no recurrence on follow-up MRI 4 years later (Fig. 15.1).

# Clinical Questions

1. What are the typical clinical and imaging findings in primary CNS lymphoma?
2. What features can help distinguish lymphoma from an inflammatory process such as ADEM?
3. What diagnostic testing needs to be conducted?
4. What are the available treatment options?
5. What is the expected course and prognosis in primary CNS lymphoma?

# Diagnostic Discussion

1. Primary CNS lymphoma (PCNSL) is a subtype of non-Hodgkin's lymphoma restricted to the CNS. It is more commonly seen in immunocompromised individuals and is rare in children [1–3]. Most PCNSL is diffuse large B-cell lymphoma, and less than 10% of cases are T-cell anaplastic large-cell lymphoma [2]. Presenting symptoms are usually multifocal and non-specific and include headache, cranial neuropathies, spinal symptoms, ataxia, encephalopathy, and seizure [1, 3]. Most patients complain of focal neurologic symptoms, while systemic symptoms such as fever and weight loss are rare [1]. Lesions are typically in supratentorial locations and adjacent to ventricular surfaces or meningeal surfaces, such as cortical convexities. Common locations include periventricular white matter, deep nuclei, and the corpus callosum [1]. There is often leptomeningeal involvement [3]. There are no pathognomonic imaging findings, but there are certain characteristic findings: lesions show homogenous contrast enhancement in the majority of cases, and on MRI they are iso- or hypointense on T1- and T2-weighted imaging [3]. Significant surrounding edema is seen in over 75% of cases, often with mass effect [1]. PCNSL typically presents as a single mass, although multiple lesions can be seen in as many as 20–40% of cases [1]. Spectroscopy shows increased choline and decreased NAA, and a lipid peak is consistently seen [1].
2. Typical clinical presentation in ADEM or tumefactive multiple sclerosis (MS) can be similar to PCNSL and includes headache, seizures, encephalopathy, cranial neuropathies, and cerebellar findings. Cord involvement is common in ADEM but not PCNSL. CSF analysis shows elevated protein and leukocytosis in both [3, 4]. However, cases of ADEM tend to have a preceding illness, usually upper respiratory; and while signs of systemic disease such as fever are rare in PCNSL, they are common in ADEM [4]. Radiological findings in PCNSL often mimic infectious or immunological etiologies, and T-cell lymphomas in general are difficult to distinguish from demyelinating disease because lymphoid cells mimic the actions of reactive T-cell processes [1, 2]. However, while lesions in PCNSL are typically periventricular and in contact with ventricular and meningeal surfaces, lesions in ADEM are predominantly in the white matter and involve deep subcortical regions with relative sparing of periventricular white

matter [1, 4]. Both ADEM and PCNSL are extremely responsive to steroid treatment in the acute phase. Although the presentation can mimic tumefactive MS at first, there is not too much overlap with a diagnosis of relapsing-remitting MS in the long term as recurrences tend to be clinically stereotyped with PCNSL, in contrast with MS. In addition, new MRI lesions develop over time in various other locations in MS.

3. Diagnosis of PCNSL may not be possible from just CSF cytology. Detecting positive cytology depends on the relative amount of malignant cells present, and spinal fluid contains malignant cells in only 25–30% of cases [3]. As such, multiple lumbar punctures over time may be needed to detect abnormalities. For imaging modalities, MRI has a much lower sensitivity of around 20–38% for detecting leptomeningeal seeding from PCNSL, as opposed to 85% for solid malignancies [3]. Brain biopsy prior to steroid treatment is the gold standard for diagnosis [1].

4. Surgical resection does not improve outcome; therefore, chemotherapy is the mainstay of treatment. It includes a combination of systemic and CSF-directed chemotherapy with or without radiation [1, 3]. The standard chemotherapy for PCNSL is methotrexate. The French-American-British Protocol includes high-dose methotrexate with cytarabine, which results in better overall survival compared to methotrexate alone [2, 5]. Other agents have also been used in combination with systemic and/or intrathecal methotrexate, such as vincristine, cyclophosphamide, and doxorubicin [2, 3]. However, trials using these agents have shown poor response rates [5]. Steroids alone, particularly dexamethasone, can produce rapid response rates up to 70%, so it is important to consider biopsy and pathological assessment *before* the findings are altered by the effects of steroid administration. Some PCNSL can appear microscopically as demyelinated areas in patients who have received steroids before biopsy, as treatment induces B-cell apoptosis. Lesions respond to radiation, but long-term survival with radiation therapy alone is rare, and the combination of chemotherapy and radiation is superior to radiation alone. There have been case reports of pediatric PCNSL treated with chemotherapy alone and the majority of these children achieve long-term remission [2].

5. In general, prognosis for PCNSL is poor, with 5-year survival ranging from 25 to 40% [5]. Without chemotherapy, average survival can be only 3 months, but with chemotherapy this average can be increased to 19 months. Median overall survival ranges from 14 to 60 months [1, 3]. Most patients achieve complete or partial clinical response, with only a quarter having progressive disease [3]. Systemic dissemination can occur in about 7–8% of cases. Chemotherapy combined with radiation improves overall survival compared to radiation alone, but survival with chemotherapy alone versus chemotherapy plus radiation is similar [2]. Relapse rate in chemotherapy plus radiation is less than with radiation alone, but relapse can occur in up to half of patients, typically within 2 years [5]. Prognosis if relapse occurs is poor, but a third of those that relapse can achieve at least a partial response to salvage therapy [3,

5]. There are no particular clinical predictors of long-term survival [3]. However, age, CSF protein concentrations, and deep brain structure involvement can be independent predictors, with young age being favorable [1, 2, 5]. There is no overall difference in the survival of patients with a single versus multiple lesions [2].

## Clinical Pearls

1. Presenting symptoms in primary CNS lymphoma are usually mono- or multifocal and non-specific, and rarely include typical systemic symptoms such as weight loss. Lesions are typically supratentorial and in contact with ventricular and meningeal surfaces with significant surrounding edema. Characteristic imaging findings include homogenous contrast enhancement and iso- or hypointensity on MRI.
2. ADEM and primary CNS lymphoma can have similar clinical presentations and diagnostic findings. ADEM can be differentiated by the tendency to have a preceding illness, presence of signs of systemic disease such as fever, and lesion location predominantly in the white matter.
3. Diagnosis of primary CNS lymphoma is difficult with CSF cytology alone, as malignant cells are often not present. Multiple lumbar punctures may be required. Brain biopsy is the gold standard for diagnosis, and it should be done before the patient is treated with steroids that can wipe out tumor cells from the lesion. Also, it should be noted that significant worsening of the lesions upon weaning IV steroid treatment should raise the clinical suspicion of primary CNS lymphoma.
4. Chemotherapy is the mainstay of treatment, and the usual regimen includes systemic and intrathecal methotrexate. Cytarabine in combination with high-dose methotrexate and the addition of radiation to chemotherapy can improve survival. Surgical resection does not improve outcome.
5. Prognosis for primary CNS lymphoma is poor without therapy, but most patients can achieve at least a partial clinical response with treatment. Relapse can occur in up to half of patients. There are no particular clinical predictors of long-term survival, but young age is favorable.

## References

1. Mansour A, Qandeel M, Abdel-Razeq H, Ali-Abu-Ali H. MR imaging features of intracranial primary CNS lymphoma in immune competent patients. Cancer Imaging. 2014;14:22.
2. Nomura M, Narita Y, Miyakita Y, Ohno M, Fukushima S, Maruyama T, Muragaki Y, Shibui S. Clinical presentation of anaplastic large-cell lymphoma in the central nervous system. Mol Clin Oncol. 2013;1(4):655–60.

3. Taylor JW, Flanagan EP, O'Neill BP, Siegal T, Omuro A, DeAngelis L, Baehring J, Nishikawa R, Pinto F, Chamberlain M, Hoang-Xuan K, Gonzalez-Aguilar A, Batchelor T, Blay J, Korfel A, Betensky RA, Lopes MS, Schiff D. Primary leptomeningeal lymphoma: international primary CNS lymphoma collaborative group report. Neurology. 2013;81(19):1690–6.
4. Dale RC, De Sousa C, Chong WK, Cox TCS, Harding B, Neville BGR. Acute disseminated encephalomyelitis, multiphasic disseminated encephalomyelitis and multiple sclerosis in children. Brain. 2000;123:2407–22.
5. Abrey LE, DeAngelis LM, Yahalom J. Long-term survival in primary CNS lymphoma. J Clin Oncol. 1998;16(3):859–63.

# Chapter 16
# Methotrexate Toxicity

Juan Ramos Canseco and Vikram V. Bhise

## Case Presentation

**Case 1:** A 21-year-old girl with a past medical history of pre-B cell acute lympho-blastic leukemia (ALL) presented to the emergency room with complaints of acute-onset expressive aphasia, left facial droop, left-sided weakness, and tongue deviation to the left side. Her family noted that the patient woke up in the morning with complaints of fatigue and trouble bending her legs. During the course of the day, she developed left-sided weakness that continued to slowly progress until she suddenly became aphasic and unable to walk. Prior to admission, her family members stated that she had been complaining of intermittent headaches and generalized fatigue. Her ALL was treated with the AALL0232 protocol which included vincristine, high-dose intrathecal methotrexate (MTX), and mercaptopurine with her most recent treatment 10 days prior to presentation.

A non-contrast CT scan of the head done in the emergency room was normal. While in the emergency room, she became more somnolent requiring prompt sedation and intubation. MRA and MRV were unremarkable, but gadolinium-enhanced brain MRI demonstrated non-enhancing bilateral symmetric white matter regions of restricted diffusion in the corona radiata on acquired diffusion coefficient (ADC) and diffusion-weighted imaging (DWI) sequences (Fig. 16.1). Lumbar puncture had

J. Ramos Canseco, M.D.
Neurology, Rutgers – Robert Wood Johnson Medical School,
125 Paterson Street, New Brunswick, NJ 08901, USA
e-mail: juanramoscanseco@gmail.com

V.V. Bhise, M.D. (✉)
Pediatrics, Neurology, Rutgers – Robert Wood Johnson Medical School, Child Health Institute, 89 French Street, Suite 2200, New Brunswick, NJ 08901, USA

Division of Child Neurology, Department of Pediatrics, New Brunswick, NJ, USA
e-mail: bhisevi@rwjms.rutgers.edu

© Springer International Publishing AG 2017
E. Waubant, T.E. Lotze (eds.), *Pediatric Demyelinating Diseases of the Central Nervous System and Their Mimics*, DOI 10.1007/978-3-319-61407-6_16

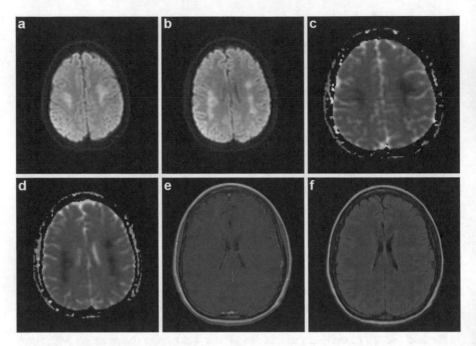

**Fig. 16.1** Bilateral restricted diffusion on MRI DWI and ADC images, without enhancement or signal change on T1 post-contrast and T2 FLAIR imaging

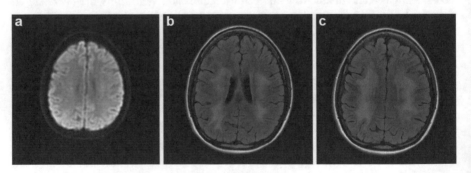

**Fig. 16.2** Repeat imaging shows development of T2 FLAIR hyperintensity in the territory previously showing restricted diffusion

0 WBC, 0 RBC, and normal protein and glucose. Stroke workup including carotid Doppler and cardiac echocardiogram was unremarkable. Routine EEG demonstrated severe diffuse bilateral slowing.

Based on the semiology, history of methotrexate treatment, and findings on MRI, she was given a presumed diagnosis of methotrexate toxicity. She was treated with dextromethorphan 30 mg every 6 h. Two days later, the patient was extubated, and her neurological exam did not show any significant abnormalities.

The next two doses of intrathecal MTX were held. The patient subsequently started delayed intensification with vincristine and doxorubicin the next month and then received her missed doses of intrathecal MTX with leucovorin rescue starting the following month without issue. Repeat MR imaging following re-dosing demonstrated resolution of restricted diffusion in the deep white matter but conversion to T2 FLAIR hyperintensity in the same distribution (Figs. 16.1 and 16.2).

**Case 2:** A 10-year-old girl with history of acute lymphoblastic leukemia (ALL) was admitted to the hospital with complaints of chills and pain in the lower extremities that progressed to the abdomen resulting in vomiting. The patient's initial imaging of the abdomen demonstrated bowel thickening which resulted in a diagnosis of typhlitis for which she was treated with bowel rest and antibiotics. One day prior to admission, the patient had received intrathecal methotrexate for treatment of her ALL. Standard treatment protocol ALL0232 was used which included vincristine and mercaptopurine.

On the second day of her admission, the patient continued to have complaints of abdominal pain and vomiting. In addition, she developed agitation and was reported to have eye deviation. Her examination revealed decreased spontaneous movements of her right upper and lower extremities. CT scan of the head did not show any significant abnormalities. EEG was not performed.

By the fourth day, along with continued abdominal pain and vomiting, she was unable to talk or move her right upper and lower extremities. She now demonstrated a left gaze preference and was able to follow commands only by blinking. An MRI brain without contrast demonstrated restricted diffusion predominately in the left frontoparietal white matter with some scattered areas in the right hemisphere. A minimal amount of T2 FLAIR intensity was also found within the same distribution. The patient was diagnosed with methotrexate toxicity and treated with aminophylline 90 mg IV every 6 h for 2 days and dextromethorphan 30 mg every 12 h for 10 days.

The patient began to improve by her sixth day of admission and could communicate with simple words. Left gaze deviation continued with some improvement of right-sided weakness. Substantial improvement was seen 10 days into her hospitalization. Her repeat MRI of the brain did not show any improvement of imaging findings despite improvement in clinical exam. Patient remained hospitalized for 30 more days for treatment of abdominal pain/typhlitis. She made a complete recovery in her neurological status.

Four months later she had transient headaches and visual changes 4 days following a methotrexate infusion (Figs. 16.3, 16.4, and 16.5).

## Clinical Questions

1. What are the typical symptoms and course found in patients with methotrexate neurotoxicity?
2. What is the proposed mechanism of action of methotrexate toxicity?

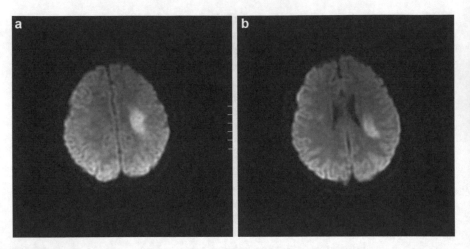

**Fig. 16.3** Bilateral (left much greater than right) restricted diffusion on MRI DWI images

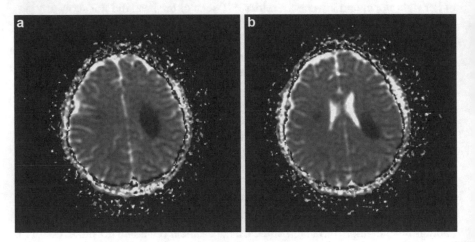

**Fig. 16.4** Corresponding bilateral (left much greater than right) restricted diffusion on MRI ADC images

3. Is methotrexate toxicity reversible or treatable?
4. What are the typical imaging findings of methotrexate toxicity?
5. How are these cases distinguished from acquired autoimmune demyelinating diseases?

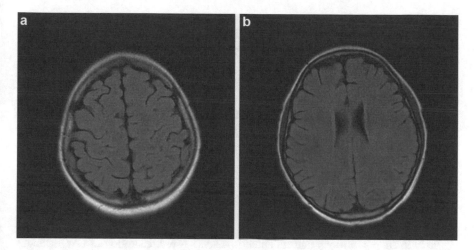

**Fig. 16.5** Corresponding T2 FLAIR images are normal

# Discussion

1. Multiple review studies show that neurotoxicity may occur 6–14 days after any form of methotrexate administration with a median of 10–11 days [1–3]. Nearly 50% of methotrexate toxicity patients present with seizures, while the remainder present with acute stroke-like symptoms. Less than 5% are reported to present with acute encephalopathy, which typically resolves in under a week [2]. These most commonly include limb paresis or plegia, aphasia, hemisensory deficits, and diplopia with ophthalmoparesis. Often the clinical signs or progression of deficits appear incompatible with conventional neurologic localization. Most patients with neurotoxicity have complete symptom resolution within 2–14 days, but some may have persistent symptoms for months. While symptoms may occur with all formulations (oral, IV, and intrathecal), the development of these symptoms empirically appears to be frequent and dose related, with a higher risk in children under the age of 10 years [3]. More severe cases may mimic an acute stroke or a severe demyelinating attack and, as in the case described above, progress into frank coma. The most devastating manifestation referred to as disseminated necrotizing leukoencephalopathy (DNL) is extremely rare but potentially fatal [4, 5]. Histologically, DNL shows multifocal coagulative necrosis, demyelination, astrocytic hypertrophy, and severe axonal swelling. Other presentations associated with MTX include aseptic meningitis, isolated or concomitant acute transverse myelopathy, posterior reversible leukoencephalopathy, cerebellopathy, optic neuropathy, and a chronic leukoencephalopathy-mineralizing angiopathy.
2. There are multiple proposed mechanisms of toxicity of methotrexate [1], but the actual cause remains poorly understood. Methotrexate functions as folate analogue

leading to inhibition of the enzyme dihydrofolate reductase which converts dihydrofolic acid to tetrahydrofolic acid (THF). THF deficiency results in deficiency of intracellular folates which in turn deplete purines and thymidine needed for cell replication. Folate deficiency presumably leads to toxicity via subsequent elevation of homocysteine levels which has been associated with infarcts via small vessel vasculopathy. MTX also impedes the conversion of homocysteine to methionine and $S$-adenosylmethionine, which participates in myelin formation through transmethylation. This mechanism is supported by the fact that individuals with higher homocysteine serum concentrations and/or MTHFR mutations are more susceptible to development of toxicity. Many studies implicate direct neuronal damage caused by local toxicity of the drug [1]. Other theories include CSF adenosine accumulation, induction of excitatory amino acids, and altered tetrahydrobiopterin metabolism. Pathology includes demyelination, white matter necrosis, oligodendrocyte apoptosis, and axonal swelling without evidence of inflammation potentially leading to atrophy and encephalomalacia. Rapid resolution of DWI changes on imaging suggests most cases involve a toxic-metabolic derangement with reversible cytotoxic edema in the myelin sheath.

3. Most patients have full resolution of symptoms within 48 h and demonstrate full recovery without any specific treatment [6]. NMDA receptor antagonists, such as dextromethorphan or memantine, may be used, or aminophylline, an adenosine agonist, may be tried [7, 8]. Other new strategies may include treatment with carboxypeptidase G2 and thymidine.

    It is not generally recommended to stop methotrexate treatments if a patient becomes neurotoxic, particularly if considered crucial to the treatment regimen. Bhojwani et al. [2] rechallenged 13 patients with high-dose methotrexate therapy who had previously been neurotoxic, and none experienced recurrence of neurotoxic symptoms. In another study [6], five neurotoxic patients were rechallenged, with four patients showing no recurrence of neurotoxicity and one patient developing a transient stroke-like event after the next methotrexate dose. High-risk patients are often prophylactically treated with leucovorin (folinic acid) prior to re-dosing of methotrexate. Treatments such as IV steroids and intravenous immunoglobulin, typically effective for immune-mediated disease, show no benefit in MTX toxicity, though do not appear to be harmful.

4. Leukoencephalopathy is often found on imaging in both symptomatic and asymptomatic patients which may worsen, remain the same, or improve and resolve [6]. In fact, nearly a quarter of patients treated with methotrexate may show findings of leukoencephalopathy, while only about 4% have symptoms of neurotoxicity. A wide range of imaging abnormalities have been identified for patients with methotrexate toxicity but primarily are described as deep white matter lesions usually in the centrum semiovale. These may include multifocal white matter lesions or, in more severe cases, demonstrate diffuse confluent bilateral subcortical white matter disease. Most patients' imaging findings show abnormalities in MRI brain DWI and ADC sequences followed later by FLAIR abnormalities, while contrast enhancement is not commonly seen. Imaging findings can persist for months as residual improving T2 or FLAIR signal changes, despite symptom resolution. Imaging findings often correlate poorly with neurological deficits on examina-

tion. It is unknown if similar preceding DWI changes would be seen in cases of MTX-induced myelopathy, but case reports describe T2 abnormalities in the dorsal columns. Cases of DNL can show symmetric multifocal white matter lesions on T2 imaging with multifocal contrast-enhancing lesions that progress rapidly.

5. The clinical history of methotrexate exposure in the days preceding clinical presentation places MTX-related toxicity as the primary differential consideration. Acquired demyelinating syndromes that might be considered in the setting of altered mental status, seizures, and polyregional neurological symptoms would include acute disseminated encephalomyelitis (ADEM) and an atypical presentation of multiple sclerosis. ADEM might be considered if the clinical syndrome begins after coincidental infection, which patients are prone to have in the midst of chemotherapy. However, the imaging findings of MTX toxicity are distinct from those of ADEM and multiple sclerosis. In addition, MS rarely presents with encephalopathy or seizures and instead manifests as relapses affecting different regions of the central nervous system at different time points.

Transverse myelopathy is a rare manifestation of MTX toxicity presenting clinically as subacute combined degeneration in the setting of normal vitamin B12 levels [9]. Pathological studies demonstrate vacuolar degeneration of white matter in the spinal cord. Cases may occur in isolation or with associated changes on brain MRI and can also be seen with coadministration of IT cytarabine. Even fewer case reports have linked reversible optic neuropathy to low-dose oral MTX [10]. As such, these cases may resemble NMO, a demyelinating disorder characterized by repeated episodes of optic neuritis and transverse myelitis. Lastly, cases with corresponding deficits to conus medullaris and cauda equina lesions have also been reported in the absence of leptomeningeal disease.

Other ancillary testing supportive for demyelinating disease would also not be present in cases of MTX toxicity. CSF oligoclonal band positivity and elevation of IgG index, typically present in MS, would be absent, as would abnormalities on optical coherence tomography showing retinal nerve fiber layer thinning. Visual evoked potential (VEP) studies would be abnormal in both eyes; however, a unilateral abnormal VEP localizes to anterior visual pathway dysfunction, seen only in MS or ADEM. There is little published data on neuropsychological profiles in MTX toxicity, but the cognitive profile in MS shows preferential impairment in processing speed. Aseptic meningitis, on the other hand, could be seen in both MTX toxicity and ADEM.

## Clinical Pearls

1. Patients exposed to high frequency and high doses of methotrexate therapy can present with subacute symptoms of toxicity characterized by encephalopathy, seizures, or stroke-like symptoms. On detailed serial neurological examinations, the findings often do not satisfy classical lesion localization.

2. Patients can show asymptomatic leukoencephalopathy ranging from 9 to 85% on neuroimaging and symptomatic toxicity in 2–10%.
3. Most cases of subacute methotrexate neurotoxicity resolve within the first 48 h with excellent recovery. Acute treatment may include aminophylline and/or dextromethorphan.
4. Patients with methotrexate toxicity during the early course of therapy can be rechallenged with methotrexate with the majority tolerating therapy without recurrence of symptoms. Pretreatment with leucovorin may further lessen the likelihood of recurrence.
5. Recent exposure to methotrexate or other chemotherapies may cause neurological symptoms suggestive of an acquired demyelinating disease. The clinical history and distinctive MRI findings help to distinguish drug toxicity from ADEM, MS, and related diseases.

# References

1. Shuper A, Stark B, Kornreich L, Cohen IJ, Avrahami G, Yaniv I. Methotrexate-related neurotoxicity in the treatment of childhood acute lymphoblastic leukemia. Isr Med Assoc J. 2002;4(11):1050–3.
2. Bhojwani D, Sabin ND, Pei D, Yang JJ, Khan RB, Panetta JC, et al. Methotrexate-induced neurotoxicity and leukoencephalopathy in childhood acute lymphoblastic leukemia. J Clin Oncol. 2014;32(9):949–59.
3. Mahoney DH, Shuster JJ, Nitschke R, Lauer SJ, Steuber CP, Winick N, Camitta B. Acute neurotoxicity in children with B-precursor acute lymphoid leukemia: an association between intermediate-dose intravenous methotrexate and intrathecal triple therapy: a Pediatric Oncology Group study. J Clin Oncol. 1998;16(5):1712–22.
4. Rubinstein LJ, Herman MM, Long TF, Wilbur JR. Disseminated necrotizing leukoencephalopathy: a complication of treated central nervous system leukemia and lymphoma. Cancer. 1975;35(2):291–305.
5. Kim JY, Kim ST, Nam DH, Lee JI, Park K, Kong DS. Leukoencephalopathy and disseminated necrotizing leukoencephalopathy following intracecal methotrexate chemotherapy and radiation therapy for central nerve system lymphoma or leukemia. J Korean Neurosurg Soc. 2011;50(4):304–10.
6. Rollins N, Winick N, Bash R, Booth T. Acute methotrexate neurotoxicity: findings on diffusion-weighted imaging and correlation with clinical outcome. AJNR Am J Neuroradiol. 2004;25(10):1688–95.
7. Sandoval C, Kutscher M, Jayabose S, Tenner M. Neurotoxicity of intrathecal methotrexate: MR imaging findings. AJNR Am J Neuroradiol. 2003;24(9):1887–90.
8. Rahiem Ahmed Y, Hasan Y. Prevention and management of high dose methotrexate toxicity. J Cancer Sci Ther. 2013;5(3):106–12.
9. Geiser CF, BIshop Y, Jaffe N, Furman L, Traggis D, Frei E. Adverse effects of intrathecal methotrexate in children with acute leukemia in remission. Blood. 1975;45(2):189–95.
10. Balachandran C, McCLuskey PJ, Champion GD, Halmagvi GM. Methotrexate induced optic neuropathy. Clin Exp Ophthalmol. 2002;30(6):440–1.

# Chapter 17
# Alexander Disease Type II

Parisa Sabetrasekh, Gulay Alper, and Adeline Vanderver

**Case 1:** A 20-year-old young woman with initially normal milestones presented with a 5-year history of progressive gait abnormalities, dysarthria, and difficulties with chewing and swallowing. The mother reported some initial concerns at the age of 5 years old when she had seemed to have some difficulty in handling her own secretions, describing her to cough and gag at times. Additionally, she had recurrent episodes of emesis at 12 years old. Both of these issues self-resolved within a short period and were not otherwise investigated. Additional concerns at the time of her presentation included nocturnal enuresis and difficulty initiating urination. There were no reported seizures.

Her past medical history was significant for orthopedic surgery to repair hammer toe deformity as a teenager and a diagnosis of gastroesophageal reflux disease.

Neurological examination demonstrated palatal myoclonus and dysarthria. She also had increased muscle tone in all four extremities but greater in the lower extremities. In association with this, she had decreased strength in flexor muscles, most notable in the proximal lower extremities. Deep tendon reflexes were increased with crossed adductor responses with an equivocal plantar response. Her gait was notable for spastic, waddling, and broad-based gait. She had dysmetria on finger-to-nose

P. Sabetrasekh, M.D.
Department of Neurology, Children's National Medical Center,
111 Michigan Avenue, NW, Washington, DC 20010, USA
e-mail: md.parisa@gmail.com

G. Alper, M.D.
Division of Child Neurology, Department of Pediatrics, Children's Hospital of Pittsburgh,
University of Pittsburgh School of Medicine, 4401 Penn Avenue, Pittsburgh, PA 15224, USA
e-mail: Gulay.Alper@chp.edu

A. Vanderver, M.D. (✉)
Children Hospital of Pennsylvania, Philadelphia, PA 19104, USA
e-mail: Avanderv@childrensnational.org

© Springer International Publishing AG 2017
E. Waubant, T.E. Lotze (eds.), *Pediatric Demyelinating Diseases of the Central Nervous System and Their Mimics*, DOI 10.1007/978-3-319-61407-6_17

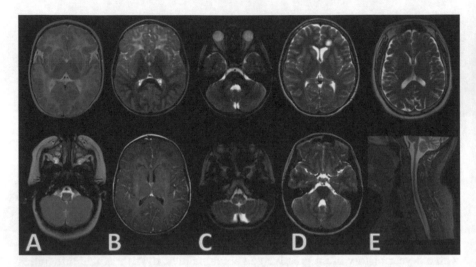

**Fig. 17.1** AxD imaging features across the lifespan. (**a**) Eleven-month-old female with encephalopathy and intractable epilepsy. *Top*: Axial T2-weighted images show diffuse white matter involvement with swollen appearance of the gyri. *Bottom*: Axial T2-weighted images demonstrate significant signal abnormality within the brainstem. (**b**) Five-year-old male child with macrocephaly, developmental delay, and seizures. *Top*: Axial T2-weighted images demonstrate frontal predominant white matter signal changes affecting the subcortical, deep, and periventricular white matter. Make note of the T2-weighted hypointensity capping the frontal horns, which is typical of AxD. There is also subtle T2-weighted hyperintensity of the caudate nuclei. *Bottom*: Contrast enhanced axial T1-weighted images demonstrate contrast enhancement of the frontal white matter and basal ganglia bilaterally. (**c**) Eight-year-old male with failure to thrive and recurrent vomiting. Axial T2-weighted images demonstrate increased signal in the pons (*top*) and the medulla (*bottom*), giving an impression of mild mass effect. These lesions were contrast enhancing. There was no change in the lesion on serial MRIs over several years. (**d**) Twelve-year-old with recurrent emesis and failure to thrive. *Top*: Axial T2-weighted images demonstrate a left frontal hyperintense lesion within normal-appearing white matter. This lesion was stable over several years on serial imaging. *Bottom*: Axial T2-weighted images demonstrate signal abnormalities in the middle cerebellar peduncles and the peri-dentate cerebellar white matter. (**e**) Fifty-five-year-old male with dysphonia, dysphagia, and progressive gait abnormalities. *Top*: Axial T2-weighted images do not show signal abnormalities in the supratentorial white matter. *Bottom*: Sagittal T2-weighted images of the spine demonstrate brainstem and spinal cord atrophy

testing and rapid alternating movements were clumsy. Her general examination was notable for a dextroconvex scoliosis.

An MRI brain revealed frontal predominant T2 hyperintense white matter disease extending from the subcortical fibers through the central white matter and involvement of the periventricular area of the frontal horns of the lateral ventricles (similar to classic presentations demonstrated in Fig. 17.1). There was contrast enhancement of the affected frontal white matter and the basal ganglia. In addition, there was T2 hyperintensity of the brainstem with atrophy of the medulla and spinal cord.

Sanger sequencing of *GFAP* revealed a de novo pathogenic mutation (p. Arg416Trp). In view of the clinical features including spasticity, scoliosis, palatal myoclonus, and recurrent vomiting along with radiological and genetic findings, the most likely diagnosis for this patient was felt to be Alexander disease.

**Case 2:** An 11-year-old girl presented with episodes of a sensation described as "having a lump" in her throat for the previous 2 years at a frequency of twice per month. This feeling was associated with a choking sensation, dry cough, and shortness of breath lasting from 5 to 30 s. She had no cyanosis or stridor and was able to breathe during the episodes. She complained of being unable to verbalize words during the attacks, but there was no change in consciousness and no abnormal movements of the extremities. There were no recognized triggers and no relation to meals or to a particular time of the day. Her past medical history was unremarkable, and developmental milestones were achieved at the appropriate age. Family history was negative for acquired and genetic neurologic disorders.

After her initial normal evaluation by pulmonology and gastroenterology, a brain MRI was ordered to evaluate for possible Arnold-Chiari malformation. The brain MRI showed multiple areas of T2 and FLAIR hyperintensity affecting the medulla oblongata, bilateral middle cerebellar peduncles, small area in the left pons, bilateral dentate nuclei of the cerebellum, and frontal periventricular white matter adjacent to the frontal horns. There was contrast enhancement in the medullary and left pontine lesions.

Based on the MRI findings, she was referred to neurology. Her neurologic examination showed normal mental status and cranial nerve examination. The patient had full ocular motility without nystagmus and normal facial and corneal sensation and no facial weakness or asymmetry. Palatal elevation was symmetric and she had active gag reflex. Tongue protruded in midline; no tongue fasciculation or atrophy was seen. Muscle strength, deep tendon reflexes, and sensory examination to all modalities were normal. She had normal coordination and gait without ataxia. No dysmetria was evident. Routine EEG captured one typical episode of abnormal throat sensation and did not reveal electrographic correlation.

Review of the MRI findings raised suspicion for late-onset Alexander disease.

Sanger sequencing of *GFAP* revealed a de novo pathogenic missense mutation (Arg239Gly) confirming the diagnosis.

Over 9 years of follow-up, she did not have progression of her symptoms and even felt some reduction in the frequency and intensity of her episodes. Her neurologic examination remained normal. Serial MRIs obtained each year did note some subtle enlargement of the brainstem and cerebellar lesions.

## Clinical Questions

1. What is Alexander disease (AxD)?
2. What are the types of Alexander disease?
3. What are the magnetic resonance imaging criteria for Alexander disease?
4. What is the molecular cause and pathogenesis of Alexander disease?

5. What are the other neurological diseases that can mimic Alexander disease?
6. What are the treatment options for Alexander disease?
7. What is the prognosis of Alexander disease?

## Diagnostic Discussions

1. Alexander disease is one of the leukodystrophies or heritable disorders of the white matter of the brain. Because this disorder seems to primarily affect astrocytes, some researchers classify it as an astrogliopathy rather than a leukodystrophy. This disease was first reported in 1949 by W. Stewart Alexander in a 15-month-old child who suffered from megalocephaly, psychomotor delay, and hydrocephalus, but the clinical spectrum has expanded significantly since then and includes patients from infancy to the fifth decade of life.

2. The old classification of Alexander disease (neonatal-infantile-juvenile-adult) was revised in 2011 into two groups based on clinical and radiologic presentation: Alexander disease Type I and Type II.

   Type I is generally more severe than Type II and characterized by early onset, typically before 4 years of age, seizures, macrocephaly, motor delay, encephalopathy, failure to thrive, developmental delay, paroxysmal deterioration, and typical neuroimaging features (see below).

   Type II is typically of later onset, with prominent bulbar symptoms, palatal myoclonus, milder neurocognitive deficits, and atypical neuroimaging features. Specifically, Type II AxD often has limited supratentorial white matter involvement, with predominant basal ganglia, brainstem, and spinal cord involvement. Pyramidal involvement, cerebellar ataxia, and urinary disturbances are common. Less frequently, obstructive sleep apnea, ocular movement abnormalities, and dysautonomia can occur.

3. In 2001, magnetic resonance imaging (MRI) criteria were suggested for Alexander disease, replacing the need for pathologic diagnosis. Four of the five following criteria are required for an MRI-based diagnosis:

   - Extensive cerebral white matter changes with frontal predominance in either extent, degree of swelling, signal change, atrophy, or cystic degeneration.
   - Periventricular rim of low signal on T2-weighted images and high signal on T1-weighted images.
   - Signal abnormality of the brainstem.
   - Signal abnormalities, atrophy, or swelling of basal ganglia and thalami.
   - Contrast enhancement of one or more of the following gray or white matter structures: ventricular lining, periventricular rim, frontal white matter, optic chiasm, fornix, basal ganglia, thalamus, dentate nucleus, cerebellar cortex, and brainstem.

Type II AxD may not have these extensive supratentorial neuroimaging findings but can show the following:

- Atrophy of the medulla and cervical spinal cord.
- T2-weighted signal abnormalities predominating in the posterior fossa including the medulla and spinal cord, in particular multifocal nodular brainstem lesions that may resemble mass lesions or multiple sclerosis. This may occur with or without supratentorial white matter changes.
- Increase in cerebellar size and cerebellar white matter abnormalities.
- Contrast enhancing garland along the ventricular wall.

In patients with very early-onset disease, MRI abnormalities may also be atypical. For example, on fetal MRI, enlarged ventricles with significant thickening of the fornices and white matter abnormalities can be seen. In neonatal cases, there may not be significant macrocephaly, and significant signal abnormalities in the basal ganglia may lead clinicians to suspect mitochondrial cytopathy and Leigh's rather than AxD.

4. AxD is caused by mutations in *GFAP*, encoding the glial fibrillary acidic protein (GFAP), on chromosome 17q21. Mutations are heterozygous and are either de novo sporadic or inherited in an autosomal dominant fashion. They are typically missense or nonsense variants and result in gain of function. AxD-causing mutations are hypothesized to result in disruption of dimerization of GFAP leading to abnormal protein aggregation and Rosenthal fibers. GFAP is an intermediate filament protein located in the mature astrocytes that is rapidly synthesized during any central nervous system injury.
   Rosenthal fibers, which are intracytoplasmic hyaline eosinophilic rod inclusions localized in astrocytes, are the pathologic hallmark in Alexander disease. These aggregates of mutated GFAP, heat shock proteins, and other proteins are found in perivascular, periventricular, and subpial spaces of the central nervous system. They can be proliferative, causing increase in cerebral volume (macrocephaly), obstructing CSF drainage (hydrocephalus), or even creating mass like lesions mistaken for malignancies.
5. Differential diagnosis is predominantly based on MRI appearance and is variable for AxD I and II.

In AxD Type I, the basal ganglia and frontal involvement with contrast enhancement can lead to radiologic overlap with features of:

- Acute disseminated encephalomyelitis (ADEM) or neuro-immune disorders of the brain, in particular in cases with significant contrast enhancement, including of the optic pathway, basal ganglia, and ependymal lining, although the often associated frontal predominant leukoencephalopathy and symmetric disease should alert the clinician to alternate diagnoses.
- Mitochondrial disease in view of the symmetric basal ganglia involvement which sometimes includes a swollen appearance of the involved basal ganglia and brainstem involvement in an almost Leigh-like presentation.

- Aicardi-Goutières syndrome (AGS) in cases with significant frontal involvement. In particular it should be noted that AxD can occasionally have associated calcifications, which are typically associated with AGS.
- Frontal variant of X-linked adrenoleukodystrophy in cases of juvenile cerebral onset. Contrast enhancement is typically seen in this condition.

In AxD II, in which predominantly brainstem lesions are seen, other disorders to consider include:

- Malignancies of the brainstem such as brainstem gliomas, in particular in those patients with asymmetric involvement or significant contrast enhancement, though signal abnormality in the basal ganglia should lead the clinician to consider alternate etiologies.
- Multiple sclerosis with a predominant posterior fossa and brainstem presentation though signal abnormality in the basal ganglia should lead the clinician to consider alternate etiologies.
- t-RNA synthetase defects including leukoencephalopathy with brainstem and spinal cord involvement and lactate elevation (LBSL), leukoencephalopathy with thalamic and brainstem involvement and high lactate (LTBL), and hypomyelination with brainstem and spinal cord and leg involvement (HBSL).
- Peroxisomal disorders which can often have predominant brainstem abnormalities.
- Mitochondrial leukoencephalopaties

6. There is no definitive treatment for Alexander disease. Symptomatic treatment should focus on management of known complications. Careful attention should be given to seizure control, particularly in the context of fever. Good rehabilitative care should be used to avoid orthopedic complications, including scoliosis and hip dislocations. In view of the significant bulbar dysfunction, the support of feeding clinics for chewing and swallowing is essential. Speech abnormalities are often present and patients should receive speech and language therapy. Evidence of obstructive sleep apnea, presumably as a result of palatal dysfunction, should be sought and treated. Recurrent vomiting and swallowing difficulties often result in weight loss, and careful attention should be given to nutrition, with placement of a gastrostomy feeding tube if necessary. Recurrent aspiration pneumonia and scoliosis can lead to significant respiratory dysfunction, and engagement of a team specialized in pulmonary function maintenance should be considered. Pharmacologic approaches and chemodenervation can be used to manage spasticity and extrapyramidal dysfunction. Attention should be given to the risk of hydrocephalus with consideration given to placement of a ventriculoperitoneal shunt when increasing ventricular size or clinical symptoms lead to concern for obstruction of CSF flow.

7. The prognosis is usually poor in Type I, and death usually occurs in the first decades of life. The later-onset AxD Type II has a more slowly progressive course, and patients are known to live for decades after diagnosis.

# Clinical Pearls

1. Presentation of AxD in adolescence or adulthood may mimic space-occupying lesions or MS due to predominant brainstem and spinal cord signal abnormalities.
2. Clinical symptoms of AxD in older patients typically include palatal myoclonus, sleep apnea, swallowing difficulties, and progressive gait abnormalities without the encephalopathy and macrocephaly seen in early-onset AxD.

# Suggested Reading

Brenner M, Johnson AB, et al. Mutations in GFAP, encoding glial fibrillary acidic protein, are associated with Alexander disease. Nat Genet. 2001;27(1):117–20.

Brenner M, Messing A. A new mutation in GFAP widens the spectrum of Alexander disease. Eur J Hum Genet. 2015;23(1):1–2.

Graff-Radford J, Schwartz K, et al. Neuroimaging and clinical features in type II (late-onset) Alexander disease. Neurology. 2014;82(1):49–56.

Hagemann TL, Connor JX, et al. Alexander disease-associated glial fibrillary acidic protein mutations in mice induce Rosenthal fiber formation and a white matter stress response. J Neurosci. 2006;26(43):11162–73.

Li R, Johnson AB, et al. Glial fibrillary acidic protein mutations in infantile, juvenile, and adult forms of Alexander disease. Ann Neurol. 2005;57(3):310–26.

Messing A, Brenner M, et al. Alexander disease. J Neurosci. 2012;32(15):5017–23.

Messing A, LaPash Daniels CM, et al. Strategies for treatment in Alexander disease. Neurotherapeutics. 2010;7(4):507–15.

Pareyson D, Fancellu R, et al. Adult-onset Alexander disease: a series of eleven unrelated cases with review of the literature. Brain. 2008;131(9):2321–31.

Prust M, Wang J, et al. GFAP mutations, age at onset, and clinical subtypes in Alexander disease. Neurology. 2011;77(13):1287–94.

Ramesh K, Sharma S, et al. Infantile-onset Alexander disease: a genetically proven case with mild clinical course in a 6-year-old Indian boy. J Child Neurol. 2013;28(3):396–8.

Rodriguez D, Gauthier F, et al. Infantile Alexander disease: spectrum of GFAP mutations and genotype-phenotype correlation. Am J Hum Genet. 2001;69(5):1134–40.

van der Knaap MS, Naidu S, et al. Alexander disease: diagnosis with MR imaging. AJNR Am J Neuroradiol. 2001;22(3):541–52.

van der Knaap MS, Ramesh V, et al. Alexander disease: ventricular garlands and abnormalities of the medulla and spinal cord. Neurology. 2006;66(4):494–8.

van der Knaap MS, Salomons GS, et al. Unusual variants of Alexander's disease. Ann Neurol. 2005;57(3):327–38.

van der Voorn JP, Pouwels PJ, et al. Unraveling pathology in juvenile Alexander disease: serial quantitative MR imaging and spectroscopy of white matter. Neuroradiology. 2009;51(10):669–75.

# Chapter 18
# Neurodegenerative Langerhans Cell Histiocytosis

Sonika Agarwal and Timothy E. Lotze

## Case Presentation

A 13-year-old right-handed Caucasian female with a 5-year history of diabetes insipidus secondary to biopsy-proven Langerhans cell histiocytosis (LCH) presented with a 10-month history of gradually progressive dysarthria, weakness of the lower extremities, and urinary retention. During these months she also developed choreiform movements involving the upper and lower extremities. She had paroxysmal episodes of expressive aphasia and behavior change lasting from 1 to 60 min with complete recovery afterward.

Neurological examination revealed a pleasant girl, fully oriented, though slow to follow commands and speak. She had slow scanning speech and bilateral horizontal nystagmus. She had increased tone in her legs, but her strength was normal (five out of five) in upper and lower extremities. She had diffuse hyperreflexia with sustained bilateral ankle clonus. Choreiform and athetoid movements were noted in all extremities. She had ataxia with dysmetria and a broad-based gait. CSF analysis was normal with one WBC, one RBC, glucose 54 mg/dL, and protein 40 mg/dL. Cytological analysis of the CSF was negative for atypical or malignant cells. Viral and bacterial cultures were negative. Long-term video EEG monitoring demonstrated the spells to be non-epileptic in nature. MRI brain revealed diffuse non-enhancing T2 hyperintense lesions in the cerebellar dentate nuclei, basal ganglia, and supratentorial white matter (Fig. 18.1).

S. Agarwal, M.D. (✉) • T.E. Lotze, M.D.
Division of Neurology and Developmental Neuroscience, Department of Pediatrics,
Baylor College of Medicine, Texas Children's Hospital,
6701 Fannin CC 1250, Houston, TX 77030, USA
e-mail: SXAgarwa@texaschildrens.org; sonikaa@bcm.edu; tlotze@bcm.edu

© Springer International Publishing AG 2017                                    137
E. Waubant, T.E. Lotze (eds.), *Pediatric Demyelinating Diseases of the Central Nervous System and Their Mimics*, DOI 10.1007/978-3-319-61407-6_18

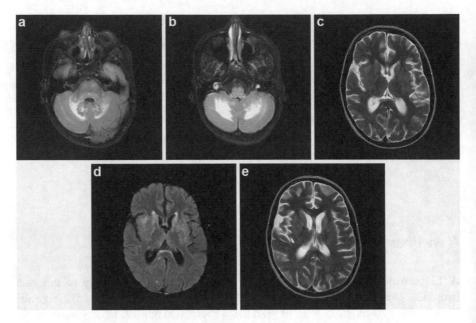

**Fig. 18.1** MRI brain demonstrating non-enhancing T2 hyperintense lesions in the cerebellar dentate nuclei, basal ganglia, and supratentorial white matter. There is evidence of generalized volume loss with ventriculomegaly

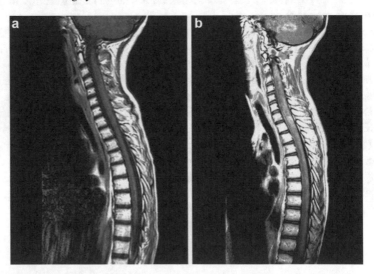

**Fig. 18.2** Contrast-enhanced MRI of the spine demonstrating nodular-enhancing lesions along the entire surface of the spinal cord as well as an enhancing intramedullary lesion in the lower thoracic and lumbar regions of the cord. In addition, there is heterogeneous T1 signal returned from the marrow of the vertebral bodies

Contrast-enhanced MRI of the spine showed nodular-enhancing lesions along the entire surface of the spinal cord as well as an enhancing intramedullary lesion in the lower thoracic and lumbar regions of the cord. There was heterogeneous T1 signal returned from the marrow of the vertebral bodies (Fig. 18.2).

The clinical history and the imaging features were felt to be consistent with neurodegenerative LCH. She received several courses of chemotherapy, followed by a combination of chemotherapy and IVIG. She subsequently had a relapsing and remitting course with gradual progression. She was additionally found to be positive for a mutation in the proto-oncogene *BRAFV600E* (gene encoding for serine/threonine-protein kinase B-Raf) and was started on vemurafenib and continued on this medication for 20 months (class 1 BRAF inhibitor). She continues to have an ataxic gait with tremors and chorea (improved with tetrabenazine), severe panhypopituitarism, nutritional challenges, episodes of behavioral arrest, and cognitive decline. She is currently on Hydrea 500 mg daily and intermittently has cycles of IVIG based on clinical worsening. It has been 3 years since her neurological symptoms started.

## Clinical Questions

1. What is Langerhans cell histiocytosis (LCH), and what are its characteristic CNS manifestations?
2. What alternative diagnoses to neurodegenerative LCH might be considered in this case?
3. What are the indications for and characteristics findings in neuroimaging of LCH?
4. What is the treatment and prognosis for neurodegenerative LCH?

## Diagnostic Discussion

1. Langerhans cell histiocytosis is a clonal proliferative disease of dendritic cells (Langerhans cells/LC) characterized by abnormal interaction of pathologic LC with T cells and associated with features of chronic inflammation. It is an extremely rare condition, and the overall incidence is 2.6–5 per million children annually [1, 2]. The disease can affect a single or multiple organ systems. Most frequently, it involves the skeleton (80%), skin (33%), and hypothalamic-pituitary region (25%). Other organs to include the spleen, liver, hematopoietic system, lungs, and lymphatics are involved in 5–15% of patients [2]. According to the European Histiocytosis Network guidelines, positive CD1a and/or CD207 (langerin) staining of lesional cells (from the skin or bony lesions) is required for definite diagnosis.

   As the hypothalamic-pituitary region is the most common CNS site affected, diabetes insipidus is the classical hallmark of CNS infiltration, and it is the most common intracranial manifestation of the disease [1]. Diabetes insipidus may manifest before, concurrently, or after a diagnosis of LCH has been made.

2. Neurodegenerative LCH (ND-LCH) occurs in 4% of patients and is the second most common manifestation of CNS disease in LCH after pituitary dysfunction. ND-LCH is a progressive disease with characteristic MRI signal changes in the cerebellar grey or white matter, pons, basal ganglia, and deep white matter of the cerebral hemispheres, with associated clinical signs. The clinical picture is very heterogeneous, ranging from headaches to subtle behavioral disturbances or from learning difficulties to severe disabilities such as psychiatric disease, psychomotor retardation, and pronounced cerebellar-pontine symptoms [1]. Neurological examination may demonstrate dysarthria, dysphagia, tremor, hyperreflexia, ataxia, gait disturbance, dysdiadochokinesis, and abnormal movements. While a pre-existing history of LCH, as in the described case, would likely lead to a rapid diagnosis for patients presenting with neurological symptoms, a broader differential diagnosis might be considered in the absence of this diagnosis or even in addition to it. Alternative diagnostic considerations might include various acquired demyelinating syndromes (acute disseminated encephalomyelitis, neuromyelitis optica, multiple sclerosis), lymphoma, CNS vasculopathy, CNS infection, autoimmune disorders (systemic lupus erythematosus), chemotherapy-related neurotoxicity, or other neurodegenerative diseases (mitochondrial, leukodystrophy, histiocytic disorders). Careful consideration of the clinical history and a directed work-up is required to rule out other causes. In particular, characteristic MRI findings and tissue diagnosis help to narrow the differential.

Diabetes insipidus with characteristic imaging of pituitary involvement (further described below in discussion point #3) in the setting of multifocal CNS involvement is a key feature raising concern for neurodegenerative LCH. However, MS (multiple sclerosis) might be considered in this context as there are rare reports of MS patients with clinical and imaging features of comorbid lymphocytic hypophysitis.

Independent of the pituitary involvement, such patients presenting with multifocal CNS symptoms as well as MRI evidence of multiple T2 hyperintense white matter lesions and a relapsing and remitting course may mimic the clinical picture of acquired demyelinating disease. The periventricular lesions may be quite similar to those seen in MS, as they can have a well-circumscribed ovoid appearance with an orientation that is perpendicular to the ventricular margins. Negative investigations for LCH, CSF supportive of MS such as increased IgG index and presence of oligoclonal bands, and ongoing monitoring of clinical and imaging features can help to distinguish the conditions. Neuromyelitis optica spectrum disorder might additionally be considered, as this condition can present with a diencephalic syndrome principally affecting the hypothalamic region and producing various endocrinopathies. Brainstem lesions in LCH are different from those encountered in MS, but could fit within the diagnostic criteria for NMO. Previously discussed investigations for LCH as well as negative serology for aquaporin 4 antibody can help to rule out NMO. Finally, a presentation with encephalopathy in the context of multifocal brain lesions could raise consideration for ADEM. However, pituitary disease, symmetric lesions of the brainstem and cerebellum, and nodular-enhancing lesions along the entire surface of the spinal cord would be atypical for ADEM, as well as MS and NMO. The clinical context and subsequent investigations would further clarify the correct diagnosis of LCH, once it has been considered.

MRI changes in CNS-LCH disease as per the Histiocyte Society CNS-LCH Study Group include tumorous/granulomatous lesions, non-tumorous/granulomatous intracerebral lesions, and atrophy [3, 4]. In the hypothalamic-pituitary region, the characteristic findings consist of enlargement of the pituitary stalk with progression to tumorous lesions in the pituitary, pineal gland, choroid plexus, meninges, or parenchyma in later stages. Loss of the posterior pituitary bright spot is characteristic of diabetes insipidus. Non-tumorous intracerebral lesions are characterized by symmetric, hyperintense signal changes on T2-weighted imaging, and hypo- or hyperintense on T1-weighted images.

3. Detailed neuroimaging of the temporal bones is indicated for all children with LCH presenting with craniofacial lesions including the maxilla or mandible or in the setting of hearing impairment or aural discharge [1]. MRI of the spine is indicated if there are complaints of back pain, progressive gait failure, or bowel and bladder dysfunction and may show lesions in the vertebrae, soft tissue, or spinal cord [1]. Neuroimaging is also indicated for any visual or neurological abnormalities or suspected endocrine abnormalities [1].

4. The treatment of active CNS disease depends on the type of CNS lesion, presence of multisystem disease, and clinical status of the patient. Tumor-like lesions of the CNS are treated with radiation or chemotherapy [5]. Treatment with a combination of monthly IVIG and chemotherapy (sometimes combined with trans-retinoic acid) has been reported to stabilize clinical and radiographic disease in a small number of patients [6]. However, no large trials have compared the various treatment modalities, and the prognosis remains poor for patients with neurodegenerative LCH. Recent studies have focused on trial with individualized treatment with BRAF inhibitors [7]. The 10-year survival varies from 40 to 90% based on location of disease and involvement of high-risk sites. Nonetheless, the course remains guarded with requirement for long-term chemotherapy and rehabilitation, and many patients continue to have residual neurologic deficits.

# Clinical Pearls

1. Neurodegenerative LCH should be considered in patients presenting with diabetes insipidus and signs, symptoms, and MRI findings of multifocal CNS involvement especially if relatively symmetrical.
2. CNS manifestations of LCH have a wide spectrum of severity from subtle neurocognitive deficits, deep tendon reflex abnormalities, or gait issues to severe neurological disability, and neuropsychiatric symptoms.

3. Prognosis for neurodegenerative LCH remains poor despite combination chemo-therapy. However, the addition of IVIG has shown to delay progression in small number of patients and is being increasingly used.

# References

1. Haupt R, Nanduri V, Calevo MG, Bernstrand B, Braier JL, Broadbent V, et al. Permanent con-sequences in Langerhans cell histiocytosis patients: a pilot study from the Histiocyte Society-Late Effects Study Group. Pediatr Blood Cancer. 2004;42:438–44.
2. Haupt R, Minkov M, Astigarraga I, Schafer E, Nanduri V, Jubran R, et al. Langerhans cell histiocytosis (LCH): guidelines, clinical work–up, and treatment for patients till the age of 18 years. Pediatr Blood Cancer. 2013;60:175–84.
3. Grois N, Fahmer B, Arceci RJ, Henter JI, McClain K, Lassman H, Nanduri V, et al. Central nervous system disease in Langerhans cell histiocytosis. J Pediatr. 2010;156:873–881.e1.
4. Prayer D, Grois N, Prosch H, Gadner H, Barkovich AJ. MR imaging presentation of intracranial disease associated with Langerhans cell histiocytosis. AJNR Am J Neuroradiol. 2004;25:880–91.
5. Abla O, Egeler RM, Wietzman S. Langerhans cell histiocytosis: current concepts and treat-ment. Cancer Treat Rev. 2010;36:354–9.
6. Idaih A, Donadieu J, Barthez MA, et al. Retinoic acid therapy in "degenerative like" neuro-Langerhans cell histiocytosis: a prospective pilot study. Pediatr Blood Cancer. 2004;43:55–8.
7. Berres ML, Lim KP, Peters T, Price J, Takizawa H, Salmon H, Idoyaga J, Ruzo A, Lupo PJ, Hicks MJ, Shih A, Simko SJ, Abhyankar H, Chakraborty R, Leboeuf M, Beltrão M, Lira SA, Heym KM, Bigley V, Collin M, Manz MG, McClain K, Merad M, Allen CE. BRAF-V600E expression in precursor versus differentiated dendritic cells defines clinically distinct LCH risk groups. J Exp Med. 2014;211:669–83.

# Chapter 19
# X-Linked Adrenoleukodystrophy

Joshua J. Bear

## Case Presentation

**Case 1:** A typically developing 6-year-old boy presented with 8 months of vision complaints. At the onset of his symptoms, his mother brought him to an optometrist for sudden outward movements of his left eye. His visual acuity was reportedly normal with no structural or functional deficits, and he was sent home. Over the next several months, he was noted to write with larger letters and worsening handwriting. A repeat optometry evaluation 4 months prior to presentation revealed difficulty focusing, for which he received corrective lenses. Despite this, his visual awareness continued to decline as he began to misjudge the position of objects in space, frequently reaching to the left of their actual location and walking into objects or tripping on steps. For 2 weeks prior to presentation, the patient started to experience nausea and emesis in the mornings. On examination, he was somnolent but arousable. His visual acuity was 20/40 on the right and 20/60 on the left with reactive pupils and full extraocular movements. He had dysmetria on finger-nose-finger that was worse on the left, and his gait had a narrow station and shuffling quality. The remainder of his neurologic examination was without deficits. Magnetic resonance imaging (MRI) of the brain was obtained and demonstrated bilateral, symmetric, and extensive T2 hyperintensity throughout much of the posterior white matter concerning for a demyelinating process (Fig. 19.1). Testing of his very long chain fatty acids (VLCFAs) demonstrated a hexacosanoic acid (C26:0) concentration of 1.3 ug/mL (normal 0.23 ± 0.09 ug/mL) and elevated ratios of C24/22 and C26/22. His adrenocorticotropic hormone (ACTH) was elevated at 146 ng/L (normal 7–50 ng/L), and an ACTH stimulation test was abnormal, with an increase in serum cortisol from 9 to

J.J. Bear, M.D., M.A (✉)
Assistant Professor of Pediatrics and Neurology, University of Colorado Denver and Children's Hospital Colorado, 505 Parnassus Avenue, Box 0114, Room M-798, San Francisco, CA 94143-0114, USA
e-mail: Joshua.bear@ucsf.edu

© Springer International Publishing AG 2017
E. Waubant, T.E. Lotze (eds.), *Pediatric Demyelinating Diseases of the Central Nervous System and Their Mimics*, DOI 10.1007/978-3-319-61407-6_19

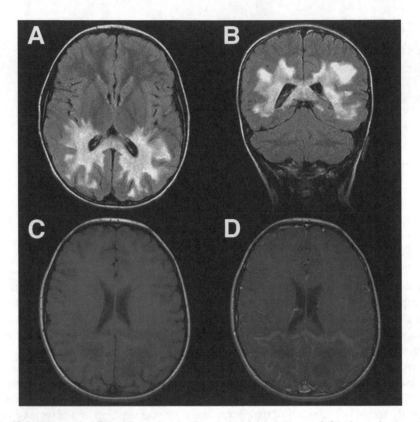

**Fig. 19.1** Diagnostic MRI of the patient in Case 1. Axial (**a**) and coronal (**b**) planes demonstrate confluent T2/FLAIR prolongation in the subcortical U fibers and deep white matter in a bilateral and posterior-predominant pattern including the parietal and occipital lobes, the splenium of the corpus callosum, the optic tracts, and the descending corticospinal tracts to the level of the medulla. Intrinsic T1 hyperintensity (**c**) and enhancement (**d**) are seen at the periphery of the white matter abnormalities, while the central areas are hypointense. There is no mass effect associated with the signal abnormalities

16 ng/L. Based on these results, he was diagnosed with X-linked adrenoleukodystrophy (X-ALD), childhood cerebral ALD (CCALD) phenotype.

The patient was started on hormone replacement therapy for adrenal insufficiency, and 2 months after diagnosis, he underwent a hematopoietic stem cell transplantation (HSCT). Despite this, his disease continued to progress to cortical blindness within the first year after diagnosis and later loss of expressive language and dysphagia requiring G-tube feeding. Four years after diagnosis, he was noncommunicative with severe episodic irritability and unresponsive to commands and had spastic quadriplegia with multiple joint contractures.

# Clinical Questions

1. What is the etiology and pathophysiology of X-ALD?
2. How is X-ALD diagnosed?
3. Why was this case considered CCALD and what are the other X-ALD phenotypes?
4. What are the imaging findings seen in cerebral X-ALD?
5. What treatment options are currently available for X-ALD?


# Diagnostic Discussion

## *What Is the Etiology and Pathophysiology of X-ALD?*

X-ALD is a peroxisomal disorder caused by a single-gene mutation in the ATP-binding cassette (ABC), subfamily D, and member 1 gene (*ABCD1*), located at Xq28. Peroxisomal disorders can be classified as disorders of biogenesis or as enzyme deficiencies with a total incidence of >1:10,000 live births. X-ALD, the most common peroxisomal disorder, has an incidence of approximately 1:17,000 in the USA. Peroxisomes are essential in several anabolic and catabolic functions including the beta-oxidation of VLCFAs and the synthesis of bile acids and plasmalogens. As a consequence, most peroxisomal disorders are characterized by the abnormal accumulation of VLCFAs, particularly those with 26 carbon atoms. The accumulation of VLCFA in cell membranes contributes to cellular dysfunction and/or cell death.

*ABCD1* encodes an ABC transporter that forms a channel through which VLCFAs enter peroxisomes for beta-oxidation. As a consequence beta-oxidation is disrupted, leading to the accumulation of VLCFAs in all tissues. The clinical consequences can be variable depending on the relative disease burden in different tissues of the brain, the spinal cord, the testes, and the adrenal glands, and this spectrum of presentations is referred to as the ALD/adrenomyeloneuropathy (AMN) complex.

The clinical symptoms are related to the location of the affected tissues. In the central nervous system (CNS), a progressive inflammatory demyelinating process typically starting in the parieto-occipital regions and progressing anteriorly results in cerebral ALD. Spinal cord involvement, often a degenerative axonopathy of the ascending and descending tracts, leads to AMN. Accumulation in the adrenal glands results in adrenal insufficiency and can present as part of the ALD/AMN complex or in isolation as Addison disease. Rarely individuals can present with other isolated symptoms such as hypogonadism and erectile dysfunction related to accumulation of VLCFA in the Leydig cells of the testes or with predominant cerebellar or pontine deficits.

## How Is X-ALD Diagnosed?

Cerebral ALD often presents as nonspecific visual or behavioral changes, as in this case, related to the typical pattern of parietal and occipital lobe involvement. Brain MRI typically provides the first clues to the diagnosis. Whether the diagnosis is suspected based on the constellation of symptoms or the results of imaging studies, the concentration of VLCFAs in the serum should be measured. By definition, a VLCFA is a fatty acid with a carbon tail with >22 carbon atoms. The laboratory evaluation will typically report the concentration of hexacosanoic acid (C26:0) as well as the ratio of C26:0 to docosanoic acid (C22:0) with additional reported values varying by laboratory. An elevated total level and elevated ratio are suggestive of a disorder of peroxisomal degradation, and this can be sufficient for the diagnosis of X-ALD if the clinical presentation is appropriate. Molecular genetic testing of *ABCD1* is useful for confirmation of the diagnosis—particularly in atypical presentations, in female patients, or in cases with borderline elevations of VLCFAs—and to aid in genetic counseling. Mutations of *ABCD1* are identified in 90% of affected individuals.

## Why Was This Case Considered CCALD and How Does It Differ from Other X-ALD Phenotypes?

The laboratory-based diagnosis of X-ALD is distinct from the spectrum of clinical phenotypes in the ALD/AMN complex. CCALD, characterized by involvement of the central nervous system during childhood, is the most common presentation in children seen in 35–40% of individuals. The age of presentation typically ranges from 3 to 15 years. The majority of patients with CCALD will also develop adrenal insufficiency during the early part of the disease.

Approximately 40–45% of affected individuals who remain symptom-free throughout childhood will develop AMN, which is characterized by spinal cord dysfunction resulting in a progressive spastic paraparesis, abnormal sphincter control, and sexual dysfunction. Although rare at the time of presentation, up to half of patients with AMN will eventually develop symptoms of cerebral involvement, and 10–20% of these individuals can experience a rapidly progressive functional decline.

Isolated Addison disease is less common, presenting in approximately 10% of patients, and can occur at any age.

Although X-ALD is typically considered a disease of male individuals, half of female carriers will also develop symptoms during their lifetime. Most commonly female individuals will develop a milder phenotype with slowly progressive neuropathy and a mild spastic paraparesis presenting in the fifth or sixth decades.

**Fig. 19.2** Axial (**a**) and coronal (**b**) FLAIR images demonstrating T2 hyperintense lesions of the corticospinal tract (*arrows*) in a patient with ADHD and a family history of X-ALD. There was no enhancement on post-gadolinium images

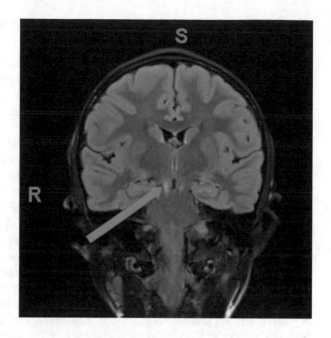

## *What Are the MRI Findings Seen in Cerebral X-ALD?*

Five distinct patterns of white matter involvement, seen best on T2 and FLAIR sequences, have been described in cerebral ALD with the vast majority of patients presenting with the first three patterns. In cases of CCALD, nearly 80% of children will have involvement of white matter in the parieto-occipital lobe and/or the splenium of the corpus callosum as seen in this case (Fig. 19.1). A further 10% will present with frontal lobe white matter involvement and/or the genu of the corpus callosum. Remaining pediatric cases might have a mixed pattern of involvement, involvement of the frontopontine and corticospinal projections, or a primary cerebellar pattern. The MRI findings are often used to calculate the Loes score, a measure of the extent of cerebral involvement ranging from 0 to 34, with 34 representing the most extensive involvement. In adult patients, most will still have involvement of either the parieto-occipital or frontal regions, but over 20% will present with isolated involvement of the frontopontine and corticospinal projections (Fig. 19.2) [1].

Not all patients will show contrast enhancement, but those who do will typically have a linear pattern of enhancement along the leading edge of demyelination. The presence of enhancement has been associated with ongoing and rapid progression of disease either radiographically, clinically, or both [2].

## What Treatment Options Are Currently Available for X-ALD?

While several pharmaceutical and dietary treatments have been and are continuing to be studied, the only therapeutic intervention shown to be effective in arresting the progression of cerebral X-ALD is allogeneic HSCT. In appropriately selected patients, HSCT can arrest disease progression and significantly improve 5-year prognosis. Unfortunately the patients most likely to benefit from HSCT are those with no or minor symptoms and with minimal cerebral involvement on MRI as measured by a Loes score ≤ 10 at the time of the procedure. Many patients have already missed the window of optimal treatment at the time of definitive diagnosis.

Because the pathological accumulation of VLCFA in affected tissues is thought to underlie the clinical symptoms, several therapeutic efforts have been targeted at reducing VLCFA concentrations. Perhaps the most well-known therapy, Lorenzo's oil, is a mixture of two monounsaturated fatty acids. The hypothesis behind Lorenzo's oil is that competitive inhibition of the biosynthesis of VLCFA with monounsaturated fatty acids, combined with dietary restriction of VLCFA, will decrease the levels of VLCFA. Several trials have demonstrated that while the treatment is effective in decreasing serum levels of VLCFA, it does not appear to have any effect on the disease course itself. Lovastatin has similarly been shown to decrease plasma VLCFA but does not seem to affect intracellular concentrations. Ongoing research is investigating other approaches including small molecules designed to inhibit the biosynthesis of VLCFA and the role of antioxidants in preventing cellular injury. Early clinical trials of gene therapy are also underway including preliminary results showing promise in autologous transplantation of lentivirally corrected CD34+ cells.

**Case 2:** The 1-year-old brother of the patient from Case 1 was developing typically with no neurologic complaints, but he was found to have elevated concentrations of C26:0 and elevated ratios of C24/22 and C26/22. He had a normal general and neurologic examination. At 18 months of age, a brain MRI was obtained that revealed no abnormalities. He has since undergone serial MRI imaging studies every 12 months and now at 4 years of age has continued to have negative imaging results including MR spectroscopy (Fig. 19.3). He is not currently receiving any medication or other therapies.

## Clinical Questions

1. What screening studies should be obtained in the siblings of patients with X-ALD?
2. Can the specific ABCD1 mutation or other factors be used to predict the clinical course?
3. What is the anticipated clinical trajectory and long-term prognosis in patients with X-ALD?

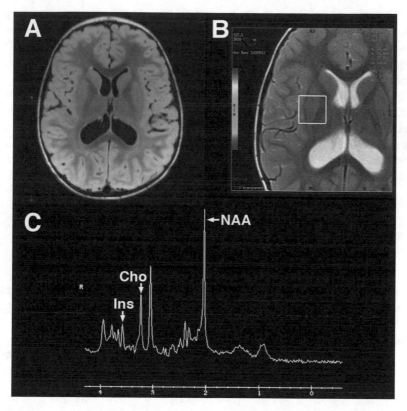

**Fig. 19.3** Screening MRI for patient in Case 2. No abnormalities of the white matter are seen on axial T2/FLAIR (**a**). MRS in the basal ganglia demonstrates NAA, choline (Cho), and myoinositol (Ins) peaks (located at 2.02, 3.2, and 3.56 ppm, respectively) within normal limits (**b**, **c**). Voxels in the white matter and CSF were also interrogated and within normal limits (not shown)

## Diagnostic Discussion

### *What Screening Studies Should Be Obtained in the Siblings of Patients with X-ALD?*

One of the challenges in the management of asymptomatic patients with laboratory evidence of X-ALD is determining treatment options. HSCT is the only treatment clearly shown to improve outcomes in CCALD variant of X-ALD, yet 60–65% of individuals with the biological findings will not develop CCALD. However, because HSCT is most likely to be beneficial before the development of clinical symptoms, identifying patients with progressive CCALD at the onset of disease is essential to improve outcomes. The MRI findings of CCALD can precede clinical symptoms by an estimated 6–12 months, and many centers recommend at least annual MRI for asymptomatic patients with X-ALD. In addition to T2/FLAIR and pre- and post-gadolinium sequences, magnetic resonance spectroscopy (MRS) has been shown to be a sensitive test for detection of cerebral involvement. T2/FLAIR changes are preceded by early markers of lesion development on MRS, which include a decreased NAA peak and elevated choline and myoinositol peaks.

In addition to screening for cerebral involvement, screening for adrenal insufficiency should be considered. Screening typically involves measurement of cortisol levels and an ACTH stimulation test performed annually. No consensus currently exists to guide when to begin screening with some institutions waiting until the individual develops clinical symptoms or exam findings of adrenal insufficiency, but ACTH is elevated in 70% of individuals with X-ALD by 2 years of age [3].

## Can the Specific ABCD1 Mutation or Other Factors Be Used to Predict the Clinical Course?

Despite the identification of over 1000 different mutations in *ABCD1*, no genotype-phenotype correlations have been identified. Irrespective of the specific mutations, individuals within the same family can present at opposite ends of the clinical spectrum. Slight differences in the incidence of CCALD among patients with X-ALD have been reported with an increased incidence in Brazilian individuals, which could suggest genetic or environmental factors that have not yet been elucidated.

## What Is the Anticipated Clinical Trajectory and Long-Term Prognosis in Patients with X-ALD?

The clinical trajectory of the ALD/AMN complex is highly variable. Approximately 35–40% of patients will develop CCALD. CCALD tends to have a rapidly progressive and devastating course resulting in severe disability and death with a 5-year survival of approximately 54% and a 10-year survival of 42%. A subset of patients presenting with CCALD seems to have spontaneous stabilization of disease, likely accounting for some of the long-term survivors. HSCT performed early in the progressive stage of CCALD results in significant reductions of mortality with 5- and 10-year survival of up to 95% [4]. The greatest benefit is seen in individuals with a Loes score of ≤10; for those with a Loes score > 10, the estimated 5-year survival drops to 60%.

For patients with AMN and isolated corticospinal ALD, the disease progression is often much slower and diagnosis does not necessitate immediate HSCT. Following the development of gait difficulties in AMN, the development of adrenal dysfunction and bladder involvement occurs near the end of the first decade from onset. Approximately half of individuals with AMN will eventually develop cerebral involvement with psychic disturbances and intellectual decline occurring nearly 15 years after diagnosis. Rarely adults with X-ALD will present with primary cerebral involvement, in which case progression is similar to the more rapid course seen in CCALD [5].

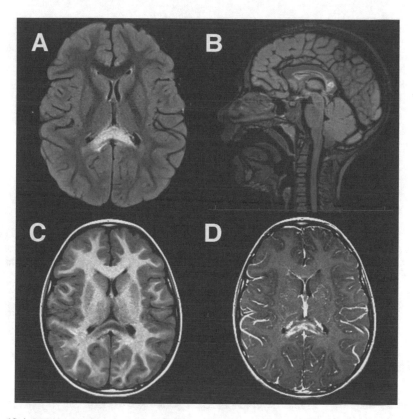

**Fig. 19.4**  MRI in a patient presenting with subacute worsening of migrainous headaches (Case 3). Axial (**a**) and sagittal (**b**) FLAIR images show a T2 hyperintense lesion involving the splenium of the corpus callosum with subtle extension into the posterior periatrial white matter. The central area of the lesion is hypointense on T1 (**c**) but shows patchy but largely peripheral enhancement after gadolinium administration (**d**)

**Case 3:**  A 6-year-old boy with 2 years of episodic migraine presented with a worsening in the frequency and severity of his headaches over 2 months. On examination, he was well appearing and behaviorally appropriate with no neurologic deficits. Given the sub-acute worsening of his symptoms, a brain MRI was obtained that revealed an enhancing T2 hyperintense lesion in the splenium of the corpus callosum (Fig. 19.4) and a lactate peak on spectroscopy. Follow-up imaging at 3 and 6 months demonstrated interval enlargement of the lesion (Fig. 19.5). A lumbar puncture was performed, and his CSF profile showed zero red blood cells, one white blood cell, a glucose of 57 mg/dL, and a protein of 19 mg/dL. The IgG index was 0.6, which is considered within normal limits, but three unique oligoclonal bands were identified. A neuropsychological evaluation showed appropriate behavior and cognition for age. Given the concern for a malignancy, a brain biopsy was obtained that demonstrated a destructive inflammatory process without evidence of malignant cells (Fig. 19.6), consistent with a chronic inflammatory process such as a demyelinating disease or infection. Subsequent metabolic studies showed a VLCFA profile consistent with a diagnosis of X-ALD.

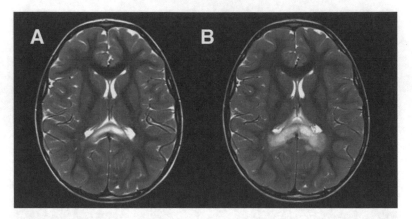

**Fig. 19.5** Axial T2 sequences on the patient presented in Case 3 at the time of presentation (**a**) and 6 months later (**b**). The T2 hyperintense lesion shows an interval increase in thickening of the splenium of the corpus callosum with extension into the fornices and along the posterior lateral ventricular margins bilaterally

## Clinical Questions

1. What diagnoses should be considered in patients with isolated lesions of the corpus callosum?
2. What are typical pathological features of X-ALD, and how do they compare to an acquired demyelinating disease like MS?
3. How does the clinical presentation of X-ALD differ from the acquired demyelinating diseases in children?

## Diagnostic Discussion

### *What Diagnoses Should Be Considered in Patients with Isolated Lesions of the Corpus Callosum?*

Isolated lesions of the corpus callosum in pediatric patients can be caused by several etiological categories. Vascular lesions can include arteriovenous malformations, which involve the corpus callosum in about 10% of cases; ischemic strokes most commonly from thromboembolic disease affecting the pericallosal or penetrating arteries can be seen in cardiothoracic surgery for congenital heart defects and

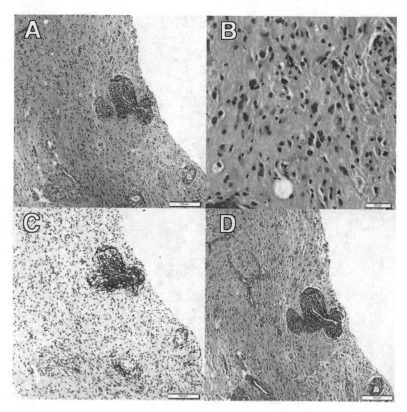

**Fig. 19.6** H&E stains at 100× (**a**) and 400× (**b**) showing perivascular and intraparenchymal chronic inflammatory cell infiltrate with reactive astrocytes, focal mineralization, and pallor. Neurofilament staining at 100× (**c**) shows a marked depletion of axonal processes. Additionally a marked depletion of myelin, which should stain a vibrant blue color, is seen on the Luxol fast blue/ periodic acid Schiff (LFB/PAS) stain (**d**) at 100× magnification. (*Image courtesy of Dr. Matthew Wood, University of California San Francisco*)

hemorrhage. Hemorrhages can be related to either a vascular anomaly or traumatic injury including non-accidental trauma putatively due to the sensitivity to shearing forces in the white matter tracts forming the corpus callosum. Although the density of the white matter fibers in the corpus callosum makes it an uncommon site of infection, the rich blood supply and position adjacent to the ventricles can lead to infections even in immunocompetent hosts, through both presumed hematogenous spread and direct invasion from ventriculitis. Figure 19.7 demonstrates a non-enhancing T2 hyperintense lesion of the splenium of the corpus callosum with restricted diffusion in an individual with meningoencephalitis. Tumors, both primary and metastatic, can involve the corpus callosum. Glioblastoma multiforme, while often extending along the white matter tracts of the corpus callosum, is rarely

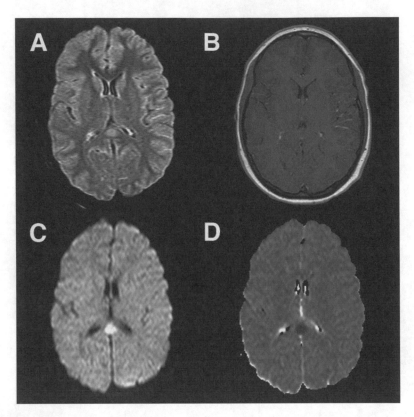

**Fig. 19.7** MRI in a patient with meningoencephalitis. An isolated T2 hyperintense lesion involving the splenium of the corpus callosum (**a**), but no signal change on T1 (**b**) demonstrates restricted diffusion on diffusion-weighted imaging (**c**) and average diffusion coefficient (**d**) sequences

isolated to the callosum. Central nervous system lymphoma, lipoma, and other tumor types can also involve the corpus callosum. Demyelinating diseases, including MS and acute demyelinating encephalomyelitis (ADEM), commonly involve the corpus callosum although typical disease presentations will also include other white matter, and rarely gray matter, lesions. In adults, particularly heavy drinkers, one should also consider Marchiafava-Bignami disease, a demyelinating disease that preferentially affects the corpus callosum. As discussed in the cases above, genetic and metabolic disorders should be considered including vanishing white matter disease and X-linked adrenoleukodystrophy as discussed in Cases 1, 2, and 3. Finally, postictal changes can be seen in the splenium of the corpus callosum with typical characteristics of T2 hyperintensity and restricted diffusion. Postictal changes and changes related to infection and acquired demyelinating diseases can be transient with partial or complete resolution on follow-up scans, a characteristic that can help differentiate these from other diagnoses [6].

## What Are Typical Pathological Features of X-ALD, and How Do They Compare to an Acquired Demyelinating Disease Like MS?

Brain biopsy in X-ALD typically shows a perivascular cuffing caused by CD8+ T-cell lymphocytic infiltration, and on electron microscopy striated trilaminar lipid inclusions can be seen in macrophages and Schwann cells. The striated trilaminar lipid inclusions are also apparent in biopsy specimens from the adrenal cortex and the testicular Leydig cells. The perivascular cuffing pattern of the lymphocytes in X-ALD is unique among the leukodystrophies but can also be seen in MS and ADEM. However, relative axonal sparing in MS and ADEM compared to the degree of myelin depletion seen can help in differentiating the underlying disease. The preferential loss of myelin is true in both active and inactive MS plaques. The pathology shown in Fig. 19.5 demonstrated a chronic inflammatory process with marked axonal and myelin loss, consistent with his ultimate diagnosis of X-ALD.

## How Does the Clinical Presentation of X-ALD Differ from the Acquired Demyelinating Diseases in Children?

As illustrated in other chapters of this book, the acquired demyelinating diseases including MS and ADEM can present with a wide variety of clinical symptoms due to the variability in areas of the brain involved. However, certain features of the history and clinical course are useful in differentiating these disorders from X-ALD. First, children with MS or their parents might report multiple nonspecific neurological complaints that often have a clear onset, frequently with gradual improvement or resolution over time. Common complaints can include fatigue, concentration difficulties, and motor and sensory phenomena. In contrast, the most common childhood form of X-ALD preferentially involves the posterior white matter and, consequently, results predominantly in a combination of visual disturbances and behavioral changes. Furthermore these symptoms are slowly progressive without periods of remission or resolution. Proper diagnosis X-ALD presenting with isolated involvement of the corticospinal tracts or spinal cord itself is more challenging, particularly in differentiating it from MS. The progressive nature without remissions still offers a clue but could also represent primary progressive MS. A careful history with a focus on symptoms of adrenal insufficiency, including skin color changes, hypogonadism in male patients, and a review of the family history can provide further guidance toward the correct diagnosis.

# Clinical Pearls

1. X-ALD can present with a spectrum of diseases ranging from isolated Addison disease, CCALD in children, and AMN in young adults that in some cases will progress to include cerebral involvement. Around 50% of female carriers will develop symptoms, typically in middle age.
2. CCALD most commonly presents with nonspecific visual complaints and behavioral changes in male school-aged children, symptoms that should prompt an MRI.
3. Characteristic MRI findings include symmetric white matter hyperintensity on T2/FLAIR in the parieto-occipital region often extending symmetrically from the splenium of the corpus callosum or in the frontal white matter sometimes involving the genu of the corpus callosum.
4. HSCT is the only therapy shown to improve outcomes in cerebral ALD. When individuals are identified early, HSCT can arrest disease progression and improve 5-year-survival rates from 54 to 95%. Given the importance of early treatment, family members should have VLCFA concentrations measured, and affected male members should have annual screening MRI, and adrenal function screening should be considered.
5. Lorenzo's oil reduces plasma VLCFA but in multiple trials has not demonstrated a benefit in CCALD. Its role in other forms of the disease remains uncertain.
6. Isolated lesions of the splenium of the corpus callosum can be seen in many different disease categories including vascular abnormalities, malignancies, infections, and demyelinating diseases, and appropriate diagnosis requires a careful review of the disease time course, family history, associated symptoms, and imaging characteristics.

**Acknowledgments** Thank you to Drs. Audrey Foster-Barber, Timothy Lotze, and Emmanuelle Waubant for helping to identify appropriate teaching cases and for their thoughtful critiques and guidance in the preparation of this manuscript. Thank you to Dr. Matthew Wood for his preparation and description of the neuropathology images.

# References

1. Loes DJ, Fatemi A, Melhem ER, Gupte N, Bezman L, Moser HW, et al. Analysis of MRI patterns aids prediction of progression in X-linked adrenoleukodystrophy. Neurology. 2003;61(3):369–74.
2. Melhem ER, Loes DJ, Georgiades CS, Raymond GV, Moser HW. X-linked adrenoleukodystrophy: the role of contrast-enhanced MR imaging in predicting disease progression. AJNR Am J Neuroradiol. 2000;21(5):839–44.
3. Dubey P, Raymond GV, Moser AB, Kharkar S, Bezman L, Moser HW. Adrenal insufficiency in asymptomatic adrenoleukodystrophy patients identified by very long-chain fatty acid screening. J Pediatr. 2005;146(4):528–32.
4. Mahmood A, Raymond GV, Dubey P, Peters C, Moser HW. Survival analysis of haematopoietic cell transplantation for childhood cerebral X-linked adrenoleukodystrophy: a comparison study. Lancet Neurol. 2007;6(8):687–92.

5. Suzuki Y, Takemoto Y, Shimozawa N, Imanaka T, Kato S, Furuya H, et al. Natural history of X-linked adrenoleukodystrophy in Japan. Brain and Development. 2005;27(5):353–7.
6. Bourekas EC, Varakis K, Bruns D, Christoforidis GA, Baujan M, Slone HW, et al. Lesions of the corpus callosum: MR imaging and differential considerations in adults and children. AJR Am J Roentgenol. 2002;179(1):251–7.

# Chapter 20
# Rapid-Onset Obesity with Hypothalamic Dysfunction, Hypoventilation, and Autonomic Dysregulation (ROHHAD)

Geetanjali Singh Rathore, Robert I. Thompson-Stone, and Leslie Benson

## Case Presentation

**Patient 1**: A 5-year-old girl was transferred to the pediatric inpatient unit with recent-onset behavioral changes in association with 1 month of significant weight gain (13.5 kg) and recurrent nocturnal fevers. Subsequently, she developed recurrent abdominal discomfort, nausea, constipation, and 2 weeks of visual hallucinations for which she was hospitalized in a psychiatric facility prior to being transferred. Admission examination showed a weight of 37 kg (far exceeding 99 percentile), a heart rate of 140 bpm, a 3 cm rectal prolapse and precocious puberty, a labile mood, a disordered thought process (hallucinations), and a depressed level of consciousness. There were no focal neurologic deficits identified. Her laboratory evaluation revealed a metabolic alkalosis, elevated creatine kinase (peak 12,000 U/L), prolactin, and CRP. Her cerebrospinal fluid (CSF) studies were normal including cell count; protein; glucose; bacterial, viral, fungal, and acid-fast bacilli cultures; *Toxoplasma*

G.S. Rathore, M.B.B.S., M.D. (✉)
Pediatric Neurology, University of Nebraska Medical Center, Children's Hospital
and Medical Center, Omaha, NE, USA
e-mail: grathore@childrensomaha.org

R.I. Thompson-Stone, M.D.
University of Rochester Medical Center, Rochester, NY, USA
e-mail: robert_stone@urmc.rochester.edu

L. Benson, M.D.
Department of Pediatric Neurology, Harvard Medical School, Boston Children's Hospital,
Boston, MA, USA
e-mail: Leslie.Benson@childrens.harvard.edu

© Springer International Publishing AG 2017
E. Waubant, T.E. Lotze (eds.), *Pediatric Demyelinating Diseases of the Central Nervous System and Their Mimics*, DOI 10.1007/978-3-319-61407-6_20

*gondii* PCR; and an encephalitis panel (including PCR for herpes simplex viruses 1 and 2, adenovirus, *Cytomegalovirus*, varicella-zoster virus, Epstein-Barr virus, human herpesvirus 6, *Eastern equine encephalitis virus*, *Enterovirus*, and *West Nile virus*). Her initial head magnetic resonance imaging (MRI) was normal, but she was found to have an enhancing right adrenal mass on abdominal MRI. Her EEG showed moderate-to-severe diffuse encephalopathy without epileptiform discharges. Over the course of a prolonged hospitalization, she experienced recurrent episodes of respiratory distress and apnea and was intubated after 22 days. She underwent a right adrenalectomy, and the mass was diagnosed as a ganglioneuroblastoma. She was not treated with any specific immunomodulatory medication. Over the next 180 days, she stayed in intensive care with frequent episodes of autonomic instability and numerous medical complications. She had a repeat MRI scan after several episodes of hypotension and was found to have bilateral basal ganglia lesions, presumed to be watershed cerebral infarctions. She eventually suffered a fatal cardiopulmonary arrest, and autopsy showed hypothalamic inflammation.

**Patient 2**: A 6.5-year-old girl with 1 year of increased appetite associated with 60–70 lb weight gain, moodiness, fatigue, esotropia, and constipation with encopresis presented with acute dyspnea due to an asthma exacerbation. During admission nocturnal hypoxia ultimately leads to the diagnoses of central and obstructive hypoventilation in sleep. Constipation workup incidentally found an adrenal mass on ultrasound, which was resected after the diagnosis of ROHHAD syndrome was made. Pathologically the mass was consistent with a ganglioneuroma with an inflammatory infiltrate which was unusual for typical ganglioneuromas. MRI brain and paired-like homeobox 2B (PHOX2B) sequencing were normal. CSF was normal except for matched oligoclonal bands in the serum and CSF. She started on IVIG 2 g/kg prior to discharge followed by 1 g/kg every 4 weeks for the following 3 years given the suspicion that ROHHAD syndrome is a paraneoplastic disease. About 6 months after treatment initiation, she began showing clear improvement with gradual resolution of hypoventilation, encopresis, and weight loss and improvement in behavior, specifically less impulsivity and inattention. After 2 years of IVIG, nightly BiPAP was discontinued. Other than elevated prolactin, she has had no other endocrinopathies or vital sign instability.

# Clinical Questions and Diagnostic Discussion

## How Does ROHHAD Typically Present?

Rapid-onset obesity with hypothalamic dysfunction, hypoventilation, and autonomic dysregulation (ROHHAD) is an extremely rare disorder [1]. As seen in both our patients, it is characterized by rapid weight gain followed by hypoventilation (central and/or obstructive), after 18 months, in a previously healthy child. Hypothalamic dysfunction may manifest as adrenal insufficiency, salt dysregulation or hyperprolactinemia, and pubertal dysfunction, as seen in our first patient. Gastric dysmotility and even rectal prolapse, as in our patients, are commonly seen due to autonomic dysfunction, in addition to impaired pain perception, temperature dysregulation, and oculomotor and pupillary defects [2].

## How Do You Establish the Diagnosis of ROHHAD and Differentiate It from Other Central Hypoventilation and Obesity Syndromes?

ROHHAD is a clinical diagnosis with variable presentation most often marked by rapid weight gain and hypoventilation. In addition to the presence of hypothalamic dysfunction, the absence of other primary neuromuscular, cardiac, lung, and central nervous system disorders and known genetic abnormalities must also be demonstrated to establish diagnosis [1]. MRI brain is essential to rule out other causes of hypothalamic dysfunction and is typically normal [1, 2].

Congenital central hypoventilation syndrome (CCHS), due to PHOX2B mutation, is the most common cause of central hypoventilation in children and must be ruled out. In contrast to ROHHAD, CCHS patients typically do not have obesity and endocrine dysfunction [1]. Autonomic dysfunction, though present in both, primarily manifests as impaired alteration in heart rate in CCHS [1].

In addition to Prader-Willi Syndrome, other less common causes of early onset obesity should be considered in the differential. Leptin deficiency due to pro-opiomelanocortin (POMC) gene mutation is characterized by childhood obesity, immunodeficiency, and red hair. Recently, mutations in the melanocortin receptor (MC4R) gene have also been identified as a cause of early onset obesity due to hyperphagia and associated hyperinsulinemia. Both conditions do not have central hypoventilation and autonomic dysfunction characteristically seen in ROHHAD patients [3].

## What Are Other Associated Neurological and Paraneoplastic Features of This Syndrome?

Neuropsychiatric features seen in both our patients have been reported in ROHHAD patients. These can vary from developmental delays, regression, attention deficit hyperactivity disorder (ADHD), autism, obsessive-compulsive disorder (OCD), bipolar disorder, and depression to even seizures, hypotonia, and encephalopathy [2].

Neural crest tumors such as ganglioneuroblastoma (patient 1) and ganglioneuroma (patient 2) have been reported in about one-third of patients with ROHHAD. These are typically found in the chest and abdomen although diagnosis is often delayed given the rarity and under-recognition of ROHHAD syndrome [1, 2].

## What Is Known About the Underlying Pathophysiology of ROHHAD?

The etiology of ROHHAD syndrome is still unknown. Due to the overlap of several features of ROHHAD and CCHS, a genetic cause was considered most likely; however, despite improved genetic technology, a gene has not been identified [1]. Patients with atypical phenotypes have been identified with alternative diagnoses [4]. Underlying autoimmune and paraneoplastic mechanisms have been entertained based on high association with neural crest tumors, identification of oligoclonal bands in the CSF, hypothalamic inflammation on autopsy, and reports of improvement in symptoms with immunosuppressive therapy [5]. The absence of a clearly identified antibody or tumor in half of the patients and mixed results with immune therapy make this mechanism controversial but still possible given similar associations in well-established paraneoplastic disorders such as NMDA receptor encephalitis and opsoclonus myoclonus ataxia syndrome.

## How Should Patients with ROHHAD Be Managed?

Being a multisystem disorder, ROHHAD patients should be managed by a multidisciplinary subspecialty team. Once the diagnosis is suspected, the patient must be monitored closely for development of additional signs and symptoms, such as hypoventilation and occult tumors that were identified in our patients. Diagnostic testing and monitoring should include an overnight sleep study to evaluate for undiagnosed hypoventilation (obstructive and central), electrocardiogram (EKG), Holter monitoring and/or telemetry and comprehensive testing of the hypothalamic pituitary axis. Imaging for neuroendocrine tumors (neuroblastic tumors) must be performed as soon as the diagnosis is considered. Abdominal ultrasound and chest x-ray can rule out large lesions, but MRI of the entire sympathetic chain and adrenal glands is often necessary to rule out smaller tumors.

Prognosis of ROHHAD is poor, as 25% patients die due to hypoventilation or cardiorespiratory arrest, and the survivors suffer from significant morbidity due to their sequelae. Immunomodulation or immunosuppression ranging from conventional steroids and intravenous immunoglobulin (IVIG) to cyclophosphamide and rituximab has shown some benefit in isolated cases [5]. Our second patient showed resolution of most symptoms when treated with long-term IVIG.

## Clinical Pearls

1. Consider the diagnosis of ROHHAD syndrome in children who have rapid weight gain and hyperphagia.

2. Rule out other primary neuromuscular, cardiac, pulmonary, central nervous system, and known genetic abnormalities prior to diagnosis of ROHHAD syndrome.
3. If considering the diagnosis of ROHHAD, monitor for other features like central and obstructive hypoventilation, neuroendocrine tumors, and hypothalamic and autonomic dysfunction.
4. Neurobehavioral and psychiatric symptoms can also be a part of the syndrome.
5. Consider immunomodulation or immunosuppression for treating ROHHAD patients. Consultation with experts in paraneoplastic disease such as neuroimmunology, rheumatology, or oncology should be considered.

# References

1. Patwari PP, Wolfe LF. Rapid-onset obesity with hypothalamic dysfunction, hypoventilation, and autonomic dysregulation: review and update. Curr Opin Pediatr. 2014;26(4):487–92.
2. Ize-Ludlow D, Gray JA, Sperling MA, Berry-Kravis EM, Milunsky JM, Farooqi IS, Rand CM, Weese-Mayer DE. Rapid-onset obesity with hypothalamic dysfunction, hypoventilation, and autonomic dysregulation presenting in childhood. Pediatrics. 2007;120(1):e179–88.
3. Kocaay P, Şıklar Z, Camtosun E, Kendirli T, Berberoğlu M. ROHHAD syndrome: reasons for diagnostic difficulties in obesity. J Clin Res Pediatr Endocrinol. 2014;6(4):254–7.
4. Thaker VV, Esteves KM, Towne MC, Brownstein CA, James PM, Crowley L, Hirschhorn JN, Elsea SH, Beggs AH, Picker J, Agrawal PB. Whole exome sequencing identifies RAI1 mutation in a morbidly obese child diagnosed with ROHHAD syndrome. J Clin Endocrinol Metab. 2015;100(5):1723–30.
5. Abaci A, Catli G, Bayram E, Koroglu T, Olgun HN, Mutafoglu K, Hiz AS, Cakmakci H, Bober E. A case of rapid-onset obesity with hypothalamic dysfunction, hypoventilation, autonomic dysregulation, and neural crest tumor: ROHHADNET syndrome. Endocr Pract. 2013;19(1):e12–6.

# Chapter 21
# ADEM Mimic with Thiamine Transporter Deficiency

Rebecca L. Holt and Keith Van Haren

## Case Presentation

A normally developing 16-month-old girl of Iranian descent born to non-consanguineous parents presented with progressive motor decline 1 week after an acute upper respiratory infection. Prior to her presentation, she was able to run and climb stairs without difficulty. Initially, she presented with falling which progressed to the point where she was unable to walk or sit unsupported over the course of 1 week. Magnetic resonance imaging (MRI) of her brain showed symmetric areas of T2-hyperintensity in the bilateral basal ganglia and subcortical white matter predominantly in the posterior temporal and parietal lobes (Fig. 21.1). Cerebrospinal fluid (CSF) analysis was normal. She was treated with 5 days of 30 mg/kg/day IV solumedrol for suspected acute disseminated encephalomyelitis (ADEM).

One week later, she had further progressive decline. She lost her ability to communicate and was no longer eating by mouth. On neurologic exam, she was awake though not speaking or following commands. Motor examination was notable for hypotonia with preserved strength in all extremities. Repeat MRI of the brain showed further extension of symmetric T2-bright signal abnormalities throughout the bilateral basal ganglia, brainstem, cerebellar hemispheres, subcortical white matter, and cortex (Fig. 21.2). Many of these lesions showed contrast enhancement. Magnetic resonance spectroscopy (MRS) showed elevated lactate doublets.

R.L. Holt, M.D.
Department of Neurology, Lucile Packard Children's Hospital at Stanford,
730 Welch Road, Palo Alto, CA 94304-1503, USA
e-mail: rkozitza@stanford.edu

K. Van Haren, M.D. (✉)
Department of Neurology, Lucile Packard Children's Hospital and Stanford University School of Medicine, 750 Welch Road, Suite 317, Palo Alto, CA 94304, USA
e-mail: kpv@stanford.edu

© Springer International Publishing AG 2017
E. Waubant, T.E. Lotze (eds.), *Pediatric Demyelinating Diseases of the Central Nervous System and Their Mimics*, DOI 10.1007/978-3-319-61407-6_21

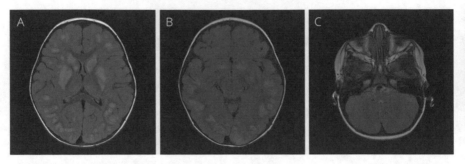

**Fig. 21.1** The initial brain magnetic resonance imaging (MRI) from a 16-month-old girl with thiamine transporter deficiency due to pathogenic mutations in SLCA19A3 reveals scattered, symmetric abnormalities of subcortical gray and white matter in a pattern that may be mistaken for more common disorders such as ADEM. Axial FLAIR sequences reveal T2 hyperintensity that is most prominent in the bilateral caudate and putamen (**a**). Numerous scattered but somewhat symmetric T2 signal abnormalities are also apparent at the medial thalami and subcortical gray-white junction in the frontal, temporal, and parietal lobes (**b**)

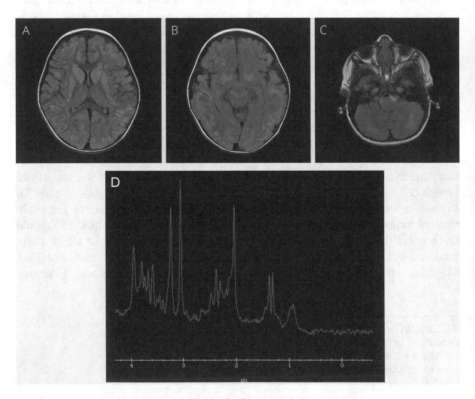

**Fig. 21.2** Three weeks later, relapse of neurological symptoms was associated with extension of previous lesions (**a**) with scattered enhancement (not shown) as well as new involvement of the cerebellum and midbrain (**b**, **c**). MR spectroscopy during the same study revealed a lactate doublet at 1.2 parts per million (**d**)

Metabolic laboratories were notable for elevated serum lactate. She was discharged home with a suspected diagnosis of Leigh syndrome.

The child regained some motor skills after her initial presentation; however, she remained nonverbal without attempts to communicate. Four months later, she returned with an upper respiratory infection accompanied by a second episode of developmental regression. Neurologic examination at that time was notable for dystonia in all extremities and significant limb ataxia bilaterally. Additional work-up during that presentation included whole-exome sequencing which showed a homozygous pathogenic mutation in SLC19A3 consistent with thiamine transporter-2 deficiency. Her parents were found to be heterozygous carriers of the same mutation. She was started on high-dose thiamine and biotin supplementation at the time of diagnosis. Six months later, she had made subtle developmental progress. She was taking steps with support and using her hands to reach for objects, though she was still nonverbal.

## Clinical Questions

1. What are the clinical features of thiamine transporter-2 deficiency?
2. What ancillary studies can be used to diagnose thiamine transporter-2 deficiency?
3. What other neurologic diseases can mimic thiamine transporter-2 deficiency?
4. What are the available treatment options?
5. What is known about the prognosis of thiamine transporter-2 deficiency?

## Diagnostic Discussion

### *What Are the Clinical Features of Thiamine Transporter-2 Deficiency?*

Thiamine transporter-2 (ThTR2) deficiency is a rare autosomal recessive disorder with childhood onset that results from mutations in the *SLC19A3* gene. This gene encodes a thiamine transporter that is highly expressed in the thalamus [1]. The disorder can affect children from all ethnic backgrounds but is most prevalent in Saudi Arabia [2]. The majority of reports describing patients with ThTR2 deficiency describe symptomatic presentation before the age of 12 years with a mean age of onset of 3.5 years and range from 1 month to 20 years [3]. Three clinical variants have been described in relation to the defect: biotin-responsive basal ganglia disease, Wernicke-like encephalopathy, and atypical infantile spasms with progressive cerebral atrophy and basal ganglia lesions [4]. The most commonly reported clinical features at onset include acute and recurrent episodes of encephalopathy, dystonia, and seizures [3]. Other symptoms frequently seen at onset include dystonia, dysarthria, dysphagia, ophthalmoplegia, and ataxia. Symptoms can progress to quadriparesis, coma, and eventually death if left untreated. Early diagnosis and administration of thiamine and biotin can reverse and prevent the progression of symptoms.

## What Ancillary Studies Can Be Used to Diagnose Thiamine Transporter-2 Deficiency?

Laboratory studies are frequently normal in older children with ThTR2 deficiency. In infants and very young children, elevated serum and CSF lactate and high excretion of urine organic acids have been reported during acute metabolic decompensations [3, 4]. The characteristic MRI pattern in ThTR2 deficiency shows bilateral, symmetric T2-bright changes in the caudate, putamen, and medial thalamic nuclei [3]. There may also be symmetric lesions in the cortex or periaqueductal gray matter. MRS may show lactate peaks in ThTR2 deficiency. A characteristic MRI pattern of injury to the dorsal striatum and medial thalamus, in association with elevated lactate and high excretion of urine organic acids in infants, suggests a diagnosis of ThTR2 deficiency. Brain pathology in a small number of patients has shown profound loss of neurons, astrogliosis, and vascular prominence, comparable to what is observed in Leigh syndrome. Whole-exome sequencing is useful in distinguishing ThTR2 deficiency from other inborn errors of metabolism with similar radiographic appearances [5]. The diagnosis can be confirmed with sequencing of the *SLC19A3* gene, though confirmatory diagnosis should not delay treatment.

## What Other Neurologic Diseases Can Mimic Thiamine Transporter-2 Deficiency?

Early in the course of disease, ThTR2 deficiency can mimic several neurologic conditions that also present with encephalopathy. In ThTR2 deficiency, recurrent episodes of encephalopathy are sometimes triggered by acute illnesses, vaccination, or trauma [4]. Similarly, episodes of acute encephalopathy often follow viral illnesses in ADEM, a much more common childhood neurologic condition. In ADEM, laboratory and cerebrospinal fluid studies may show evidence of inflammation, though these studies can also be normal. Lactate and urine organic acids are normal in ADEM. Magnetic resonance imaging lesions in ADEM are often bilateral, though not typically symmetric as seen in inborn errors of metabolism, such as ThTR2 deficiency. In ADEM, lesions are usually concentrated in deep and subcortical white matter though they can affect the basal ganglia and thalami.

   Mitochondrial DNA (mtDNA)-associated Leigh syndrome is another mimic that has both similar clinical and radiological features. Unlike ThTR2 deficiency, neurologic deficits in mtDNA-associated Leigh syndrome are irreversible. Children with mitochondrial disorders often have elevated serum and CSF lactate similar to ThTR2 deficiency. Magnetic resonance imaging in mtDNA-associated Leigh syndrome can be similar in appearance to ThTR2 deficiency with bilateral, symmetric involvement of the basal ganglia and thalami. In ThTR2 deficiency, lesions may be more concentrated in the dorsal striatum and medial thalamus [3]. MRS can show lactate peaks in patients with a variety of disorders, including ThTR2 deficiency as well as mtDNA-associated Leigh syndrome. Given the similarities between these disorders and the relative safety of the intervention, an empiric trial of high-dose thiamine and biotin should be considered in any patient with a subacute encephalopathy and MRI abnormalities that include prominent bilateral T2 lesions of the caudate and putamen, particularly if elevated lactate levels are confirmed in the blood or brain during the acute event. Although this might include incidental treatment of patients with similar appearing disorders (e.g., Leigh syndrome, maple syrup urine disease, glutaric acidemia, Wilson disease), the subsequent diagnostic work-up should include genetic testing to determine the presence or absence of ThTR2-associated mutations, thereby clarifying the need for continued biotin and thiamine supplementation.

## What Are the Available Treatment Options?

Several reports suggest that high-dose biotin and thiamine supplements may improve neurologic recovery among patients with ThTR2 deficiency. Outcomes are better with dual therapy [2, 6]. Currently there is no standardized dosing regimen, with the documented doses of thiamine and biotin ranging from 100 to 900 mg per day and from 2 to 12 mg/kg per day, respectively [3]. Treatment should be initiated as early in the disease course as possible and continued lifelong [3]. Higher doses may be required when potential triggers such as illness or trauma are present.

## What Is Known About the Prognosis of Thiamine Transporter-2 Deficiency?

Although prospective data are somewhat limited, the available evidence suggests that biotin and thiamine supplements should be started (and continued) as early as possible.. Patients treated within the first days of encephalopathy can show complete or near complete resolution of symptoms within days [2, 3]. Late treatment has been associated with profound cognitive impairment, quadriparesis, and refractory epilepsy. Patients who do not receive treatment demonstrate continued deterioration and early death [2, 6].

## Clinical Pearls

1. Thiamine transporter-2 deficiency typically presents in childhood with acute and recurrent episodes of encephalopathy often triggered by illness or trauma. Commonly associated symptoms include dystonia and seizures.
2. Magnetic resonance imaging shows bilateral, symmetric T2-bright changes in the caudate, putamen, and medial thalamus. Elevated serum and CSF lactate and high excretion of urine organic acids may be seen in very young children.
3. A diagnosis of ThTR2 deficiency should be considered in any patient presenting with acute encephalopathy or dystonia, and empiric treatment with high-dose thiamine and biotin should be considered. Early treatment with high-dose thiamine and biotin may reverse symptoms and prevent progression of disease. Untreated, children typically demonstrate continued deterioration and early death.
4. Whole-exome sequencing is useful in distinguishing ThTR2 deficiency from other metabolic disorders with similar clinical and radiographic appearances and should be considered in the diagnostic work-up of any patient with a suspected inborn error of metabolism.

## References

1. Kono S, Miyajima H, et al. Mutations in a thiamine-transporter gene and Wernicke's-like encephalopathy. N Engl J Med. 2009;260(17):1792–4.
2. Tabarki B, Al-Shafi S, et al. Biotin-responsive basal ganglia disease revisited: clinical, radiologic, and genetic findings. Neurology. 2013;80(3):261–7.
3. Ortigoza-Escobar JD, Serrano M, et al. Thiamine transporter-2 deficiency: outcome and treatment monitoring. Orphanet J Rare Dis. 2014;9:92.
4. Perez-Duenas B, Serrano M, et al. Reversible lactic acidosis in a newborn with thiamine transporter-2 deficiency. Pediatrics. 2013;131(5):e1670–5.
5. Kevelam SH, Bugiani M, et al. Exome sequencing reveals mutated SLC19A3 in patients with an early-infantile, lethal encephalopathy. Brain. 2013;136(5):1534–43.
6. Majid A, Makki A, et al. Biotin-responsive basal ganglia disease should be renamed biotin-thiamine-responsive basal ganglia disease: a retrospective review of the clinical, radiological and molecular findings of 18 new cases. Orphanet J Rare Dis. 2013;8:83.

# Part II
# Diseases That Affect the Brainstem

# Chapter 22
# Acute Disseminated Encephalomyelitis: Brainstem and Cerebellar Presentation

Gulay Alper

## Case Presentation

A 10-year-old boy developed fever, mouth sores, and vomiting with decreased oral intake over a 1-week period. He was diagnosed with herpetic gingivostomatitis and admitted for treatment with IV fluids, acyclovir, and pain medications. During the first days of his hospitalization, he developed right-sided facial numbness, double vision, and ataxia requiring neurological consultation.

His neurological examination was remarkable for bilateral dysmetria (left worse than right) and gait ataxia to the extent that he was not able to stand or walk without support. He reported diminished light touch sensation on both sides of his face. Although the patient described intermittent horizontal diplopia, his ocular movements appeared full on examination. His mental status examination was normal.

A gadolinium-enhanced brain MRI was performed and showed T2 hyperintense lesions involving bilateral middle cerebellar peduncles, the pons, and the medulla with extension down into the cervical cord ending at the level of C2. In addition, there was involvement of bilateral anterior basal ganglia and the hypothalamic region (Fig. 22.1). None of the foci demonstrated enhancement or restricted diffusion. The spine MRI demonstrated abnormal increased T2 signal in the central aspect of the cord at the C2 level which seemed to be a continuation of brainstem lesion. In addition there was also a subtle area of increased T2 signal seen at the T7–T9 level. No areas of abnormal enhancement were seen in these regions. CSF showed a white cell count of 2, glucose of 97 mg/dL, and protein of 13 mg/dL. The IgG index was elevated at 0.85 (normal < 0.7), but there were no oligoclonal bands. CSF cultures were negative, as were PCRs for HSV, EBV, *Enterovirus*, HHV6, and HHV7.

G. Alper, M.D. (✉)
Division of Child Neurology, Department of Pediatrics, Children's Hospital of Pittsburgh,
University of Pittsburgh School of Medicine, 4401 Penn Avenue, Pittsburgh, PA 15224, USA
e-mail: Gulay.Alper@chp.edu

© Springer International Publishing AG 2017                                                     173
E. Waubant, T.E. Lotze (eds.), *Pediatric Demyelinating Diseases of the Central
Nervous System and Their Mimics*, DOI 10.1007/978-3-319-61407-6_22

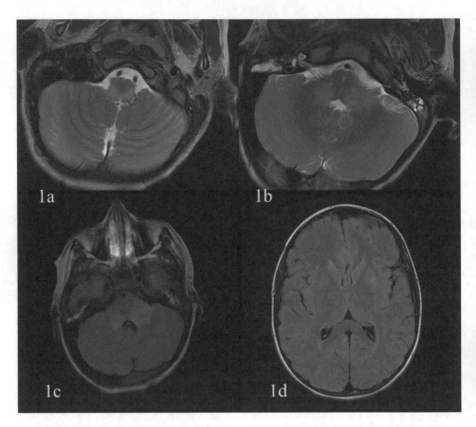

**Fig. 22.1** (**a**) T2-weighted image showing abnormal signal which is seen in the medulla dorsally bilaterally. (**b**) There is also involvement of the brainstem tegmentum involving the rostral pons on the left side and the bilateral inferior pons. (**c**) The imaging demonstrates abnormal T2 FLAIR hyperintensity which is seen in the bilateral middle cerebellar peduncles left greater than right. (**d**) There is also abnormal signal which is seen in the area of the anterior left basal ganglia

Additional studies included negative serum and CSF aquaporin-4 IgG antibody, negative ANA, and other rheumatological markers. Serum lactate pyruvate and angiotensin-converting enzyme were normal. Infectious work-up for Lyme disease, *Bartonella henselae*, *West Nile virus*, Coxsackie A 16, *Listeria monocytogenes*, influenza A and B viruses, and adenovirus was negative. HSV1 IgM was elevated in the serum consistent with his diagnosis of herpetic gingivostomatitis.

After review of the MRI, ADEM was suspected, and he was treated with methylprednisolone 30 mg/kg/dose IV for 5 days. His examination improved steadily each day, so that by the end of his IV steroid course, he had only minimal left-sided dysmetria. He was discharged on an oral prednisone taper over 6 weeks. Three months after discharge, a repeat brain MRI showed complete resolution of the lesions and no new lesions. His neurological examination at that time was normal.

## Clinical Questions

1. What are common brainstem syndromes associated with demyelinating disease?
2. Aside from acquired demyelinating syndromes, what are other differential diagnostic considerations of acute ataxia in childhood?
3. Why is ADEM the most likely acquired demyelinating syndrome diagnosis for this patient?

## Diagnostic Discussion

1. Combinations of symptoms including diplopia, facial numbness, ataxia, and dysmetria localize the problem to the brainstem, to the cerebellum, or to the pathways connecting the brainstem and cerebellum such as the cerebellar peduncles. Numerous studies have reported that the MRI of patients with ADEM, MS, and NMO can show cerebrum, brainstem, cerebellum, and spinal cord lesions. Brainstem lesions on MRI have been reported in 37.5–65.0% of patients with ADEM, 23.0–44.8% of patients with NMO, and 29.0–58.0% of patients with MS [1]. Some brainstem syndromes have been associated with specific diseases such as internuclear ophthalmoplegia (INO) with MS and hiccups and persistent emesis with NMO.

   Few studies have focused on imaging characteristics that might distinguish ADEM, MS, and NMO brainstem lesions on MRI, especially in pediatric patients. One adult study found that lesion size in patients with MS was typically smaller than that in patients with ADEM (1). Patients with NMO had a significantly higher frequency of medulla oblongata lesions than did patients with ADEM. On axial sections of brain MRI, the majority of patients with ADEM showed lesions in the ventral aspect of the brainstem, while the lesions in NMO were typically located in the dorsal aspect of the brainstem. Lesions in patients with MS were found in both the ventral and dorsal aspects. Lesions in patients with ADEM and NMO had poorly defined margins, contrary to the lesions in patients with MS which showed well-defined margins. Furthermore, brainstem lesions in patients with ADEM were usually bilateral, while lesions in patients with NMO and MS were usually unilateral.

   Neuromyelitis optica (NMO) is a CNS inflammatory demyelinating autoimmune disease characterized by relapsing attacks that target the optic nerves and spinal cord, as well as aquaporin-4 (AQP4)-enriched periventricular brain regions [2]. Aquaporin-4 IgG is a specific autoantibody marker for NMOSDs. It binds selectively to aquaporin-4 (AQP4). Brainstem involvement, especially in the medulla oblongata, has been reported in neuromyelitis optica spectrum disorders (NMOSDs). The distribution of NMO-characteristic brainstem lesions corresponds to sites of high aquaporin-4 protein expression [2]. Current studies have demonstrated pathological abnormalities in the caudal medulla at the floor of the fourth ventricle, and the area postrema [3]. Area postrema is one of the brain regions of high AQP4 expression, and it is the most frequently involved area in NMOSDs [3]. This frequency corresponds to clinical episodes of intractable nausea/vomiting and hiccups. Neuropathologic findings suggest the area postrema, the emetic reflex center, may be a selective target of the disease process in NMO. These symptoms may accompany or precede NMO relapses [3].

Disturbance of brainstem function is frequently found in patients with MS and may be the presenting symptoms. While diplopia, ataxia, and vertigo are relatively frequent initial manifestations of the disease, hearing loss, facial paralysis, and trigeminal neuralgia are uncommon [4]. Eye movement abnormalities in MS are often the result of damage to the interconnections between the brainstem neural integrators and the gaze-holding centers of the cerebellar tonsils and demyelination and conduction slowing along these pathways, which is common in MS, sufficiently disrupts their normal function, and leads to abnormal, spontaneous firing patterns [5]. Detailed neuro-ophthalmic examination of patients with MS with visual complaints often yields a diagnosis with highly specific neuroanatomic localization. A focal injury of the brainstem commonly involves one or more cranial nuclei and corticospinal and/or the spinothalamic pathways. Internuclear ophthalmoplegia (INO) is a distinctive ocular motor disorder resulting from dysfunction of the medial longitudinal fasciculus, which lies in the pontine tegmentum. INO is one of the most localizing brainstem syndromes in patients with MS and has been observed in 17% and 41% of the patients [6]. INO is characterized by adduction slowing with and without eye movement limitation and abduction nystagmus in the fellow eye during the horizontal saccades. This characteristic abnormality is related to a lesion in the medial longitudinal fasciculus (MLF) in the pontine or midbrain tegmentum which is most commonly caused by MS. The MLF is highly myelinated to support the rapid neural transmission necessary for abduction of one eye and adduction of the fellow eye to be nearly synchronous. Many patients have been shown to have lesions on T2-weighted images, but not all of the patients have characteristic lesions. Frohman et al. studied the medial longitudinal fasciculus (MLF) in 58 patients with MS and chronic internuclear ophthalmoparesis. All patients studied had evidence of an MLF lesion hyperintensity on proton density imaging (PDI), whereas T2-weighted imaging and FLAIR imaging showed these lesions in 88% and 48% of patients, respectively. With PDI, dorsomedial tegmentum lesions were seen in the pons in 93% of patients and in the midbrain of 66% of patients. This suggests that proton density imaging best shows the MLF lesions with MS and INO [6].

Less common brainstem syndromes include trigeminal neuralgia, which is present in no more than 1% of MS cases at onset. Intrapontine "peripheral" facial palsy may represent up to 4% of the cases. Few cases of MS starting with hemifacial spasm have been reported [4]. Sensorineural deafness is considered rare in MS. Vestibulocerebellar symptoms and signs such as vertigo, ataxia, and dizziness can be seen in 15% of the patients.

The clinical manifestations, locations of brainstem lesions, morphological features, and recognition of specific syndromes might be helpful in the diagnosis and management strategies of acquired demyelinating disorders.

2. In addition to ADEM, acute cerebellar ataxia (also known as postinfectious cerebellar ataxia) commonly presents following a viral illness. Postinfectious acute cerebellar ataxia represents a benign condition that is characterized by acute truncal and gait ataxia, variably with appendicular ataxia, nystagmus, dysarthria, and hypotonia. It occurs mostly in young children, presents abruptly, and recovers over weeks. Neuroimaging is normal. Cerebrospinal fluid examination often shows a lymphocytic pleocytosis. In contrast, the term "acute cerebellitis" is generally used selectively for more severe cases, specifically with abnormal neuroimaging, and it has a less favorable long-term prognosis. Severe cases of acute cerebellitis may additionally have altered consciousness secondary to cerebellar swelling resulting in raised intracranial pressure, hydrocephalus, and even herniation. Neuroimaging is abnormal with findings of diffuse cerebellar edema and extension of the cerebellar tonsils through the foramen magnum in the setting of herniation. In a few cases, an infectious agent has been isolated from the cerebrospinal fluid suggesting a direct infectious etiology [7].

ADEM may be confused with acute cerebellitis when the clinical findings are predominantly cerebellar, but lesions on neuroimaging are more widespread and not confined to the cerebellum.

There are infectious agents with known predilection to brainstem and/or cerebellum. Viral encephalitides specifically enterovirus serotypes 68 and 71 are known to cause lesions of the brainstem, dorsal tegmentum, and cerebellum. EV71 mostly affects children, manifesting as hand, foot, and mouth disease, aseptic meningitis, brainstem encephalitis, and poliomyelitis-like acute flaccid paralysis [8]. *Listeria monocytogenes* causes rhombencephalitis involving both the brainstem and cerebellum. Bickerstaff brainstem encephalitis is ill-defined inflammatory disease of unknown origin. Most of its pathological, clinical, and analytical characteristics are similar to those observed in Miller Fisher syndrome. This spectrum includes ataxia, ocular paresis, and impaired reflexes. Infectious brainstem encephalitis is unlikely on the basis of CSF findings, negative PCRs, bacterial cultures, and viral serology studies. Furthermore the patient responded to the steroid treatment which does not support the infectious etiology.

In general, a metabolic disorder is less likely because this patient presented acutely. There was no pre-existing developmental delay or other neurological problems to suggest gradually progressing course. Some metabolic disorders may present acutely, but lesion characteristics are different than those seen in this patient. Mitochondrial disorders such as Leigh's disease typically involve brainstem structures with a highly symmetric pattern and frequently associated with restricted diffusion reflecting cytotoxic injury. CNS involvement of connective tissue disorders and other vasculitides (systemic lupus erythematosus, neuro-Behcet disease, neurosarcoidosis, primary CNS vasculitis) is not the likely diagnoses due to complete resolution of lesions and no further relapsing course. Clinical and radiological characteristics were not consistent with central pontine myelinolysis, ischemic lesions, neoplasm, or genetic disorders such as Alexander disease.

Opsoclonus myoclonus ataxia syndrome in young children most often is a paraneoplastic, immune-mediated encephalopathy associated with an occult neural crest cell tumor. Brain MRI is normal without any findings to suggest brainstem or cerebellar inflammation. As seen in other immune-mediated disorders, OMS may also present following a viral infection, in the absence of a tumor.

3. The clinical presentation of multiple cranial nerve deficits and ataxia is consistent with a brainstem and cerebellar syndrome. Asymptomatic lesions were present supratentorially and in the spinal cord. Wide spread lesions support the diagnosis of ADEM, which is the most common acquired demyelinating syndrome in this age group.

Among the acquired demyelinating syndromes, NMO is unlikely because the NMO aquaporin-4 antibody was negative and lesion distribution was not typical for NMO.

The differential diagnosis of ADEM is most challenging when it comes to distinguishing from the first attack of MS especially in young children. This could be the first presenting episode of MS, defined as CIS, although a monophasic course with a full recovery, complete resolution of lesions, and no new lesions with serial MRIs favor an ADEM diagnosis in this child.

One can argue that this child did not have encephalopathy; therefore this case would not meet consensus criteria for ADEM. Encephalopathy was proposed to be a required criterion for acute disseminated encephalomyelitis [9]. Children with polyfocal onset but no encephalopathy are usually categorized as a clinically isolated syndrome (CIS) to better identify those children at higher risk for multiple sclerosis. However some studies have shown that a substantial number of patients with *polyfocal onset demyelination without encephalopathy* remained monophasic for longer than 2 years [10, 11]. Therefore, the presented case could represent an atypical variant of ADEM without encephalopathy. Alternatively, these patients could be considered as having a clinically isolated syndrome at onset, implying a possible future risk of multiple sclerosis, but they should not be categorized as CIS indefinitely. ADEM is the most likely diagnosis in children, such as the one described here, who present with widespread polyfocal demyelination and remain monophasic for several years, although confirmation of ADEM is retrospective and requires prolonged observation.

Long-term outcome studies are needed in children who clinically present only with brainstem and cerebellar symptoms without encephalopathy, and the pathogenesis of encephalopathy in ADEM needs to be better understood. Furthermore, a marker more specific than encephalopathy is needed to allow for a more reliable method of distinction between acute disseminated encephalomyelitis and the first attack of multiple sclerosis in children.

## Clinical Pearls

1. Neuroimaging plays a key role in the diagnosis of ADEM because there is no biomarker available. ADEM can present predominantly with brainstem and cerebellar lesions. ADEM should be considered in all cases of unexplained encephalitis.
2. ADEM is a treatable disease, but delay in treatment may cause complications such as axonal loss and further progression of disease, which can be catastrophic, particularly if lesions involve crucial locations such as the brainstem. Once ADEM is diagnosed, the therapeutic aim is to abbreviate the CNS inflammatory reaction as quickly as possible and to speed up clinical recovery.

## References

1. Lu Z, Zhang B, Qiu W, et al. Comparative brainstem lesions on MRI of acute disseminated encephalomyelitis, neuromyelitis optica, and multiple sclerosis. PLoS One. 2011;8:e22766.
2. Pittock SJ, Weinshenker BG, Luchinetti CF, et al. Neuromyelitis optica brain lesions localized at sites of high aquaporin 4 expression. Arch Neurol. 2006;63:964–8.
3. Popescu BF, Lennon VA, Parisi JE, et al. Neuromyelitis optica unique area postrema lesions: nausea, vomiting, and pathogenic implications. Neurology. 2011;76:1229–37.
4. Zaffaroni M, Baldini SM, Ghezzi A. Cranial nerve, brainstem and cerebellar syndromes in the differential diagnosis of multiple sclerosis. Neurol Sci. 2001;22:S74–8.
5. Prasad S, Galetta SL. Eye movement abnormalities in multiple sclerosis. Neurol Clin. 2010;28:641–55.
6. Frohman EM, Zhang H, Kramer PD, et al. MRI characteristics of the MLF in MS patients with chronic internuclear ophthalmoparesis. Neurology. 2001;57:762–8.
7. Desai J, Mitchell WG. Acute cerebellar ataxia, acute cerebellitis, and opsoclonus-myoclonus syndrome. J Child Neurol. 2012;27:1482–8.
8. Ooi MH, Wong SC, Lewthwaite P, et al. Clinical features, diagnosis, and management of enterovirus 71. Lancet Neurol. 2010;9:1097–105.
9. Krupp LB, Tardieu M, Amato MP, et al. for the International Pediatric Multiple Sclerosis Study Group. International Pediatric Multiple Sclerosis Study Group criteria for pediatric multiple sclerosis and immune-mediated central nervous system demyelinating disorders: revisions to the 2007 definitions.
10. Dale RC, Pillai SC. Early relapse risk after a first CNS inflammatory demyelination episode: examining international consensus definitions. Dev Med Child Neurol. 2007;49:887–93.
11. Neuteboom RF, Boon M, Catsman Berrevoets CE, et al. Prognostic factors after a first attack of inflammatory CNS demyelination in children. Neurology. 2008;71:967–73.

# Chapter 23
# Multiple Sclerosis with Brainstem Presentation

William Hong, Carla Francisco, and Timothy E. Lotze

## Case Presentation #1

A 14-year-old girl without prior history of neurological problems or recent illness presented with a 2-week history of double vision, vertigo, tinnitus, sensory changes in her left hand, and difficulty walking. She had additional constitutional symptoms of photophobia, nausea, and vomiting.

Her general examination was normal. On neurological exam, she had normal mental status. There was decreased sensation in the lower part of her left face and left arm. She had internuclear ophthalmoplegia with impaired adduction in her left eye in right lateral gaze and normal abduction of her right eye with horizontal nystagmus. She had left-sided dysmetria and an ataxic gait, tending to fall toward the left side. On ophthalmic exam, she complained of pain with extraocular movements but showed normal visual acuity, visual fields, and normal optic disks.

MRI of the brain showed numerous T2 hyperintense lesions to include the dorsal aspect of the pons and middle cerebellar peduncles with gadolinium enhancement in a lesion affecting the right and left middle cerebellar peduncles. There was a hyperintense T2 lesion in the region of the left medial longitudinal fasciculus (Fig. 23.1). Additional lesions were noted in the frontal subcortical white matter and

W. Hong, M.D., M.S.E. • T.E. Lotze, M.D. (✉)
Division of Neurology and Developmental Neuroscience, Department of Pediatrics, Baylor College of Medicine, Houston, TX, USA
e-mail: William.Hong@bcm.edu; WH3@bcm.edu; tlotze@bcm.edu

C. Francisco, M.D.
Multiple Sclerosis and Neuroinflammation Center, University of California, San Francisco, San Francisco, CA, USA
e-mail: Carla.Francisco@ucsf.edu

© Springer International Publishing AG 2017
E. Waubant, T.E. Lotze (eds.), *Pediatric Demyelinating Diseases of the Central Nervous System and Their Mimics*, DOI 10.1007/978-3-319-61407-6_23

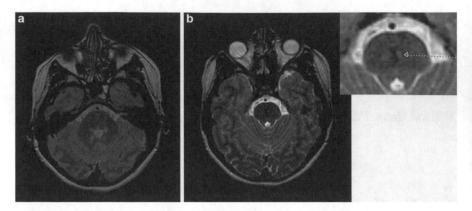

**Fig. 23.1** MRI of the brain. MRI of the brain demonstrating bilateral T2 hyperintense lesions in the pontine tegmentum and middle cerebellar peduncles (**a**) with a discrete punctate hyperintense T2 lesion in the region of the left medial longitudinal fasciculus, magnified in inset (**b**)

corpus callosum. MRI of the spine showed T2 hyperintense lesions in the cervical cord that did not enhance. CSF studies noted 1 WBC, normal protein (43 mg/dL), and normal glucose (52 mg/dL) but were significant for greater than two oligoclonal bands on isoelectric focusing and an elevated IgG index. Opening pressure was within normal limits and cytology was negative for malignancy.

The history and findings were concerning for multiple sclerosis, but she did not meet the 2010 McDonald diagnostic criteria for separation in time, as she was symptomatic from the only enhancing lesions identified on the MRI in the cerebellar peduncles and did not have any asymptomatic enhancing lesions. She was treated with methylprednisolone 1000 mg IV daily for 5 days followed by a 2-week oral prednisone taper. She had complete resolution of almost all of her symptoms over the course of the subsequent month but remained with right sensorineural hearing loss, for which she was fitted with a hearing aid. A second MRI brain performed 2 months after this initial event demonstrated the accrual of a new hyperintense T2 periventricular lesion, confirming a diagnosis of multiple sclerosis.

She initiated disease-modifying drug therapy with glatiramer acetate but did not tolerate treatment after 6 months due to side effects and injection-related anxiety. She was changed to dimethyl fumarate but did not tolerate side effects of facial flushing despite slow titration of the dose and addition of aspirin. She was subsequently switched to fingolimod, and she remained on this treatment without side effects and no clinical relapse or new MRI lesions for the subsequent 12 months.

## Case Presentation #2

A 15-year-old right-handed previously healthy African American female presented with 7 days of generalized headache and double vision. An optometrist initially noted impaired horizontal eye movements and nearly normal visual acuity of 20/30 in both eyes. With the subsequent development of slurred speech and difficulty walking the following day, she was brought to the emergency room. Upon presentation, mother also noted that she was having difficulty hearing. Her initial examination noted inability to abduct or adduct both eyes, ptosis of right eye, flattening of her right nasolabial fold, and substantially decreased hearing to finger rub bilaterally. Strength and sensation were intact. She had dysmetria noted on the right compared to left as well as a wide-based gait.

MRI brain with and without contrast noted >20 T2 hyperintense areas in the deep white matter, including the corpus callosum and posterior fossa; some of these lesions were asymptomatic. There were multiple enhancing and nonenhancing lesions, including a number involving the dorsal pons in the region of the medial longitudinal fasciculus. Given her clinical event and dissemination in space and time on the initial MRI, she was diagnosed with multiple sclerosis. Cerebrospinal fluid (CSF) analysis demonstrated 11 white blood cells that were predominantly lymphocytic, 1 red blood cell, normal glucose (64 mg/dL), and normal protein (17 mg/dL). IgG index was elevated (0.9), and there were 5 oligoclonal bands present in the CSF that were not present in the serum.

She received methylprednisolone 30 mg/kg/day IV for 5 days with minimal improvement in abduction/adduction of her eyes and persistent ataxia. EDSS was 4.0. She then underwent five rounds of plasmapheresis with moderate improvement in ataxia and horizontal eye movements. She was placed on natalizumab as an outpatient. Ten months after the initial event, her EDSS had improved to 2.0, and repeat brain MRI scan after four infusions of natalizumab showed five new, nonenhancing lesions compared to previous MRI.

## Clinical Questions

1. What are the most common features of brainstem or cerebellum syndromes in MS?
2. What is the differential diagnosis of acute brainstem or cerebellum syndromes in children?
3. Does brainstem demyelinating disease affect disability prognosis in MS?

## Clinical Discussion

### What Are the Most Common Features of Brainstem or Cerebellum Syndromes in MS?

Various brainstem symptoms have been identified to occur in 10% of patients with MS. Due to the close anatomical and functional interaction between the brainstem and the cerebellum, symptoms are often discussed as a brainstem and/or cerebellum syndrome.

Symptoms related to brainstem involvement typically seen in MS include *bilateral* internuclear ophthalmoplegia, sixth nerve palsy, and facial numbness. Ataxia, vertigo, and multidirectional nystagmus may be signs of isolated or additional cerebellum involvement. Those that occur less commonly are *unilateral* internuclear ophthalmoplegia, facial palsy, or facial myokymia, deafness, one-and-a-half syndrome, trigeminal neuralgia, and paroxysmal tonic spasms. In one adult prospective study, diplopia was the most common presentation (68%), followed by facial sensory symptoms (32%), unstable gait (30.7%), and vertigo (18.7%). In the pediatric population, patients with multiple sclerosis typically have a polysymptomatic presentation and frequent complaints with coordination (37%).

The patient described in the vignette had unilateral internuclear ophthalmoplegia. This condition can be attributed to a demyelinating lesion in the medial longitudinal fasciculus disrupting ascending fibers between the contralateral paramedian pontine reticular formation abducens nucleus complex and the ipsilateral oculomotor nucleus.

The patient also experienced tinnitus with residual high-frequency sensorineural hearing loss. While not common in multiple sclerosis, tinnitus and hearing loss are reported in approximately 9% of MS patients and are related to demyelinating lesions in the auditory pathways. As hearing loss is uncommon in MS, alternative causes should be investigated, especially if this symptom is isolated.

### What Is the Differential Diagnosis of Acute Brainstem or Cerebellum Syndromes in Children?

The diagnosis of multiple sclerosis requires elimination of other likely diagnosis. Evaluation should begin with thorough history and neurologic examination. Symptoms that are not typically associated with multiple sclerosis and thus suggestive of other causes include complete ophthalmoplegia, vertical gaze palsies, vascular territory syndrome, isolated third nerve palsy, progressive trigeminal sensory neuropathy, focal dystonia, and torticollis.

There is a wide range of etiologies that mimic brainstem/cerebellum syndromes seen in multiple sclerosis (Table 23.1). Brain tumors, the second most common oncologic process in the pediatric population, mostly occur in the infratentorial area. These present with more insidious progression of brainstem and/or cerebellar

**Table 23.1** Differential diagnosis for brainstem and cerebellum syndromes in multiple sclerosis

| *Oncologic* |
| --- |
| Medulloblastoma |
| Pontine glioma |
| Cerebellar astrocytoma |
| *Vascular* |
| Lateral medullary syndrome (posterior inferior cerebellar artery) |
| Lateral pontine syndrome (anterior inferior cerebellar artery) |
| Cavernous angioma |
| *Infectious* |
| Lyme disease, *Borrelia burgdorferi* |
| Syphilis, *Treponema pallidum* |
| Cerebellitis, *Coxiella burnetii* |
| Cerebellitis, viral |
| Cerebellitis, postinfectious |
| *Autoimmune* |
| Sarcoidosis |
| Behcet's |
| *Congenital/metabolic* |
| Mitochondrial disorders |
| Amino acid metabolism disorders |
| Lysosomal storage disorders |
| Ataxia-telangiectasia |
| Friedreich's ataxia |
| *Toxic* |
| Drug ingestion (barbiturates, benzodiazepines, alcohol) |
| Heavy metal poisoning (lead or mercury) |
| Solvent poisoning (paint thinner) |
| *Other demyelinating diseases* |
| Acute disseminated encephalomyelitis |
| Miller fisher syndrome[a] |

[a]Disease of the peripheral nervous system

symptoms. Medulloblastoma, pontine glioma, and cerebellar astrocytoma are notable examples. The lesions can be identified and distinguished with brain MRI.

Vascular events affecting the brainstem present with acute symptoms. Classically, lateral medullary syndrome and lateral pontine syndrome due to stroke in the posterior inferior cerebellar artery and anterior inferior cerebellar artery, respectively, can cause cranial nerve deficits with ataxia. Rarely, vascular lesions such as a cavernous angioma of the brainstem might clinically mimic an acute MS relapse following hemorrhage. Imaging with susceptibility sequences for blood products on MRI should readily distinguish cavernous angioma from a demyelinating plaque.

When patients with brainstem dysfunction also have systemic signs such as fever and meningismus, an infectious process affecting the brainstem should be considered. Tuberculosis produces a basilar meningitis with associated cranial neuropathies and communicating hydrocephalus. Lyme disease can also produce facial nerve palsy and other cranial neuropathies. In addition, many viruses can cause brainstem and cerebellum dysfunction as either brainstem encephalitis, cerebellitis, or postinfectious cerebellitis. Miller Fisher syndrome is an acute inflammatory demyelinating disease characterized by ophthalmoplegia, ataxia, and areflexia linked to a gastrointestinal *Campylobacter jejuni* infection with related anti-GM1 and anti-GQ1b antibodies. Miller Fisher syndrome is a disease of the peripheral nervous system, and CSF findings are similar to these in Guillain-Barré syndrome with a cytoalbuminologic dissociation, helping to distinguish it from a demyelinating disease of the central nervous system.

Other rare autoimmune non-demyelinating diseases such as sarcoidosis, Wegener's granulomatosis, and Behcet's disease are also important differentials. Neuro-sarcoidosis and Wegener's granulomatosis often present with multiple cranial nerve deficits, thus a CSF angiotensin-converting enzyme level or serum antineutrophil cytoplasmic antibody (ANCA) titers, respectively, as well as chest radiography for both conditions are important diagnostic studies. Patients with established neuro-Behcet can occasionally meet McDonald criteria for multiple sclerosis which may challenge differentiating the two autoimmune diseases in some.

Other diseases such as those related to inborn error of metabolism and genetic disorders (mitochondrial or amino acid metabolism disorders) will often present with a comorbid history of developmental delay, altered mental status, and even seizures. Imaging will demonstrate symmetric lesions through the brainstem, in contrast to the asymmetric appearance of acquired inflammatory demyelinating syndromes, such as multiple sclerosis.

Other inflammatory demyelinating diseases than multiple sclerosis should be considered. Acute disseminated encephalomyelitis may be a more likely disease when there is an associated encephalopathy although encephalopathy can accompany first events of multiple sclerosis, especially in those younger than 12. ADEM will more typically demonstrate large poorly circumscribed lesions in the supratentorial white and gray matter. Neuromyelitis optica can also present with brainstem syndromes such as intractable vomiting or hiccoughs related to area postrema involvement. MRI findings of hyperintense T2 lesions in the area postrema and along the ventricular margins, as well as positive aquaporin-4 IgG serology, would distinguish neuromyelitis optica from MS.

## *Does Brainstem Demyelinating Disease Affect Disability Prognosis in MS?*

The involvement of multiple anatomic systems is a negative prognostic factor in relapsing-remitting MS. Brainstem dysfunction at MS onset is associated with higher number of relapses and disability progression in adults with the disease. Onset of multiple sclerosis with initial brainstem symptoms has been associated with increased long-term morbidity. Residual deficits in extraocular movements, hearing, and balance can impair significantly daily activities. Very rarely, sudden unexpected deaths due to cardiac arrhythmia and pulmonary edema due to impaired autonomous respiration have been reported in patients with MS lesions in the medulla.

## Clinical Pearls

1. Brainstem dysfunction including bilateral internuclear ophthalmoplegia, sixth nerve palsy, and facial numbness is one of the most common initial symptoms in patients with pediatric MS.
2. Differential diagnosis of brainstem and cerebellum dysfunction in the pediatric population includes various forms of demyelinating disease that require the application of diagnostic criteria to distinguish. Alternative diseases should be considered when the clinical context and imaging features are not typical of acquired demyelinating conditions.
3. Involvement of the brainstem in MS may indicate higher risk for subsequent disease progression and disability in adults, but this has not been confirmed in children.

## Suggested Reading

1. Confavreux C, Vukusic S, Moreau T, Adeleine P. Relapses and progression of disability in multiple sclerosis. N Engl J Med. 2000;343(20):1430–8.
2. Miller DH, Weinshenker BG, Filippi M, Banwell BL, Cohen JA, Freedman MS, Galetta SL, Hutchinson M, Johnson RT, Kappos L, Kira J, Lublin FD, McFarland HF, Montalban X, Panitch H, Richert JR, Reingold SC, Polman CH. Differential diagnosis of suspected multiple sclerosis: a consensus approach. Mult Scler. 2008;14(9):1157–74.
3. Sastre-Garriga J, Tintoré M. Multiple sclerosis: Lesion location may predict disability in multiple sclerosis. Nat Rev Neurol. 2010;6(12):648–9.
4. Belman AL, Krupp LB, Olsen CS, Rose JW, Aaen G, Benson L, Chitnis T, Gorman M, Graves J, Harris Y, Lotze T, Ness J, Rodriguez M, Tillema JM, Waubant E, Weinstock-Guttman B, Casper TC; US Network of Pediatric MS Centers. Characteristics of children and adolescents with multiple sclerosis. Pediatrics. 2016;138(1).
5. Akman-Demir G, Mutlu M, Kiyat-Atamer A, Shugaiv E, Kurtuncu M, Tugal-Tutkun I, Tuzun E, Eraksoy M, Bahar S. Behçet's disease patients with multiple sclerosis-like features: discriminative value of Barkhof criteria. Clin Exp Rheumatol. 2015;33(6 Suppl 94):S80–4.
6. Degenhardt A, Ramagopalan SV, Scalfari A, Ebers GC. Clinical prognostic factors in multiple sclerosis: a natural history review. Nat Rev Neurol. 2009;5(12):672–82.
7. Tintore M, Rovira A, Arrambide G, Mitjana R, Río J, Auger C, Nos C, Edo MC, Castilló J, Horga A, Perez-Miralles F, Huerga E, Comabella M, Sastre-Garriga J, Montalban X. Brainstem lesions in clinically isolated syndromes. Neurology. 2010;75(21):1933–8.
8. Bramow S, Faber-Rod JC, Jacobsen C, Kutzelnigg A, Patrikios P, Sorensen PS, Lassmann H, Laursen H. Fatal neurogenic pulmonary edema in a patient with progressive multiple sclerosis. Mult Scler. 2008;14(5):711–5.

# Chapter 24
# Neuromyelitis Optica Spectrum Disorder with Brainstem Presentation

Sona Narula and Amy T. Waldman

## Case Presentation

A 15-year-old African American male presented with one week of intractable nausea and vomiting and difficulty swallowing. He was initially evaluated for gastroenteritis as he also reported several days of preceding abdominal pain. Due to his persistent symptoms, he was ultimately evaluated by gastroenterology, and an endoscopy was performed. The study was notable for severe esophagitis, gastritis, and a Mallory-Weiss tear. With his swallowing complaints, a barium swallow was also done and revealed trace silent aspiration with thin liquids. The remainder of his gastroenterology workup was unrevealing. The patient was previously healthy aside from intermittent complaints of dry mouth and dry eye.

During the course of his hospital admission, the patient developed persistent hiccups. He also developed a headache, which prompted further evaluation with brain magnetic resonance imaging (MRI). The MRI revealed an enhancing lesion in the dorsal medulla, near the cervicomedullary junction (Fig. 24.1). The remainder of his brain and spine imaging was unremarkable. Cerebrospinal fluid analysis including cell counts, protein, and glucose was normal. Oligoclonal band testing was negative. As a result of the patient's imaging findings, antibody testing for neuromyelitis optica (anti-aquaporin 4 immunoglobulin G) was sent from serum and cere-

S. Narula, M.D. (✉)
Division of Neurology, The Children's Hospital of Philadelphia, Philadelphia, PA 19104, USA

Departments of Pediatrics and Neurology, Perelman School of Medicine, University of Pennsylvania, Philadelphia, PA, USA
e-mail: narulas@email.chop.edu

A.T. Waldman, M.D., M.S.C.E.
Division of Neurology, The Children's Hospital of Philadelphia, Philadelphia, PA 19104, USA
e-mail: WALDMAN@email.chop.edu

© Springer International Publishing AG 2017
E. Waubant, T.E. Lotze (eds.), *Pediatric Demyelinating Diseases of the Central Nervous System and Their Mimics*, DOI 10.1007/978-3-319-61407-6_24

189

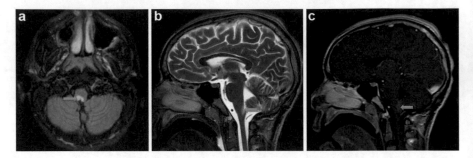

**Fig. 24.1** Isolated lesion in the dorsal medulla in a patient with neuromyelitis optica spectrum disorder presenting with an area postrema clinical syndrome. (**a**) Axial T2-weighted fluid-attenuated inversion recovery (FLAIR) image. (**b**) Sagittal T2-weighted image. (**c**) Sagittal T1-weighted image with gadolinium

brospinal fluid, and both were found to be positive using a cell-binding assay. The patient was diagnosed with neuromyelitis optica spectrum disorder (NMOSD).

Upon review of the patient's MRI and initial cerebrospinal fluid results, he was treated with intravenous corticosteroids and had complete resolution of his gastrointestinal symptoms within days. Upon learning that he was seropositive for the anti-aquaporin 4 immunoglobulin G, he was started on preventative immuno-suppressive therapy with mycophenolate mofetil and was titrated to a dose of 1 g twice daily. He has not had any further demyelinating attacks or accrual of new lesions on MRI since starting treatment 4 years ago.

Additional blood work done at the time of hospitalization was notable for a positive antinuclear antibody (1:640), anti-ribonucleoprotein (RNP) antibody (114, range 0–19 units), and anti-SSA (93, range 0–19 units) and anti-SSB antibodies (55, range 0–19 units). A lip biopsy was subsequently performed and confirmed a diagnosis of Sjogren's syndrome. The patient's Sjogren's symptoms have since been well controlled with mycophenolate mofetil.

## Clinical Questions

1. How do the patient's presenting signs and symptoms relate to his underlying neurologic condition?
2. What additional serologic workup should be done in cases of neuromyelitis optica spectrum disorder?
3. What other etiologies should have been considered at the time of initial presentation?
4. What are the treatments available for pediatric neuromyelitis optica spectrum disorder?
5. What do we know about the anticipated course and prognosis of pediatric neuromyelitis optica spectrum disorder?

# Discussion

1. Neuromyelitis optica spectrum disorder (NMOSD) is a central nervous system inflammatory disorder in which an autoantibody is thought to attack aquaporin 4, a water channel found in astrocytic foot processes in the blood-brain barrier. Though this disorder has been historically identified in patients presenting with repeated relapses affecting the optic nerves and spinal cord, it has recently been noted that patients with NMOSD may develop characteristic brain lesions in regions where aquaporin 4 is highly expressed, such as the hypothalamus and the area postrema, a medullary structure located at the floor of the fourth ventricle. In fact, the 2015 update to the diagnostic criteria for NMOSD [1] now includes area postrema, brainstem, and diencephalic syndromes as core clinical features of the disorder, and allows for the diagnosis of NMOSD in the absence of optic neuritis and myelitis in certain clinical scenarios if one of these syndromes is present and the anti-aquaporin 4 antibody is detected (Table 24.1).

   As the area postrema encompasses the chemoreceptor trigger zone, patients with NMOSD and brain lesions involving the dorsal medulla can present with intractable nausea, vomiting, and hiccups. In fact, one retrospective study reported that intractable vomiting was the first presentation of NMOSD in about 12% of cases [2]. It has also been reported that approximately 40% of cases of NMOSD demonstrate selective loss of aquaporin 4 in the medullary floor of the

**Table 24.1**  Current diagnostic criteria for neuromyelitis optica spectrum disorder (NMOSD) [3]

| |
|---|
| *Diagnostic criteria for NMOSD with anti-aquaporin 4 immunoglobulin seropositivity:* |
| 1.   At least one core clinical characteristic[a] |
| 2.   Detection of the anti-aquaporin 4 immunoglobulin using best available method |
| 3.   Exclusion of alternative diagnoses |
| *Diagnostic criteria for NMOSD without anti-aquaporin 4 immunoglobulin seropositivity or if anti-aquaporin 4 immunoglobulin status is unknown:* |
| 1.   At least two core clinical characteristics[a] occurring as a result of one or more clinical attacks and meeting all of the following requirements:<br>  –  At least one core clinical characteristic must be optic neuritis, acute myelitis with longitudinally extensive transverse myelitis, or an area postrema syndrome<br>  –  Dissemination in space<br>  –  Fulfillment of additional MRI requirements, as applicable |
| 2.   Negative test for anti-aquaporin 4 immunoglobulin using best available detection method, or testing is unavailable |
| 3.   Exclusion of alternative diagnoses |

[a]Core Clinical Characteristics
- Optic neuritis
- Acute myelitis
- Area postrema syndrome: episode of otherwise unexplained hiccups or nausea and vomiting
- Acute brainstem syndrome
- Symptomatic narcolepsy or acute diencephalic clinical syndrome with NMOSD-typical diencephalic MRI lesions
- Symptomatic cerebral syndrome with NMOSD-typical brain lesions

fourth ventricle/area postrema when examined pathologically [3]. Lesions that involve the dorsal medulla in NMOSD patients are often small and bilateral and can be contiguous with lesions in the upper cervical spinal cord [1].

Patients with NMOSD may also present with bulbar symptoms, such as swallowing dysfunction, if brainstem lesions are present. Characteristic brainstem lesions in NMOSD typically involve the periependymal surfaces of the fourth ventricle [1].

2. In a cohort of 75 children who were found to be seropositive for the anti-aquaporin 4 antibody, additional autoantibodies were detected in 76% of patients, and 42% were ultimately diagnosed with at least one comorbid autoimmune disorder such as Sjogren's syndrome, systemic lupus erythematosus, Graves' disease, or juvenile rheumatoid arthritis [4]. Similarly, adults with NMOSD have also been reported to develop associated autoimmune disorders. As a result, it is recommended that patients with NMOSD are screened for autoantibodies, including an antinuclear antibody (ANA) profile, anti-neutrophil cytoplasmic antibody (ANCA), anti-SSA/SSB antibodies, and thyroid studies, especially if they endorse associated symptoms. Children with NMOSD should be followed by a multidisciplinary team that includes neurology, ophthalmology, and rheumatology (if needed).

3. The differential diagnosis for an isolated brainstem lesion in a child is broad and includes infection, inflammation, and neoplasm. If an infectious etiology is suspected based on a history of recent exposure, prodromal symptoms, or examination findings, a lumbar puncture should be done for further evaluation. Brain tumors may be difficult to distinguish from isolated areas of demyelination at the time of initial diagnosis and may require further evaluation with cerebrospinal fluid studies, magnetic resonance spectroscopy, or serial brain MRI. An open-ring pattern of lesion enhancement, characterized by incomplete enhancement typically in the shape of a crescent or open ring, has been historically associated with demyelination, though is not a specific sign, and has also been reported in cases of malignancy and infection. A "cloud-like" enhancement pattern (multiple areas of patchy enhancement with blurred margins with adjacent areas) has also been reported in NMOSD and requires further study [5]. Granulomatous disease, macrophage activation syndromes, mitochondrial disease, and central nervous system vasculitis may also rarely present as isolated brain lesions and should be considered in the differential if the patient's history and clinical scenario are compatible.

Cerebrospinal fluid (CSF) analysis can be helpful when evaluating a case of suspected NMOSD. A pleocytosis has been reported in more than half of children with NMOSD (greater than 50 cells/m$^3$ in some cases), and patients may have either a lymphocytic or neutrophilic predominance [4]. CSF protein levels are also usually elevated in NMOSD. Oligoclonal bands are typically negative but have been reported in up to 5–10% of children with NMOSD [4].

4. As there have been no randomized controlled trials studying optimal treatment of pediatric and adult NMOSD, therapy is based on the results of observational studies in both age groups. First-line treatment of an acute attack typically

involves use of high-dose corticosteroids, such as methylprednisolone 20–30 mg/kg up to 1 g per day for 3–5 days. If the attack is severe or a patient is not improving with high-dose corticosteroids, secondary therapies such as plasma exchange or occasionally intravenous immunoglobulin may also be required. Most children will also require a preventative therapy when their diagnosis of NMOSD is confirmed as attacks in NMOSD can be severe (on occasion lethal) and may result in permanent sequelae and disability.

Medications including rituximab, azathioprine, and mycophenolate mofetil have been used as preventative therapies with success in pediatric NMOSD, with each medication differing slightly with regard to potential side effects and monitoring protocols [6]. Rituximab can be dosed at 750 mg/m$^2$/dose (maximum of 1 g) and administered as two doses 2 weeks apart, or at 375 mg/m$^2$/dose weekly for 4 weeks. As NMOSD patients are at high risk for relapse, they are generally re-dosed with rituximab approximately every 6 months or based on early B-cell (CD19+) repopulation. Adverse events associated with rituximab use in children include infusion-related hypersensitivity reactions, infection, and a reduction in immunoglobulin levels, all of which should be closely monitored [7]. Dosing of azathioprine is based on weight and can range from 1 to 3 mg/kg/day based on tolerability and side effects. Nausea, elevated transaminases, leukopenia, diarrhea, bone marrow suppression, and fatigue have all been reported with azathioprine in NMOSD patients [6]. Thiopurine methyltransferase (TPMT) activity should be measured before starting azathioprine as patients with reduced activity are more susceptible to toxicity and will need closer monitoring. Mycophenolate mofetil dosing is also limited by tolerability in children and is typically titrated to a dose of 40 mg/kg/day divided twice daily (typically up to 1 g twice daily). Side effects reported with mycophenolate mofetil include headache, diarrhea, and leukopenia [6]. A potential long-term risk of chronic immunosuppression with azathioprine or mycophenolate mofetil is the development of secondary malignancies.

Other factors that may influence choice of a particular drug include the severity of the patient's disease, and whether the patient has a comorbid rheumatologic disorder that also requires treatment. NMOSD does not typically respond to multiple sclerosis-directed immunomodulatory therapy, and there have been reports of beta interferon possibly triggering NMOSD exacerbations.

5. If not treated expediently, children with NMOSD are at risk for permanent disability as clinical exacerbations can be severe and patients may have incomplete recovery from attacks [4]. Ideally, patients should be started on one of the above-mentioned preventative therapies when a diagnosis of NMOSD is confirmed, with the choice of therapy based on patient comorbidities, medication side effects, monitoring requirements, and patient and family's expectations. Though long-term prospective studies are needed to fully assess the effect of early initiation of therapy on disability in pediatric NMOSD patients, one small cohort study recently reported benefit with regard to limiting disability progression when early treatment with rituximab was implemented [8]. Better understanding of cognitive outcomes in children with NMOSD is also needed, and such long-term studies are now underway.

# Clinical Pearls

1. Consider the diagnosis of NMOSD in a child with intractable vomiting or hiccups, especially if there is no clear gastrointestinal etiology.
2. Consider the diagnosis of NMOSD in a child who is found to have isolated lesions in the dorsal medulla/area postrema even if he does not have a history of optic neuritis or myelitis; a brainstem syndrome may be the presenting attack in a patient with NMOSD.
3. Patients with pediatric NMOSD are commonly found to have comorbid autoimmune disorders, and additional autoantibody studies should be sent.
4. Initial treatment of acute exacerbations in pediatric NMOSD typically involves use of high-dose corticosteroids. Additional therapies such as plasma exchange or intravenous immunoglobulin may be needed in severe or refractory cases.
5. Disability in pediatric NMOSD can be severe and can accrue rapidly. Once a diagnosis of NMOSD is confirmed, early initiation of preventative therapy with rituximab, azathioprine, or mycophenolate mofetil is important for prevention of further relapses. Additional studies are needed to assess the long-term impact of these medications on disease course and prognosis in children.

# References

1. Wingerchuk DM, Banwell B, Bennett JL, et al. International consensus diagnostic criteria for neuromyelitis optica spectrum disorders. Neurology. 2015;85(2):177–89.
2. Apiwattanakul M, Popescu BF, Matiello M, et al. Intractable vomiting as the initial presentation of neuromyelitis optica. Ann Neurol. 2010;68(5):757–61.
3. Popescu BF, Lennon VA, Parisi JE, et al. Neuromyelitis optica unique area postrema lesions: nausea, vomiting, and pathogenic implications. Neurology. 2011;76(14):1229–37.
4. McKeon A, Lennon VA, Lotze T, et al. CNS aquaporin-4 autoimmunity in children. Neurology. 2008;71(2):93–100.
5. Ito S, Mori M, Makino T, et al. "Cloud-like enhancement" is a magnetic resonance imaging abnormality specific to neuromyelitis optica. Ann Neurol. 2009;66(3):425–8.
6. Kimbrough DJ, Fujihara K, Jacob A, et al. Treatment of neuromyelitis optica: review and recommendations. Mult Scler Relat Disord. 2012;1(4):180–7.
7. Dale RC, Brilot F, Duffy LV, et al. Utility and safety of rituximab in pediatric autoimmune and inflammatory CNS disease. Neurology. 2014;2(2):142–50.
8. Longoni G, Banwell B, Filippi M, Yeh EA. Rituximab as a first-line preventive treatment in pediatric NMOSDs: Preliminary results in 5 children. Neurol Neuroimmunol Neuroinflamm. 2014;1(4):e46.

# Chapter 25
# Infection Mimics with Brainstem Presentation

Dana Marafi and Timothy E. Lotze

## Case Presentation

A 16-year-old previously healthy male presented with 2 months of progressive right-sided weakness. His examination was notable for mild right-sided hemiparesis and hyperreflexia. Fundoscopic examination was normal. MRI of the brain showed a T1 hypointense, T2 hyperintense intra-axial ring-enhancing round lesion measuring 18 mm × 18 mm × 18 mm (Fig. 25.1a). CSF studies demonstrated an opening pressure of 20 cmH$_2$O, protein of 53 mg/dl, glucose of 52 mg/dl, with only one WBC and no RBCs. IgG index was normal, and oligoclonal bands were not present. CSF gram stain and culture, mycobacterial and fungal cultures, cryptococcus antigens, and cytology were negative. Blood aerobic and fungal cultures, cryptococcus and histoplasma antigens, histoplasma antibodies, QuantiFERON gold test, mycobacteria PCR, HIV test, fungal complement fixation test, beta-D-glucan and galactomannan, and NMO IgG were all negative. C3, C4, and ACE were normal. Spine MRI and CT chest/abdomen/pelvis were unremarkable.

Without evidence for an infectious or other etiology, a demyelinating lesion was considered. The patient received a course of methylprednisolone 1000 mg IV daily for 5 days with significant improvement of the right-sided weakness. Repeat brain MRI (Fig. 25.1b) showed an interval decrease in the size of the lesion. He was diagnosed with a clinically isolated syndrome and discharged on an oral prednisone taper for 6 weeks. Eight weeks after the initial presentation, he presented with recurrent right-sided weakness. Brain MRI showed mild increase in the size of the lesion.

D. Marafi, B.M.B.Ch. (✉)
Department of Neurology, Baylor College of Medicine, Houston, TX, USA
e-mail: Dana.Marafi@bcm.edu

T.E. Lotze, M.D.
Division of Neurology and Developmental Neuroscience, Department of Pediatrics,
Baylor College of Medicine, Texas Children's Hospital, Houston, TX, USA

© Springer International Publishing AG 2017
E. Waubant, T.E. Lotze (eds.), *Pediatric Demyelinating Diseases of the Central Nervous System and Their Mimics*, DOI 10.1007/978-3-319-61407-6_25

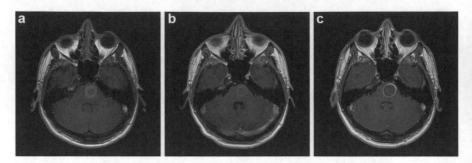

**Fig. 25.1** T1 with contrast sequence of brain MRI imaging at the level of the pons. (**a**) At the initial presentation. (**b**) After 1 week from initial presentation and following a steroid trial. (**c**) After 8 weeks from the initial presentation

He was given a second course of methylprednisolone 1000 mg IV daily for 5 days, and steroid taper was resumed again at discharge.

Within 48 h of discharge, the patient was readmitted again with headache, recurrent vomiting, and photophobia. No optic nerve edema or meningeal signs were noted on examination. His right-sided hemiparesis was stable. Repeat brain MRI (Fig. 25.1c) was unchanged. Repeat CSF analysis showed an opening pressure of 50 cmH$_2$O, protein of 11 mg/dl, and glucose of 56 mg/dl, with 660 WBC and 1150 RBC. CSF cryptococcal antigen was positive, and *Cryptococcus* was isolated on CSF culture. Quantitative cryptococcal antigen was elevated at 4086. HIV testing was negative. Treatment with antifungals was initiated for cryptococcal meningitis with a primary brainstem cryptococcoma. Lymphocyte phenotyping showed severe CD4 lymphopenia. He was thus diagnosed with idiopathic CD4 lymphopenia.

## Clinical Questions

1. Why was the diagnosis of cryptococcoma initially missed?
2. How did this patient proceed to having cryptococcal meningitis?
3. How can infections mimic demyelinating lesions and what are the common infection mimics of demyelinating lesions of the brainstem and cerebellum?
4. Are there any radiological features that distinguish demyelinating lesions from infection mimics?
5. What should a clinician consider when is it difficult to establish a diagnosis of a brainstem or cerebellar lesion by radiological features alone?

# Diagnostic Discussion

1. This patient had a cryptococcoma of the brainstem at his initial presentation that later ruptured giving rise to cryptococcal meningitis. Cryptococcoma is a rare localized fungal infection of central nervous system. It has been described to affect both immunocompromised and immunocompetent children and adults. Risk factors include chronic steroid use, diabetes, sarcoidosis, and immunosuppression. The infection usually presents with progressive focal neurological deficits and a ring-enhancing lesion on contrast imaging. Affected individual rarely manifests with fever. The lesion is usually T1 hypointense and T2 hyperintense on MRI. Since the lesion is encapsulated, specific CSF and serum titers can be negative and the infection can be easily missed. In these cases, the diagnosis is dependent on obtaining pathology samples. Since more than 50% of the cases affect the brainstem and cerebellum, biopsy of these deep-seated lesions is very challenging [1].
2. Diagnosis of a clinically isolated syndrome was suggested based on the MRI features with a negative infectious workup. Known for their anti-inflammatory properties, steroids can improve the symptoms of various conditions including infections, tumors, and demyelinating disorders. The use of steroid trials should be avoided unless tumors and serious infections are ruled out as the initial improvement can be falsely reassuring, causing delays in the establishment of an accurate diagnosis and potentially leading to serious complications. When in doubt, a biopsy should be considered.
3. Infectious lesions can mimic multiple sclerosis and other demyelinating diseases in both distribution and appearance [2]. When inflammation involves the hindbrain, i.e., the pons, medulla, and cerebellum, it is usually referred to as rhombencephalitis or brainstem encephalitis. Rhombencephalitis can be caused by infections or autoimmune disorders. Common autoimmune causes of rhombencephalitis include Behcet's disease, systemic lupus erythematosus, and paraneoplastic syndromes. The brainstem and cerebellum are also commonly involved in multiple sclerosis. Infections that have strong propensity to affect the brainstem include *Listeria*, enteroviruses, and herpes viruses. Other infections such as flaviviruses, *Brucella*, and *Toxoplasma* can also cause rhombencephalitis but are uncommon [3].
4. Typical acute demyelinating lesions appear well defined, hyperintense on T2 imaging, and hypointense on T1 imaging with rim enhancement on contrast imaging. Rim enhancement is highly specific for demyelinating lesions; however, the same pattern of rim enhancement can be seen in multiple infectious lesions such as tuberculosis, neurocysticercosis, toxoplasmosis, cryptococcosis, and histoplasmosis [2]. Tuberculosis and neurocysticercosis can be seen in both immunocompetent and immunocompromised individuals, while toxoplasmosis, cryptococcosis, and histoplasmosis typically affect immunocompromised individuals. The distribution and size can help narrow the differential although the diagnosis is rarely established based on imaging alone. Tuberculomas usually appear as irregularly shaped solid lesions that are more than 20 mm in size. They are often associated with severe perifocal edema. Magnetic resonance spectroscopy

of tuberculomas has been described to show increase in choline/creatine ratio and decreases in *N*-acetylaspartate (NAA) but is not specific. Neurocysticercosis (NCC) lesions on the other hand are round and small (usually less than 20 mm in size) and can be single or multiple without any surrounding edema [4]. There is often a DWI hyperintense eccentric dot within the NCC lesions representing the scolex [5]. All these infectious lesions have been reported to affect multiple areas in the brain including the brainstem and cerebellum, making the distinction sometimes difficult. Diffusion restriction, when present, can be a useful feature to differentiate demyelination lesions from infection. While abscesses commonly exhibit central diffusion restriction due to the presence of pus and proteinaceous material at the center, peripheral diffusion restriction is more commonly seen in acute demyelinating lesions as a result of preischemic conditioning, intramyelinic edema, and hypercellular inflammatory infiltrate at the rim [6]. In contrast to abscesses, the pattern of diffusion restriction in demyelinating lesions is heterogeneous due to rapid evolution from one stage to another in demyelination. Diffusion restriction is rare in tumors and metastasis and when present indicates high cellularity.

5. Due to the wide range of pathology that can affect the brainstem and cerebellum, it is often difficult to arrive on a diagnosis based on clinical and radiological features alone. Since lesions of the brainstem and cerebellum are deeply seated in a location with a critical function, surgical biopsy of these lesions is associated with some morbidity and mortality and thus is typically avoided. Stereotactic biopsy of the brainstem (SBB), although controversial, is a feasible option. SBB can help establish histopathological confirmation of diagnosis and allows for early initiation of appropriate treatment. The procedure can be done under local or general anesthesia and is generally guided by CT or MRI. Diagnosis can be established in up to 90% of the cases with minimal morbidity and mortality. Management of brainstem lesions often requires multidisciplinary team of neurologists, neurosurgeons, oncologists, and infectious disease specialists. The decision to proceed with stereotactic biopsy studies should be carefully considered. It is important to remember that early initiation of appropriate treatment can prevent various complications and lower associated morbidity and mortality [7].

## Clinical Pearls

- Clinically isolated syndrome is a diagnosis of exclusion. There are various infection mimics of multiple sclerosis and other demyelinating lesions of the brainstem and cerebellum. A clinician must be highly vigilant, and a complete workup must be pursued prior to initiating steroids.
- Rhombencephalitis is the inflammation of the hindbrain, i.e., the pons, medulla, and cerebellum. Rhombencephalitis can be caused by infections or autoimmune conditions. Common autoimmune causes include Behcet's disease, systemic lupus erythematosus, paraneoplastic syndromes, and multiple sclerosis. *Listeria*,

enteroviruses, and herpes viruses are the three most common infections known to cause rhombencephalitis.

- Several infectious lesions share the same characteristic rim enhancement seen in demyelinating lesions. Although the location and size of these lesions and the pattern of diffusion restriction are usually very helpful in distinguishing between them, it may be impossible to arrive on a diagnosis based on imaging alone.
- Stereotactic biopsy of the brainstem is a feasible option that should be carefully considered when a diagnosis of brainstem lesion cannot be established based on clinical and radiological features alone. This procedure remains controversial, and thus risk and benefit should be discussed within the members of the team. Early initiation of appropriate treatment can prevent significant morbidity and mortality.

# References

1. Li Q, You C, Liu Q, Liu Y. Central nervous system cryptococcoma in immunocompetent patients: a short review illustrated by a new case. Acta Neurochir. 2010;152(1):129–36.
2. Rocha AJ, Littig IA, Nunes RH, Tilbery CP. Central nervous system infectious diseases mimicking multiple sclerosis: recognizing distinguishable features using MRI. Arq Neuropsiquiatr. 2013;71(9B):738–46.
3. Jubelt B, Mihai C, Li TM, Veerapaneni P. Rhombencephalitis/brainstem encephalitis. Curr Neurol Neurosci Rep. 2011;11(6):543–52.
4. Shetty G, Avabratha KS, Rai BS. Ring-enhancing lesions in the brain: a diagnostic dilemma. Iran J Child Neurol. 2014;8(3):61–4.
5. Santos GT, Leite CC, Machado LR, McKinney AM, Lucato LT. Reduced diffusion in neurocysticercosis: circumstances of appearance and possible natural history implications. AJNR Am J Neuroradiol. 2013;34(2):310–6.
6. Abou Zeid N, Pirko I, Erickson B, Weigand SD, Thomsen KM, Scheithauer B, Parisi JE, Giannini CL, Lucchinetti CF. Diffusion-weighted imaging characteristics of biopsy-proven demyelinating brain lesions. Neurology. 2012;78(21):1655–62.
7. Manoj N, Arivazhagan A, Bhat DI, Arvinda HR, Mahadevan A, Santosh V, Devi BI, Sampath S, Chandramouli BA. Stereotactic biopsy of brainstem lesions: techniques, efficacy, safety, and disease variation between adults and children: a single institutional series and review. J Neurosci Rural Pract. 2014;5(1):32–9.

# Chapter 26
# Chronic Lymphocytic Inflammation with Pontine Perivascular Enhancement Responsive to Steroids

Jason S. Gill and Timothy E. Lotze

## Case Presentation

A 16-year-old right-handed Caucasian female with a prior suspected diagnosis of conversion disorder presented for a second opinion regarding her 5-year history of progressive lower extremity weakness. She described her course beginning 5 years earlier with gait instability and "stiff" legs. This progressed over the course of 2 years to being unable to arise unassisted when seated on the floor. Over the subsequent 3 years, this weakness continued to progress, so that she eventually required a wheelchair for mobility. In conjunction with lower extremity weakness, the patient reported intermittent dysarthria and urinary incontinence. She was reported to have had a number of previously normal investigations at another institution including MRI brain, serum electrolytes, renal function, liver enzymes, CBC, and inflammatory indices.

On her presenting examination for a second opinion, her cranial nerves and upper extremity sensory and motor exam were unremarkable, including no finding of dysarthria at the time of presentation. Power examination of her lower extremities revealed no movement against gravity bilaterally. She had hyperreflexia in her patellar deep tendon reflexes with crossed adductors and clonus bilaterally at the ankles. There was a Babinski sign bilaterally. She had a sensory level at T6, and stage III pressure ulcers were noted on both heels.

MRI brain and spine with contrast demonstrated multifocal punctate T2 hyperintense lesions scattered throughout the brainstem to include the pons and the full extent of the spinal cord; retrospective analysis of previously obtained MRI brain

J.S. Gill, M.D., Ph.D. (✉) • T.E. Lotze, M.D.
Division of Neurology and Developmental Neuroscience,
Department of Pediatrics Baylor College of Medicine, Texas Children's Hospital,
6701 Fannin St, Houston, TX 77035, USA
e-mail: jg30@bcm.edu

© Springer International Publishing AG 2017                                          201
E. Waubant, T.E. Lotze (eds.), *Pediatric Demyelinating Diseases of the Central Nervous System and Their Mimics*, DOI 10.1007/978-3-319-61407-6_26

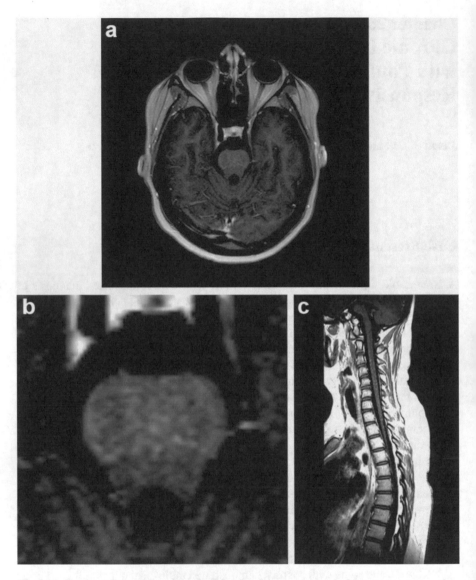

**Fig. 26.1** Post-gadolinium T1-weighted MRI. (**a**) Axial cut at the level of the *cisterna interpeduncularis* highlighting the characteristic pontine predominant punctate and curvilinear gadolinium-enhancing lesions. (**b**) *Inset*: magnified image of the pons from (**a**). (**c**) Sagittal slice showing midline view of the spinal cord from rostral T spine to pons. Image shows hyperintense gadolinium-enhancing lesions "peppering" the spinal cord. (**a**–**b**) Of note, lesions are evident primarily on post-contrast imaging

with and without contrast showed similar findings several months prior. All of these lesions demonstrated a curvilinear enhancement pattern (Fig. 26.1).

Subsequent investigations included negative serum studies for infectious agents (*Bartonella*, *Ehrlichia*, syphilis, TB, *Schistosoma*, *Cryptococcus*), paraneoplastic antibodies, and autoimmune disease (ESR, CRP, ANCA, ACE, AQP4-IgG, antiphospholipid antibodies, NMDAR antibodies, RF, ANA, NMO). CSF demonstrated four white cells with normal leukocyte cytology, elevated protein of 85 mg/dL, and normal glucose of 48 mg/dL. There were no oligoclonal bands, and the IgG index was normal at 0.5.

With negative investigations for an alternate rheumatologic disease, infection, or malignancy and in consideration of the MRI pattern of signal change, a diagnosis of chronic lymphocytic inflammation with pontine perivascular enhancement responsive to steroids (CLIPPERS) was made. She was started on methylprednisolone 1000 mg IV daily for a 5-day course followed by ongoing monthly infusions of methylprednisolone 1000 mg. Acute response to steroid therapy included a subjective improvement in sensory changes. She was additionally started on mycophenolate mofetil progressively up to 1000 mg twice daily. Repeat MRI immediately after her initial 5-day course of methylprednisolone-noted reduction in the enhancement of the spinal cord and pontine lesions. As the duration of follow-up at the time of this writing is only 2 months, the recovery of her deficits remains modest with ongoing need for wheelchair mobility (Fig. 26.1).

## Questions

1. What is CLIPPERS?
2. What alternative diagnoses can be considered with this presentation?
3. What are the hallmarks of a CLIPPERS diagnosis?
4. What is known of the pathogenesis of this novel clinical entity?
5. What are the treatment options and prognosis for CLIPPERS diagnosis?

## Discussion

1. Chronic lymphocytic inflammation with pontine perivascular enhancement responsive to steroids (CLIPPERS) is a pontine predominant encephalomyelitis that was first described in 2010. This clinical entity was initially defined by episodic facial paresthesias or diplopia and subsequent brainstem or myelopathic symptoms presenting in a subacute course. Patients exhibit characteristic MRI findings of symmetric curvilinear-enhancing pontine lesions, with variable extension into surrounding brain parenchyma and spinal cord. CLIPPERS clinical presentation can include focal cranial nerve and cerebellar deficits, usually in combination rather than in isolation, along with possible associated long-tract or spinal cord signs, pseudobulbar affect, or cognitive dysfunction. One of the more common features of this entity is rapid response to glucocorticosteroid treatment, with both clinical and radiographic improvement, and relapse in the absence of continued immunosuppressive therapy. Response to steroids may

depend on how promptly treatment is initiated (i.e., in the case of our patient, CNS injury may have occurred over the years that may not be fully reversible).

2. The differential diagnosis for a patient presenting with cranial nerve deficits, ataxia, and/or long-tract findings is broad. CNS infectious workup, including fungal, mycobacterial, and rickettsial studies in addition to the more common viral and bacterial studies, should be thorough. Neoplastic/paraneoplastic processes should also be considered including evaluation of CNS lymphoma, histiocytosis (Langerhans, malignant), lymphomatoid granulomatosis, and glioma. Finally, the differential for alternative inflammatory etiologies must not be overlooked, with particular attention paid to neuro-Behcet, neurosarcoidosis, or lupus and Sjogren's with CNS involvement.

3. The diagnosis of CLIPPERS requires the exclusion of more common CNS pathologies as well as typical imaging findings and, possibly, typical findings of predominant T-lymphocyte infiltrations on brain biopsy. Due to the relative novelty of this clinical entity, validated criteria for the diagnosis of CLIPPERS do not yet exist. However, proposed criteria include four core features: (1) clinical course, (2) radiographic findings, (3) response to glucocorticoids, and (4) confirmatory histopathology. In general, a patient with CLIPPERS will present with a subacute course of progressive gait ataxia and diplopia or subacute neurological findings that localize to the brainstem or spinal cord. There will be the characteristic radiographic findings, as highlighted in the described case, which include punctate-enhancing lesions bilaterally with predominance in the pons and brainstem ("peppered" feature of the enhancement). Given an appropriate clinical course and radiographic findings consistent with CLIPPERS, a trial of glucocorticosteroids can be initiated. However, if upon thorough workup there is continued question as to the appropriate diagnosis, a biopsy should be performed to differentiate from alternative diagnostic possibilities; there are reported cases in which biopsy was crucial in identifying alternative underlying pathologies, including CNS neoplasms.

4. The pathogenesis of CLIPPERS is not well understood; however, several clues exist that aid in our understanding of its pathogenesis. In cases where brain biopsy was performed, the consistent finding with CLIPPERS was that of a CD4+ predominant T-lymphocytic infiltration of the pontocerebellar parenchyma. This, coupled with the finding of clinical response to immunosuppressive therapy, suggests an autoimmune or inflammatory process. The striking localization of focal deficits and gadolinium-enhancing lesions on MRI may offer further clues to the pathogenesis. Several hypotheses have been proposed for brainstem localization of the infiltrative pathology of CLIPPERS, including immune-mediated attack on the intra-axial venous drainage system that is predominant in the brainstem or the known susceptibility of the brainstem to autoimmune and paraneoplastic processes.

5. The efficacy of high-dose glucocorticosteroids in inducing clinical improvement and resolution of MRI findings is a hallmark of the diagnosis. Initial treatment should consist initially of high-dose IV methylprednisolone 30 mg/kg/dose (maximum of 1000 mg) for 5–7 days. This should be followed by maintenance

glucocorticosteroids sometimes used in conjunction with a steroid-sparing immunosuppressant. Pulse infusions of IV methylprednisolone can be considered as an initial alternative to lessen potential side effects of daily oral treatment. Long-term therapy is a necessity in CLIPPERS, with taper or withdrawal of steroid treatment often being associated with clinical and radiographic relapse. Early identification and initiation of treatment is a critical component of the management of CLIPPERS. As the number of cases reported has grown, alternatives to long-term steroid therapy have emerged, including common steroid-sparing agents such as methotrexate and mycophenolate. More recently, reports of efficacy with biologics, such as rituximab and interferon beta-1a, have been published as well. As CLIPPERS is a relatively novel diagnosis, evidence for efficacy of targeted therapies should become increasingly available.

6. Despite the subacute presentation and the rapid response to glucocorticoids, CLIPPERS is not a benign disease. Failure to identify this disease or to initiate and maintain appropriate treatment is associated with persistent focal deficits as well as atrophy of involved structures.

## Clinical Pearls

1. CLIPPERS can be diagnosed with subacute presentation of intermittent dysarthria, ataxia, and/or diplopia and characteristic-enhancing MRI lesions "peppering" the pontocerebellar or brainstem regions. Spinal cord disease can additionally occur and produce gait failure.
2. CLIPPERS is responsive to short course, high-dose IV glucocorticosteroids and long- term maintenance therapy with steroids with possible adjunct of a steroid-sparing agent. Relapse often occurs in the absence of therapy.
3. In cases where diagnosis is uncertain or response to glucocorticosteroids is poor, consideration should be made for brain biopsy to rule out a neoplastic or chronic infectious process.

## Suggested Reading

1. Chronic lymphocytic inflammation with pontine perivascular enhancement responsive to steroids (CLIPPERS). Pittock SJ, Debruyne J, Krecke KN, Giannini C, van den Ameele J, De Herdt V, McKeon A, Fealey RD, Weinshenker BG, Aksamit AJ, Krueger BR, Shuster EA, Keegan BM. Brain. 2010;133(9):2626–34. Epub 2010 Jul 17.
2. CLIPPERS: chronic lymphocytic inflammation with pontine perivascular enhancement responsive to steroids. Review of an increasingly recognized entity within the spectrum of inflammatory central nervous system disorders. Dudesek A, Rimmele F, Tesar S, Kolbaske S, Rommer PS, Benecke R, Zettl UK. Clin Exp Immunol. 2014;175(3):385–96.

3. Expanding the clinical, radiological and neuropathological phenotype of chronic lymphocytic inflammation with pontine perivascular enhancement responsive to steroids (CLIPPERS). Simon NG, Parratt JD, Barnett MH, Buckland ME, Gupta R, Hayes MW, Masters LT, Reddel SW. J Neurol Neurosurg Psychiatry. 2012;83(1):15–22. Epub 2011 Nov 5.
4. Long-term outcomes of CLIPPERS (chronic lymphocytic inflammation with pontine perivascular enhancement responsive to steroids) in a consecutive series of 12 patients. Taieb G, Duflos C, Renard D, Audoin B, Kaphan E, Pelletier J, Limousin N, Tranchant C, Kremer S, de Sèze J, Lefaucheur R, Maltête D, Brassat D, Clanet M, Desbordes P, Thouvenot E, Magy L, Vincent T, Faillie JL, de Champfleur N, Castelnovo G, Eimer S, Branger DF, Uro-Coste E, Labauge P. Arch Neurol. 2012;69(7):847.

# Part III
# Diseases That Affect the Spinal Cord

# Chapter 27
# Acute Disseminated Encephalomyelitis with Spinal Cord Presentation

Hsiao-Tuan Chao, Kimberly M. Houck, and Timothy E. Lotze

## Case Presentation

A 3-year-old, right-handed, previously healthy girl presented with a several-day history of progressive fatigue, irritability, and left hemiparesis. Two weeks prior to presentation, she had an upper respiratory infection characterized by cough, congestion, and rhinorrhea that subsequently improved. Four days prior to presentation, she had elevated temperature (Tm 100.1F) and decreased appetite. Over the next few days, she became increasingly fatigued and irritable. She was sleeping more and talking less than usual, and she subsequently developed pain and numbness in the left leg with unsteady gait and progressive left-sided weakness, including a left-sided facial droop. She had two episodes of urinary incontinence and developed constipation.

Neurologic examination was significant for a left lower facial droop, left upper and lower extremity weakness (2/5) that was more pronounced in the lower extremity with difficulty bearing weight, and truncal ataxia. CSF analysis revealed leukocytosis (41 WBC/mm$^3$) with lymphocytic predominance (69% lymphocytes, 23% monocytes/macrophages, and 0% neutrophils), normal IgG index, and negative oligoclonal banding. CSF erythrocyte (1/mm$^3$), glucose (78 mg/dL), and protein (35 mg/dL) composi-

H.-T. Chao, M.D., Ph.D. (✉)
Jan and Dan Duncan Neurological Research Institute, Texas Children's Hospital, 1250 Moursund St, Suite 1125, Houston, TX 77030, USA

Division of Neurology and Developmental Neuroscience, Department of Pediatrics, Baylor College of Medicine and Texas Children's Hospital, 6701 Fannin St, CCC Suite 1250, Houston, TX 77030, USA
e-mail: hxchao@texaschildrens.org

K.M. Houck, M.D. • T.E. Lotze, M.D.
Division of Neurology and Developmental Neuroscience, Department of Pediatrics, Baylor College of Medicine and Texas Children's Hospital, 6701 Fannon CC 1250, Houston, TX 77030, USA
e-mail: khouck@bcm.edu; tlotze@bcm.edu

© Springer International Publishing AG 2017
E. Waubant, T.E. Lotze (eds.), *Pediatric Demyelinating Diseases of the Central Nervous System and Their Mimics*, DOI 10.1007/978-3-319-61407-6_27

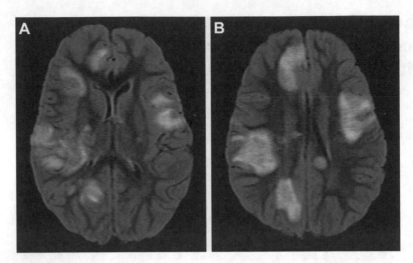

**Fig. 27.1** Representative MRI brain axial T2-weighted FLAIR images. (**a** and **b**) Bilateral, multi-focal, patchy areas of FLAIR hyperintense signal within the cerebral hemispheres, predominantly involving the white matter although with some cortical involvement. There is also involvement of the right posterior limb of the internal capsule. Axial sections showing the (**a**) level of the basal ganglia and thalamus, (**b**) level of the body of the corpus callosum

tion was normal. CSF culture and viral studies were negative. The brain MRI showed multifocal, patchy areas of FLAIR hyperintense signal within the cerebral hemispheres, predominantly in the white matter but with some cortical involvement (Fig. 27.1). There were also FLAIR hyperintensities in the right posterior limb of the internal capsule, left superior cerebellar peduncle, and right medulla. The spine MRI with gadolinium revealed longitudinally extensive, nonenhancing central cord signal abnormality with mild cord expansion extending from T6 into the conus medullaris (Fig. 27.2).

She was treated with a 5-day course of IV methylprednisolone (30 mg/kg/day) and physical therapy, after which symptoms and focal neurologic deficits resolved. At the time of discharge, she was able to ambulate without assistance, void spontaneously, and returned to baseline mentation. On follow-up 4 months after presentation, she remained clinically stable with residual subtle left hemiparesis and occasional urinary incontinence.

## Questions

### What Clinical Findings in ADEM Are Suggestive of Spinal Cord Versus Brain Involvement?

ADEM includes "encephalomyelitis," which suggests concomitant involvement of both brain and spinal cord, and the clinical presentation can be predominantly related to spinal cord symptoms. The clinical presentation of bilateral extremity

**Fig. 27.2** Representative
MRI spinal cord
T2-weighted images. (**a**
and **b**) Midsagittal
cervical, thoracic, and
lumbar spine image
showing T2 hyperintense
signal within the spinal
cord beginning at the level
of T6 and extending
inferiorly into the conus
medullaris. There is mild
enlargement of the affected
spinal cord, particularly in
the distal cord and conus.
Axial images from boxed
areas are shown in (**c**) and
(**d**) panels. (**c** and **d**)
Representative axial
thoracic spine images
showing T2-weight
hyperintensity at (**c**) level
T8 and (**d**) level T10

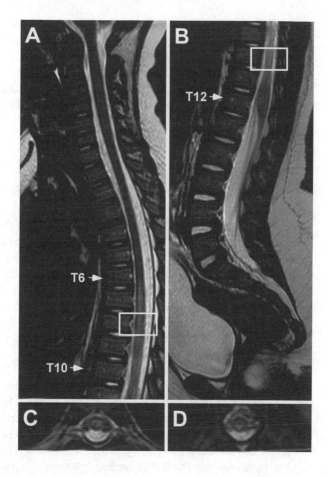

weakness, predominantly affecting legs more than arms, sensory changes consistent
with a dermatomal level, and impairment of bowel and bladder function, are signs
concerning for spinal cord involvement, especially bilateral myelitis. Unilateral, or
partial, myelitis can present with left- or right-sided extremity weakness and associated ipsilateral dorsal column dysfunction and contralateral spinothalamic dysfunction. Bowel and bladder impairment can occur with unilateral myelitis but may not
be as pronounced as with bilateral involvement [1]. Features suggestive of brain
involvement include encephalopathy, seizures, headaches, cranial nerve palsies,
ataxia, and sometimes unilateral deficits.

Up to 40% of all ADEM cases are reported to have spinal cord involvement on
imaging in studies that included patients with myelopathic symptoms as well as incidental spinal cord MRI findings in patients without clinical cord involvement [1–4].
Myelitis in ADEM tends to predominantly affect the thoracic cord with typically

minimal patchy contrast enhancement [1]. Spinal cord involvement in ADEM can be focal and segmental, contiguous, or longitudinally extensive, sometimes involving the entire cord [1]. The lesions on imaging can have a characteristic flame-shaped appearance, but when considered in isolation, this can raise concern for intrinsic cord tumors [5]. Therefore, imaging features alone are insufficient to diagnose ADEM with myelitis and need to be interpreted in the context of the clinical setting.

## What Are the Clinical Differences Between ADEM-Related Transverse Myelitis and Idiopathic Transverse Myelitis?

Acute transverse myelitis (TM) is a focal inflammatory disorder of the spinal cord resulting in motor, sensory, or autonomic dysfunction with signs and symptoms of bilateral involvement [6]. Acute TM is either idiopathic or associated with systemic inflammatory disease, multiple sclerosis, neuromyelitis optica, or ADEM. ADEM-associated TM requires meeting the ADEM clinical diagnostic criteria that include encephalopathy and multifocal inflammation [6]. About 5–16% of all acute TM pediatric cases occur in association with ADEM [7, 8]. Distinguishing idiopathic TM from ADEM-associated TM prior to diagnostic imaging may be challenging. Both may have a prodromal illness in the weeks prior to symptom onset. In addition, for infants and younger children, myelopathic pain related to idiopathic TM may produce nonspecific inconsolable irritability. ADEM-related central encephalopathy may be difficult to differentiate from a primary painful myelopathy in the pediatric population. Imaging of the brain and spinal cord is therefore critical to distinguish these entities. In the absence of brain MRI findings suggestive of ADEM, a diagnosis of idiopathic TM can be made once systemic inflammatory disorders are excluded.

One pediatric case series compared symptoms between idiopathic TM and ADEM-associated myelitis. Headaches and fever were more commonly observed in children with ADEM-associated myelitis (67% vs. 14% in idiopathic TM for headaches and 75% vs. 45% in idiopathic TM for fever). In contrast, sensory level with areflexia was more common in idiopathic TM (55% vs. 8% in ADEM-associated myelitis), but this may be underreported in ADEM, as an encephalopathic patient is less likely to voice a sensory level [9].

## What Is the Treatment for ADEM with Spinal Cord Involvement, and How Does the Presence of Transverse Myelitis Affect ADEM Outcome?

Treatment for ADEM with spinal cord involvement is similar to treatment for ADEM in general and other inflammatory demyelinating disorders. High-dose intravenous corticosteroids (30 mg/kg/dose up to 1000 mg per daily dose) for 3–5 days are used as a first-line agent to resolve acute inflammation. In case of lack of improvement after steroids or contraindication to steroid treatment, intravenous immunoglobulins (IVIg) or plasmapheresis (PLEX) can be considered depending on the severity of illness. While corticosteroids have been shown to be beneficial for treatment of myelitis in the setting of MS and NMO, it may not be equally beneficial to all forms of myelitis [10]. There has been no randomized controlled trial of IVIg or PLEX for acute idiopathic TM, and as such, their respective benefits are unclear. Corticosteroid-refractory myelitis associated with ADEM may improve after IVIg therapy based on one retrospective study showing that 10 of 19 patients who did not improve substantially after IV methylprednisolone therapy exhibited improved motor function following IVIg treatment [10]. However, it is unclear whether recovery was related to treatment effect or to natural recovery.

While spinal cord lesions tend to be more longitudinally extensive in ADEM, this does not necessarily correlate with clinical outcome. Children across all ages with ADEM-associated TM have overall better outcome compared with idiopathic TM [9]. At 12 months after symptom onset, nearly 100% of ADEM-associated TM will have normal or near-normal outcome. Less than 10% of ADEM-associated TM cases continue to have mild motor deficits and mild urinary sequelae [9]. In contrast, about 70% of acute TM cases will have normal or good global outcome. Of the other 30% of acute TM cases, there is about 10% with moderate motor deficits, 14% with mild urinary sequelae, and 5% with moderate to severe urinary sequelae [9]. Poor prognostic factors for functional recovery in children with acute myelitis, either acute idiopathic TM or ADEM-associated myelitis, include flaccid paraparesis at presentation, age less than 6 months, and respiratory failure requiring ventilatory support [9]. Spine neuroimaging features such as contrast enhancement, T1 hypointensity, cord expansion, or axial T2 hyperintensity patterns are not prognostic [9].

## Clinical Pearls

1. Clinical encephalopathy can be difficult to distinguish from myelopathic pain or discomfort, especially in young children and infants. MRI of the brain and spinal cord should be performed in all children with clinical suspicion of ADEM or transverse myelitis to better define the underlying diagnosis and extent of disease. The extent to which ADEM is associated with clinically silent spinal cord lesions remains to be elucidated.
2. Acute transverse myelitis can be seen as an initial presenting feature of ADEM. Prognosis for good recovery is better for ADEM with spinal cord involvement compared to acute idiopathic transverse myelitis.
3. Treatment for ADEM with spinal cord involvement is similar to other acute demyelinating disorders. Corticosteroid-refractory ADEM with spinal cord involvement may improve after IV immunoglobulin therapy or PLEX.

# References

1. Cree BA. Acute inflammatory myelopathies. Handb Clin Neurol. 2014;122:613–67.
2. Dale RC, et al. Acute disseminated encephalomyelitis, multiphasic disseminated encephalo-myelitis and multiple sclerosis in children. Brain. 2000;123(Pt 12):2407–22.
3. Hynson JL, et al. Clinical and neuroradiologic features of acute disseminated encephalomyeli-tis in children. Neurology. 2001;56:1308–12.
4. Erol I, Ozkale Y, Alkan O, Alehan F. Acute disseminated encephalomyelitis in children and adolescents: a single center experience. Pediatr Neurol. 2013;49:266–73.
5. Sheerin F, Collison K, Quaghebeur G. Magnetic resonance imaging of acute intramedul-lary myelopathy: radiological differential diagnosis for the on-call radiologist. Clin Radiol. 2009;64:84–94.
6. Roman GC. Proposed diagnostic criteria and nosology of acute transverse myelitis. Neurology. 2003;60:730–731.; author reply 730–1.
7. O'Mahony J, et al. Recovery from central nervous system acute demyelination in children. Pediatrics. 2015;136:e115–23.
8. Mikaeloff Y, et al. First episode of acute CNS inflammatory demyelination in childhood: prog-nostic factors for multiple sclerosis and disability. J Pediatr. 2004;144:246–52.
9. Yiu EM, Kornberg AJ, Ryan MM, Coleman LT, Mackay MT. Acute transverse myelitis and acute disseminated encephalomyelitis in childhood: spectrum or separate entities? J Child Neurol. 2009;24:287–96.
10. Ravaglia S, et al. Severe steroid-resistant post-infectious encephalomyelitis: general features and effects of IVIg. J Neurol. 2007;254:1518–23.

# Chapter 28
# Post-infectious Acute Transverse Myelitis

Anusha K. Yeshokumar and Emmanuelle Waubant

## Case Presentation

**Case 1** A 13-year-old previously healthy Hispanic boy presented with progressively worsening bilateral leg weakness and urinary and bowel incontinence for 10 days, culminating in flaccid lower extremity paralysis. There had been no preceding upper respiratory symptoms or recent vaccinations. There were no vision changes or mental status alterations. His neurologic examination demonstrated full 5/5 power with normal reflexes in the bilateral upper extremities and 2/5 power reduction with hyperreflexia with spread in the bilateral lower extremities. Sensation was intact to all modalities in the arms but was globally impaired in both legs. There was a sensory level at T6 to pinprick testing.

Gadolinium-enhanced MRI of the spine showed a non-enhancing T2 hyperintense intramedullary lesion from C4 to the conus medullaris, mostly involving the central cord (Fig. 28.1). Gadolinium-enhanced MRI of the brain showed no abnormalities. Lumbar puncture revealed a lymphocytic pleocytosis (112 white blood cells, 86% lymphocytes) with normal protein and glucose (Table 28.1). There were no oligoclonal bands, and IgG index was 0.6 (normal <0.8). Aquaporin-4 (AQP4) antibodies from both serum and CSF were negative. Complete blood count results were within normal limits. Chest X-ray was clear. Serum ANA, ACE, *Borrelia* serologies, HTLV-1 and HTLV-2, HIV, and RPR were also negative, as was HSV

A.K. Yeshokumar, M.D. (✉)
Mount Sinai in NYC, Jamaica, NY, USA
e-mail: ayeshok1@jhmi.cdu

E. Waubant, M.D., Ph.D.
Clinical Neurology and Pediatrics, Regional Pediatric MS Clinic at UCSF,
University of California San Francisco, 675 Nelson Rising Lane, Suite 221,
San Francisco, CA 94158, USA
e-mail: Emmanuelle.waubant@ucsf.edu

© Springer International Publishing AG 2017
E. Waubant, T.E. Lotze (eds.), *Pediatric Demyelinating Diseases of the Central Nervous System and Their Mimics*, DOI 10.1007/978-3-319-61407-6_28

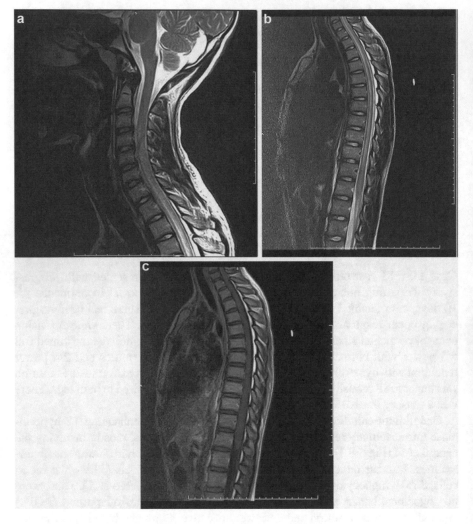

**Fig. 28.1** T2-weighted sagittal cervical (**a**) and thoracic (**b**) spine as well as post-contrast T1-weighted (**c**) sagittal thoracic spine MRI images of Case 1, mycoplasma-associated post-infectious acute transverse myelitis (TM), showing a non-enhancing T2 hyperintense intramedullary lesion from C4 to the conus medullaris

PCR. CMV IgG was positive while IgM was negative. *Mycoplasma* IgM and IgG levels resulted positive (IgM = 1295, positive >950; IgG = 2.77, positive ≥1.10), raising the possibility of a post-infectious acute transverse myelitis (TM). Sputum PCR testing for *Mycoplasma* was negative. Bladder function was not objectively assessed.

The patient was treated with high-dose methylprednisolone (1 g/day) for 5 days and concurrently underwent five daily cycles of plasmapheresis (PLEX) to optimize shortened hospital admission duration. Antimicrobial medications were not given,

**Table 28.1** CSF results from case presentations

| Case | WBC (differential) | Protein (mg/dL) | Glucose (mg/dL) | IgG index | Oligoclonal bands |
|------|--------------------|-----------------|-----------------|-----------|-------------------|
| 1 | 112 (87% lymphocytes, 1% polymorphonuclear, 12% monocytes) | 60 | 97 | 0.6 (normal) | 0 (normal) |
| 2 | 3 (33% lymphocytes, 67% PMNs) | 18 | 89 | 0.7 (normal) | 0 (normal) |

as was suspected to be a post-infectious rather than acute infectious process. Follow-up *Mycoplasma* IgM titers drawn 6 weeks after hospitalization were negative, but IgG levels increased to four times (23.09) those drawn during acute illness. Rehabilitation therapy was initiated during his hospital admission and continued as an outpatient after hospital discharge. Functionally, the patient recovered completely within about 3 months, regaining full strength in the legs, ambulation without difficulty, and normal bladder function. Repeat gadolinium-enhanced MRI of the cervical and thoracic spine performed 5 months later were both normal. There had been no recurrence of neurologic symptoms at the last neurology follow-up, 12 months after initial presentation.

**Case 2** A 3-year-old previously healthy African-American girl presented with 1 day of difficulty walking along with intermittent falling and one episode of urinary incontinence. There were no vision changes or mental status alterations. Her neurologic examination demonstrated 2/5 power reduction with absent reflexes in the bilateral upper extremities (right worse than left) and complete paralysis with absent flexes in the bilateral lower extremities. Sensation was intact to all modalities in the bilateral arms and legs. Of note, 10 days prior to presentation, she developed fever to 40.5 °F and otitis media for which she was treated with oral amoxicillin for 7 days. Her fever resolved within 48 h, and she had no residual fever or infectious symptoms at the time neurologic symptoms developed.

Gadolinium-enhanced MRI of the spine showed cord edema and an enhancing T2 hyperintense intramedullary lesion from C1 to C6, mostly involving the central and posterior cord (Fig. 28.2). Gadolinium-enhanced MRI of the brain showed no abnormalities. Lumbar puncture revealed no pleocytosis with normal protein and glucose (Table 28.1). There were no oligoclonal bands, and IgG index was 0.7 (normal <0.8). AQP4 antibodies from serum were negative. Multiple bladder ultrasounds, done to evaluate for urinary retention, were normal. Complete blood count results were within normal limits. HSV, EBV, CMV, VZV, and West Nile virus PCRs were negative. Serum rheumatologic panel (including ANA, ANCA, anti-Ro (SS-A) Ab, anti-La (SS-B) Ab, anti-RNP/Smith (Sm) Ab, anti-double-stranded DNA Ab, cardiolipin antibody panel, and C3/C4) was unremarkable. Lyme and *Mycoplasma* IgM and IgG levels were normal, as was sputum PCR testing for *Mycoplasma*. Chest X-ray revealed a left lower lobe infiltrate, and sputum culture was positive for *Haemophilus influenzae*. Together, these findings were suggestive of a post-infectious acute transverse myelitis (TM).

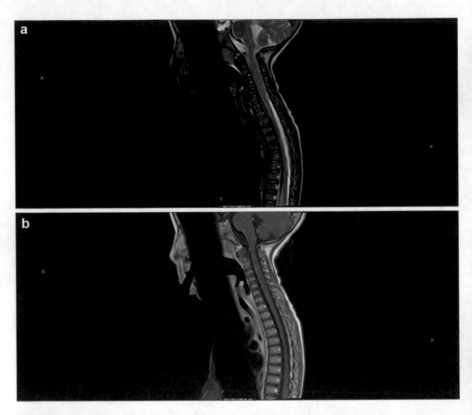

**Fig. 28.2** T2-weighted (**a**) and post-contrast T1-weighted (**b**) sagittal cervical spine MRI images of Case 2, post-infectious acute transverse myelitis (TM), showing cord edema and an enhancing T2 hyperintense intramedullary lesion from C1 to C6

**Table 28.2** Diagnostic criteria for post-infectious and idiopathic acute TM [6] (all criteria must be fulfilled)

| | |
|---|---|
| 1. Sensory, motor, or autonomic dysfunction attributable to the spinal cord | 4. No evidence of compressive cord lesion |
| 2. Bilateral signs or symptoms (can be symmetric or asymmetric) | 5. Inflammation defined by CSF pleocytosis, CSF elevated IgG index, and/or gadolinium enhancement on MRI |
| 3. Clearly defined sensory level | 6. Progression to symptom nadir between 4 h and 21 days |

The patient was treated with high-dose methylprednisolone (20 mg/kg/day) for 5 days followed by a 4-week oral steroid taper. In addition, she received a total of five cycles of PLEX, which were performed every other day. Her pneumonia was treated with a 10-day course of intravenous ceftriaxone. Rehabilitation therapy was initiated during her hospital admission. She was transferred to an inpatient rehabilitation center, where she was admitted for 7 weeks, and subsequently received outpatient rehabilitation therapy. Functionally, the patient recovered completely within about 6 months, regaining full strength in the legs, ambulation without difficulty, and normal bladder function. Repeat gadolinium-enhanced MRI of the spine performed 5 weeks later demonstrates residual patchy T2 hyperintensity in the C1–C6 region with improved edema and no contrast enhancement. There had been no recurrence of neurologic symptoms at the last neurology follow-up, 8 months after initial presentation.

## Clinical Questions

1. What is transverse myelitis, and how does it typically present?
2. What diagnostic tools assist in confirming the diagnosis?
3. What other etiologies should be considered in the differential diagnosis?
4. What treatment modalities should be employed in the acute phase?
5. What short-term outcomes can be expected for patients following acute treatment?

## Diagnostic Discussion

### What Is Transverse Myelitis, and How Does It Typically Present?

Transverse myelitis (TM) is a broad term encompassing acute and subacute infectious, post-infectious, and inflammatory diseases of the spinal cord. About 20% of all cases of TM occur in childhood [1], equating to an annual incidence of two new cases/million per year [2]. There is a bimodal distribution of disease in children with clustering in toddlers less than 2 years of age and in preadolescence 10–12 years of age [3]. Gender predilection is unclear, though one study has suggested a male predominance in children under 10 years and a slight female predominance in children over 10 years [4].

In cases associated with clinical and biological evidence for a recent infection, acute TM is thought to occur as a direct consequence of the infection or as a result of a post-infectious syndrome (i.e., not directly caused by the infectious organism). In some cases, definitive evidence of an infectious agent or process may be missing, making the absolute causal relationship between systemic infection and TM difficult to confirm.

Approximately 50% of all patients with acute TM report a preceding symptomatic infection, most commonly upper respiratory tract symptoms, within the preceding month [5]. There are several case reports of acute TM following administration of a vaccine, namely, against hepatitis B (HBV) and measles-mumps-rubella (MMR), but again causality has been difficult to clearly establish [2].

Children with acute TM present with rapid onset of symptoms including bilateral leg and sometimes arm weakness, often accompanied by bowel and/or bladder dysfunction as well as sensory symptoms, predominantly paresthesia, numbness, and back pain [6]. A transverse sensory level related to the myelitis is typically noted in the thoracic region (50%), though cervical (25%) and lumbar (5%) sensory levels are not infrequently seen [4]. Typically, deep tendon reflexes below the level of the lesion are increased, but this may not be seen in very severe cases, particularly early on in the clinical course. This phenomenon, referred to as spinal shock, can lead clinicians to incorrectly assume a peripheral nerve process and miss a spinal cord etiology.

Exam findings can be consistent with a complete or incomplete cord injury. Complete cord lesions present with relatively symmetric loss of motor and sensory function bilaterally caudal to the level of the lesion with sphincter involvement. These are more typically seen in idiopathic transverse myelitis and neuromyelitis optica. Conversely, partial cord lesions present with patchy or asymmetric findings typically milder in nature and are more commonly seen in patients with multiple sclerosis (MS).

## What Various Diagnostic Tools Assist in Confirming the Diagnosis?

MRI of the entire spine and brain should be obtained urgently to identify and characterize disease-causing lesions. Presence of an intramedullary white and/or gray matter cord lesion noted on sagittal and axial cuts with enhancement on post-gadolinium sequences supports the diagnosis of myelitis, and there may be accompanying spinal cord swelling. Longitudinally extensive TM (LETM) is defined as presence of a lesion that extends over three or more vertebral segments.

MRI of the brain will identify clinically relevant and silent lesions, which may suggest another entity causing myelitis. Multiple abnormal foci suspected to have arisen at different time points (determined by presence of some lesions which enhance and others which do not) are suggestive of MS, while lesions in the brain stem or optic nerve may raise consideration for NMO.

Lumbar puncture assesses for an inflammatory state in the cerebrospinal fluid (CSF) and may diagnose an infectious etiology through various antibody titers and viral PCRs. Abnormal CSF findings can include pleocytosis with lymphocytic predominance and/or elevated protein levels in approximately 50% of children with acute TM [4]. A normal CSF profile is seen in about 25% of cases.

Oligoclonal bands (OCBs) are typically absent in the CSF of children with monophasic acute TM. Studies in adult patients demonstrate that the presence of OCBs in the CSF at the first presentation of acute TM suggests a higher risk of developing MS, though it is noteworthy that OCBs can be present in patients with monophasic acute TM as well [3]. Autoimmune serology, namely, to detect aquaporin-4 (AQP4) antibodies associated with NMO, should also be obtained.

In some cases, cerebral angiogram may be pursued when the history or initial evaluation is concerning for a vascular etiology. Spinal cord biopsy is not often required and is reserved for cases with concern for neoplastic or otherwise unclear etiology. Should biopsy be indicated, clinicians should first evaluate for possible systemic targets for biopsy. If one is not identified, consideration must be given to the significant risk of further neurologic deficit that may result from spinal cord biopsy.

## What Etiologies Should Be Considered in the Differential Diagnosis?

One of the most recognized infections resulting in post infectious TM is *Mycoplasma pneumoniae*. This is thought to result from molecular mimicry, wherein immunologic mechanisms targeted against the infectious organism systemically may also attack native central nervous system (CNS) tissue because of structural similarities between the microbial cellular wall components and neuronal receptors [7]. Other viruses implicated in post-infectious TM include varicella zoster (VZV), herpes simplex (HSV), Epstein-Barr (EBV), cytomegalovirus (CMV), and the enteroviruses [8].

Infectious TM, caused by direct CNS invasion of infectious organisms, can also occur from a number of systemic viral, bacterial, and fungal infections including *Mycoplasma pneumoniae*, VZV, HSV, EBV, CMV, enteroviruses, influenza, human T-cell lymphotropic virus 1 (HTLV-1), syphilis, Lyme, and tuberculosis. In many TM cases, no etiology is identified, leading to the diagnosis of idiopathic TM or post-infectious TM, in the cases with presumed preceding infection.

Acute TM can be the initial presentation of acquired demyelinating diseases, including MS and NMO. Lesions of short segment length and partial cord pattern, positive oligoclonal bands in CSF, and brain MRI with multiple demyelinating lesions suggest a diagnosis of MS. NMO lesions are more classically longitudinally extensive (though this is not always the case), are located centrally within the cord, and may be accompanied by extensive cord swelling. These patients may also present with optic neuritis or lesions in the high cervical and brain stem areas. Systemic autoimmune disorders, including systemic lupus erythematosus (SLE) and sarcoidosis, can also produce acute TM.

Other disorders can present with myelopathy and must be differentiated from post-infectious TM. Spinal cord infarction (from hypercoagulable disorder or anterior spinal artery thrombosis), vascular malformation, and spinal cord tumors (including astrocytomas and ependymomas) can appear as intramedullary lesions similar in appearance on imaging to TM. Other potential mimics include neurosurgical emergencies such as spinal cord compression from epidural abscesses or traumatic hematomas.

## What Treatment Modalities Should Be Employed in the Acute Phase?

There have been no randomized controlled trials regarding acute treatment of acute TM in children; therefore, the following recommendations are based on multiple case reports and series.

After evidence for an inflammatory etiology is gathered, and concern for compressive as well as vascular etiologies is eliminated with imaging, treatment should be initiated first with a trial of methylprednisolone IV (i.e., 20–30 mg/kg once daily to a maximum 1 g for 3–5 days) [ 9]. This is typically done while additional test results for infectious and malignant etiologies may be pending. Should initial presentation be severe or should patients not significantly improve with corticosteroids, IVIg, plasma exchange, or pulse cyclophosphamide may be considered.

Attention must also be paid to symptomatic management as appropriate. This may include urinary bladder catheterization, bowel regiments, gastrointestinal prophylaxis (while on corticosteroids), deep venous thrombosis prophylaxis, and pain management. Physical therapy and family psychosocial support are also invaluable aspects of longer-term care. The Transverse Myelitis Association (www.myelitis. org) provides resources including podcasts, newsletters, and support group information for patients and their families, including information specifically for children.

## What Short-Term Outcomes Can Be Expected for Patients Following Acute Treatment?

Prognosis for children with post-infectious acute TM is generally quite variable. Small case series have demonstrated that without immunomodulatory therapy, 60% of children with acute TM of varying causes have full or good recovery [4]. With therapy, children typically experience rapid improvement, with many regaining ambulation within 2 weeks following maximal deficits [3]. However, approximately 20% of children with acute TM do not recover completely, typically left with persistent ambulatory difficulties though sensory disturbances and abnormal bladder function are also reported.

Factors suspected to be associated with better functional outcome include older age at time of diagnosis, shorter time to diagnosis, lower sensory and anatomic levels of spinal injury, absence of T1 hypointensity on spinal MRI at that time of acute presentation, lack of white blood cells in the CSF, and fewer affected spinal cord segments [5]. Other studies have also noted incomplete cord syndromes, cases reaching maximal symptom severity in less than 24 h from onset, and persistent upper motor neuron signs including increased deep tendon reflexes as factors associated with inability to regain independent ambulation [3].

The recovery process typically begins quickly over days to weeks first with improved motor function followed by slower improvement in bladder and bowel function. Complete recovery to the new baseline may require many months to over 1 year. Post-infectious acute TM typically has a monophasic course, and recurrence is thought to be extraordinarily unlikely.

Close neurologic and MRI follow-up is recommended to assess for recurrence, which would suggest the presence of an acquired demyelinating disease, such as MS, and therefore potential need for extended immunomodulatory therapy.

## Clinical Pearls

1. Acute transverse myelitis (TM) is a disease of the spinal cord defined by [1] sensory, motor, or autonomic dysfunction attributable to the spinal cord; [2] bilateral signs or symptoms; [3] clearly defined sensory level; [4] no evidence of compressive cord lesion; [5] inflammation defined by CSF pleocytosis, CSF elevated IgG index, and/or gadolinium enhancement on MRI; and [6] progression to symptom nadir between 4 h and 21 days [5].
2. In up to 50% of cases of idiopathic cases, an ongoing or preceding systemic infection is documented, but its causal role in the pathophysiology of this disease is unclear. Post-infectious acute TM is thought to be an autoimmune process triggered at least in part by post-infectious inflammation.
3. Urgent neuroimaging followed by comprehensive evaluation with lumbar puncture and autoimmune serology is required to confirm an inflammatory etiology and to rule out mimics such as infection, infarction, vascular malformation, tumor, or disease-related TM (from a systemic autoimmune disorder or an acquired demyelinating disease).
4. After evidence for an inflammatory etiology is gathered, treatment should be initiated first with high-dose intravenous corticosteroids. Should initial presentation be severe or should patients not significantly improve with corticosteroids, plasma exchange, IVIg, or pulse cyclophosphamide may be considered.
5. Other important aspects of treatment include symptomatic management, physical therapy, and patient/family psychosocial support. The Transverse Myelitis Association (www.myelitis.org) provides resources including podcasts, newsletters, and support group information for patients and their families, including information specifically for children.
6. Prognosis for children with post-infectious acute TM is quite variable. While the majority of children do have full or good recovery, many are left with residual neurologic deficits including persistent ambulatory difficulties, sensory disturbances, and/or abnormal bladder function.

# References

1. Kaplin AI, Krisnan C, Deshande DM, Pardo CA, Kerr DA. Diagnosis and management of acute myelopathies. Neurologist. 2005;11(1):2–18.
2. Borchers AT, Gershwin ME. Transverse myelitis. Autoimmun Rev. 2012;11(3):231–48.
3. Verhey LH, Banwell BL. Inflammatory, vascular, and infectious myelopathies in children. Handb Clin Neurol. 2013;112:999–1017.
4. Banwell B, Kennedy J, Sadovnick D, Arnold DL, Magalhaes S, Wambera K, Connolly MB, Yager J, Mah JK, Shah N, Sebire G, Meaney B, Dilenge ME, Lortie A, Whiting S, Doja A, Levin S, MacDonald EA, Meek D, Wood E, Lowry N, Buckley D, Yim C, Awuku M, Guimond C, Cooper P, Grand'Maison F, Baird JB, Bhan V, Bar-Or A. Incidence of acquired demyelination of the CNS in Canadian children. Neurology. 2009;72(3):232–9.
5. Pidcock FS, Krishnan C, Crawford TO, et al. Acute transverse myelitis in childhood: center-based analysis of 47 cases. Neurology. 2007;68(18):1474–80.
6. Transverse Myelitis Consortium Working Group. Proposed diagnostic criteria and nosology of acute transverse myelitis. Neurology. 2002;59(4):499–505.
7. Tsiodras S, Kelesidis T, Kelesidis I, Voumbourakis K, Giamarellou H. *Mycoplasma pneumoniae*-associated myelitis: a comprehensive review. Eur J Neurol. 2006;13(2):112–24.
8. West TW, Hess C, Cree BA. Acute transverse myelitis: demyelinating, inflammatory, and infectious myelopathies. Semin Neurol. 2012;32(2):97–113.
9. Dale RC, Brilot F, Banwell BL. Pediatric central nervous system inflammatory demyelination: acute disseminated encephalomyelitis, clinically isolated syndromes, neuromyelitis optica, and multiple sclerosis. Curr Opin Neurol. 2009;22(3):233–40.

# Chapter 29
# Complete Transverse Myelitis (Idiopathic)

Sita Paudel and Jayne M. Ness

## Case Presentation

A 16-year-old African-American young man with no preceding illness or history of immunization in prior month but with history of poorly controlled type 1 diabetes diagnosed at age 6 awoke at 4:00 AM with left arm and neck pain. Two hours later, he developed right arm weakness but was still able to walk. Within 3 h of symptom onset, he had severe numbness below his neck, left > right. Three hours later, he had progressed to quadriplegia with neurogenic bladder. Neurologic examination demonstrated complete left hemiplegia and severe right-sided paresis worse proximally (2/5 strength in right deltoid and triceps and 4/5 in right quadriceps muscles). There was a T4 sensory level, and all sensory modalities were severely impaired from the neck down, left > right. Reflexes were 1+ in patella but absent elsewhere with negative Babinski sign. The patient also had left ptosis. His mentation and speech were normal. MRI spine (Fig. 29.1) obtained within 12 h of symptoms onset showed subtle linear T2 signal in the cord at the C3–C5 vertebral levels with faint enhancement. Lumbar puncture showed increased protein but no pleocytosis (Table 29.1). Brain MRI was normal. He was treated with methylprednisolone, 1 g daily for 5 days (without a subsequent taper due to his diabetes) for suspected diagnosis of transverse myelitis. As he showed no improvement after high-dose steroids, he underwent plasmapheresis (1 volume) for seven cycles followed by 2 g/kg of IVIG. Four weeks after symptom onset, the patient was still quadriplegic with

S. Paudel, M.D. (✉)
Pediatric Neurology, Sanford Children's Hospital,
1600 West 22nd Street, Sioux Falls, SD 57117, USA
e-mail: drsitapaudel@gmail.com

J.M. Ness, M.D., Ph.D. (✉)
The Division of Neurology, University of Alabama at Birmingham,
1600 7th Ave. S., CHB Suite 314, Birmingham, AL 35233, USA
e-mail: JNess@peds.uab.edu

© Springer International Publishing AG 2017        225
E. Waubant, T.E. Lotze (eds.), *Pediatric Demyelinating Diseases of the Central Nervous System and Their Mimics*, DOI 10.1007/978-3-319-61407-6_29

**Fig. 29.1** Cervical MRI
obtained <12 h after
symptom onset;
T2-weighted sagittal view
(**a**) with axial section (**b**)
and T1-weighted,
post-contrast (**c**) with axial
section (**d**). Note
T2-weighted
hyperintensity involving
gray matter, best seen on
axial section (**b**) with only
scant contrast enhancement
(**d**). Although the patient
was quadriplegic when this
MRI was obtained, cord
edema is not present

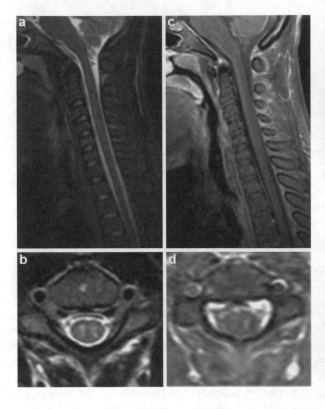

severe sensory impairment. As repeat MRI at that time (Fig. 29.2) showed marked
cord swelling with gadolinium enhancement, a 6-week steroid taper was started at
60 mg daily, and cyclophosphamide 750 mg/m² was given monthly for 3 months.
The patient developed hypertension with steroid treatment and required antihypertensive medications (amlodipine and labetalol).

One year after symptom onset, he remained paraplegic with severe leg spasticity.
He had slowly regained patchy areas of strength and sensation in his arms and was
able to lift both arms to about shoulder level. Follow-up MRI (Fig. 29.3) showed
myelomalacia, decreased T2 hyperintensity, no enhancement, and no new lesions.

The patient continued to require intermittent catheterization plus oxybutynin for
neurogenic bladder, baclofen for spasticity, gabapentin for neuropathic pain, and
carbamazepine for ephaptic spasms. He continues to get physical and occupational
therapy.

## Clinical Questions

- Does this patient fulfill criteria for idiopathic TM?
- What was the explanation for his ptosis?

**Table 29.1** Laboratory results

| Test | | Results |
|---|---|---|
| CSF | WBC | 3 (3% segs, 91% lymphs, 6% monos, 0% eos) |
| | RBC | 33 |
| | Protein | 66 |
| | Glucose | 144 |
| | IgG index | Negative |
| | Oligoclonal bands | Negative |
| | NMO AB | Negative |
| Serum | Glucose | 426 |
| | HBA1C | 14 |
| | Epstein-Barr serology | Negative IgG, IgM, EBNA |
| | TSH | Normal |
| | T4 | Normal |
| | ESR | Normal |
| | CRP | Normal |
| | ANA | Negative |
| | CK | Normal |
| | Anti-cardiolipin AB | Negative |
| | Phosphatidylethanolamine | Negative |
| | Oligoclonal bands | Negative |
| | Gad-65 | Normal |
| | Lupus anticoagulant | Negative |
| | NMO AB | Negative |
| | ACE level | Normal |

- Were there any other treatments that could have been used to improve his outcome?
- Was there any disease-modifying therapy indicated in this patient?
- What is the likelihood of relapse/recurrence after idiopathic acute TM?
- What is the outcome/prognosis of acute idiopathic TM?
- What are the other differential diagnostic considerations, and how do you distinguish between these conditions?

# Diagnostic Discussion

1. This patient meets the diagnostic criteria for transverse myelitis that include:

   - Sensory, motor, or autonomic dysfunction attributable to the spinal cord
   - Bilateral signs and/or symptoms
   - Clearly defined sensory level
   - No evidence of compressive cord lesion

**Fig. 29.2** Cervical MRI obtained 1 month after symptom onset; T2-weighted sagittal view (**a**) with axial section (**b**) and T1-weighted, post-contrast (**c**) with axial section (**d**). The patient had minimal recovery at this point despite treatment with high-dose methylprednisolone, plasmapheresis, and IVIG. There is edema of the lower cervical cord with T2-hyperintense signal throughout the cervical cord and upper thoracic cord. Regions of hypointense T1 signal within central gray matter are surrounded by linear contrast enhancement

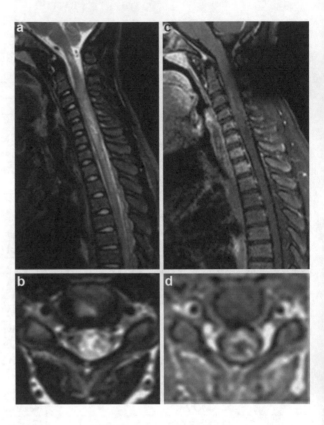

- Inflammation defined by cerebrospinal fluid pleocytosis, elevated IgG index, or gadolinium enhancement on MRI
- Progression to nadir between 4 h and 21 days

This patient had idiopathic complete TM. TM is divided into two main types: idiopathic vs. secondary. Idiopathic TM is defined by its occurrence without a definitive etiology despite a thorough work-up, suggesting an immune basis, and it is essentially a diagnosis of exclusion. Secondary TM is attributable to an underlying process including chronic demyelinating condition (multiple sclerosis, neuromyelitis optica), or a systemic autoimmune condition (systemic lupus erythematosus and Sjogren's syndrome), and an infectious/parainfectious etiology (West Nile virus, herpes, Lyme disease, mycoplasma).

TM also can be differentiated on the basis of the clinical severity and radiologic extent of the spinal cord lesion. These include:

- Acute partial TM (refers to spinal cord dysfunction that is mild or grossly asymmetric with an MRI lesion extending one to two vertebral segments)
- Acute complete TM (refers to spinal cord dysfunction that causes symmetric, complete, or near-complete neurologic deficits below the level of the lesion with an MRI lesion extending one to two vertebral segments)

**Fig. 29.3** Cervical MRI obtained 1 year after symptom onset; T2-weighted sagittal view (**a**) with axial section (**b**) and T1-weighted, post-contrast (**c**) with axial section (**b**). Myelomalacia is most prominent in left cervical cord

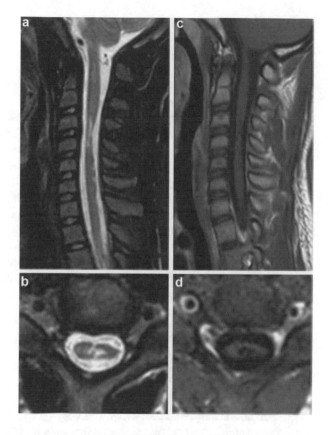

- Longitudinally extensive TM (refers to complete or incomplete spinal cord dysfunction with a lesion on MRI that extends three or more vertebral segments)

2. Lesions or injury of the sympathetic tracts in the cervicothoracic spinal cord can produce a Horner's syndrome. The signs and symptoms occur on the same side as the lesion of the sympathetic trunk. Signs and symptoms of Horner's syndrome include ptosis, miosis, enophthalmus, and anhidrosis.

3. The first-line therapy in idiopathic acute transverse myelitis is high-dose corticosteroids, such as methylprednisolone (20–30 mg/kg/day, maximum dose 1 g/day) for 3–5 days. For patients who fail to respond to methylprednisolone therapy, plasma exchange, IVIG, and broad-spectrum immunosuppression such as cyclophosphamide can help in some cases, if used during the acute phase.

4. Chronic immunomodulatory or disease-modifying therapy must be considered in a patient with recurrent disease in the same location or in patients with MS or NMO with dissemination in space and time. Treatment for recurrent TM not related to MS or NMO can include azathioprine, methotrexate, mycophenolate, or cyclophosphamide. Since this patient had not developed any recurrent disease

and had no evidence of dissemination in space and time on imaging, disease-modifying therapy was not indicated.

5. The majority of patients with TM experience monophasic disease. Recurrence has been reported in approximately 25–33% of patients with idiopathic TM. Features present at the time of initial acute onset that may predict recurrence include the following: female sex, multifocal or longitudinally extensive lesions in the spinal cord on MRI, brain lesions on MRI, presence of one or more autoantibodies (ANA, dsDNA, phospholipid, c-ANCA), underlying mixed connective tissue disease, presence of oligoclonal bands in the cerebrospinal fluid, and seropositivity for NMO-IgG (anti-aquaporin-4) antibody.

6. Most patients with idiopathic TM have at least a partial recovery, which usually begins within 1–3 months and continues with exercise and rehabilitation therapy. Recovery can proceed over years. Some degree of persistent disability is common, occurring in about 40%. Factors associated with poor outcome include female sex, severe ASIA (American Spinal Injury Association) impairment scale at onset, gadolinium enhancement on spinal MRI, absence of pleocytosis, very rapid onset with complete paraplegia, and spinal shock. The most common long-term complications of acute TM are urinary, motor, and sensory dysfunction.

7. The differential diagnosis of idiopathic TM is:

   – Conditions that cause other types of myelopathy which can be further divided into compressive (e.g., disc herniation, epidural masses or blood, vertebral body compression fractures, spondylosis, and tuberculosis of spine) and non-compressive (includes infectious, parainfectious, toxic, nutritional, and vascular)

   – Conditions that cause secondary TM which are chronic demyelinating conditions (multiple sclerosis, neuromyelitis optica), infection of the nervous system (e.g., West Nile virus, herpes, central nervous system Lyme disease, mycoplasma), and a systemic rheumatologic disease (e.g., systemic lupus erythematosus, Sjogren's syndrome)

   – Conditions that mimic TM but involve the peripheral nerve, such as Guillain-Barre syndrome (GBS)

   – GBS can be differentiating from a myelopathy by clinical examination, normal spinal cord MRI, and CSF study which usually will show cyto-albumino-logic dissociation. Electrodiagnostic studies may show conduction block or slowed conduction of peripheral nerves in GBS. Patients with spinal cord ischemia show no CSF pleocytosis, which could be a useful marker to differentiate inflammatory myelopathies from spinal cord infarcts. Spinal MRI imaging usually shows lesion in myelopathy. Electrodiagnostic studies are usually normal in myelopathies.

# Clinical Pearls

1. Complete transverse myelitis is an acute inflammatory disease of the spinal cord, characterized by rapid onset of bilateral neurological symptoms referable to the spinal cord, including weakness, sensory disturbance, and autonomic dysfunction evolving to maximal clinical severity between 4 h and 21 days. The lower limit of a 4-h onset is designed to prevent cases of cord infarction or cord arteriovenous malformations (AVM), which are typically of abrupt onset, from being erroneously diagnosed as transverse myelitis.
2. The causes of a transverse myelopathy include compressive myelopathies, such as neoplasm and AVM. The differential diagnosis of noncompressive myelopathy is broad and includes infectious, parainfectious, toxic, nutritional, vascular, and systemic disease; however, diagnostic work-up in many cases is negative, and so these cases are considered idiopathic.
3. The diagnostic evaluation of acute transverse myelopathy first requires emergent spine MRI to exclude acute cord compression which requires surgical intervention.
4. An active inflammatory process is defined by the presence of either a cellular infiltrate or elevated protein on CSF analysis or contrast enhancement on MRI of the spinal cord.
5. In the setting of normal initial MRI brain, acute partial transverse myelitis has a 10% risk of conversion to MS over 5 years of follow-up. Longitudinally extensive transverse myelitis is associated with a very low rate of conversion to MS (<2%), but up to 60% will be diagnosed with NMO.

# Suggested Reading

1. Deiva K, Absoud M, Hemingway C, Hernandez Y, Husssou B, Maurey H, Niotakis G, Wassmer E, Lim M, Tardieu M, United Kingdom Childhood Inflammatory Demyelination (UK-CID) Study and French Kidbiosep Study. Acute idiopathic transverse myelitis in children: early predictors of relapse and disability. Neurology. 2015;84(4):341–9.
2. Transverse Myelitis Consortium Working Group. Proposed diagnostic criteria and nosology of acute transverse myelitis. Neurology. 2002;59(4):499–505.
3. Goh C, Desmond PM, Phal PM. MRI in transverse myelitis. J Magn Reson Imaging. 2014;40(6):1267–79.
4. Greenberg BM, Thomas KP, Krishnan C, Kaplin AI, Calabresi PA, Kerr DA. Idiopathic transverse myelitis: corticosteroids, plasma exchange, or cyclophosphamide. Neurology. 2007;68(19):1614–7.
5. Cree BA. Acute inflammatory myelopathies. Handb Clin Neurol. 2014;122:613–67.

# Chapter 30
# Transverse Myelitis with Acute Inflammatory Polyradiculoneuropathy

Aaron L. Cardon and Timothy E. Lotze

## Case Presentation

A 15-year-old previously healthy female presented with lower extremity weakness and numbness shortly after a gastrointestinal illness. Twelve days prior to admission, she had a self-limited episode of presumed viral gastroenteritis, with abdominal pain, diarrhea, and vomiting, but no reported fever, lasting 3 days. She recovered and was symptom-free until 5 days prior to admission, when she developed fever and malaise. Urinalysis was consistent with infection and she was treated with cefdinir and famotidine. Her malaise worsened and she developed intractable vomiting, however, so she was admitted for intravenous fluids and antibiotics. Upon admission, she began complaining of back pain and tingling in her feet. A few hours later, she described numbness and tingling in a band around her ribs that rapidly progressed to complete loss of sensation below the level of the nipple and paralysis of both legs. She had not urinated in over 24 h and had not had a bowel movement in 3 days. Following Foley catheterization, 1.5 L of urine was collected.

Examination revealed flaccid paraparesis with absent patellar, ankle, and plantar reflexes. She had a T10 sensory level with loss of all modalities (light touch, pinprick, temperature, and proprioception) in both lower extremities. All neurologic testing was intact in the cranial nerves and upper extremities. She had a microcytic anemia, elevated sedimentation rate of 113 (normal range 0–20), and elevated C-reactive protein of 5.6 (normal range 0–1.0) on admission labs. Serum chemistries, urinalysis, NMO antibody testing, CT, and ultrasound of the abdomen were normal. MRI of the spine and brain (Fig. 30.1a) demonstrated multiple sites of

A.L. Cardon, M.D., M.Sc • T.E. Lotze, M.D. (✉)
Division of Neurology and Developmental Neuroscience, Department of Pediatrics,
Baylor College of Medicine, Texas Children's Hospital, 6701 Fannon CC 1250,
Houston, TX 77030, USA
e-mail: aaron.cardon@bcm.edu; tlotze@bcm.edu

© Springer International Publishing AG 2017                                              233
E. Waubant, T.E. Lotze (eds.), *Pediatric Demyelinating Diseases of the Central Nervous System and Their Mimics*, DOI 10.1007/978-3-319-61407-6_30

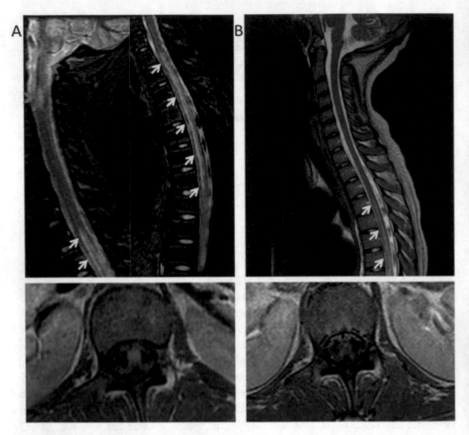

**Fig. 30.1** (a) Initial spinal and brainstem imaging—(*top*) sagittal T2-weighted images demonstrating dorsal medulla T2 hyperintensity (*green arrowhead*), expansion of the C2–C3 region with T2 hyperintensity (*green arrowhead*), and longitudinally extensive expansion and hyperintensity (*yellow arrows*) of the thoracic cord from the level of T1 downward. Each lesion also demonstrated enhancement on T1 post-gadolinium contrast imaging (not shown); (*bottom*) axial T1 post-contrast image from the lumbar spine, showing representative lack of enhancement or involvement of nerve roots. (b) Follow-up (day 21) spinal imaging—(*top*) sagittal T2-weighted images demonstrating resolution of cervicomedullary changes and improved thoracic hyperintensity (*yellow arrows*); (*bottom*) representative enhancement of ventral greater than dorsal lumbar nerve roots (*green arrows*), extensive throughout the lumbar spinal region.

enhancement restricted to the spinal cord and brainstem. Lumber puncture revealed neutrophilic pleocytosis, elevated protein and hypoglycorrhachia, and no oligoclonal banding (Table 30.1).

She was diagnosed with acute transverse myelitis and concurrently treated with 7 days of intravenous methylprednisolone (1 g daily) and six rounds of plasmapheresis, followed by an oral steroid taper. MRI of the spine repeated 3 weeks after presentation (Fig. 30.1b) revealed new enhancement of the cauda equina, dorsal and ventral lumbar nerve roots. Lumbar puncture was repeated with similar results but improved pleocytosis (Table 30.1). She was additionally found to have positive

**Table 30.1** Initial and follow-up testing in transverse myelitis with AIDP. Initial (admission) and follow-up (day 21) CSF and serum testing demonstrating CSF pleocytosis, hypoglycorrhachia, and negative oligoclonal banding consistent with transverse myelitis

|  | Admission | Day 21 | Normal range |
|---|---|---|---|
| Serum |  |  |  |
| Glucose | **150** | 77 | 70–100 |
| Vitamin D 25-OH (ng/mL) | **17** |  | ≥20 |
| C-reactive protein (mg/dL) | **5.6** | <0.5 | <1.0 |
| Sedimentation rate (mm/h) | **113** | 23 | 0–20 |
| ANA profile |  |  |  |
| Ds-DNA titer | **1:80** |  | Negative |
| FANA | **>1:1280** |  | Negative |
| SS-A antibody | Negative |  | Negative |
| SS-B antibody | Negative |  | Negative |
| Antiphospholipid antibodies |  |  |  |
| IgG cardiolipin | **High positive** |  | Negative |
| IgG phosphatidic acid | **High positive** |  | Negative |
| Cerebrospinal fluid |  |  |  |
| Glucose | **30** | **32** | >100 (2/3 × serum) |
| Protein | **240** | **153** | 15–45 |
| White blood cells (#/mm³) | **1225** | **14** | 0–5 |
| Neutrophils (%) | **90** | **5** | 0–2 |
| Red blood cells (#/mm³) | 595 | 220 |  |
| Oligoclonal bands | Negative | Negative | Negative |
| NMO antibody | <1.6 |  | <1.6 |

anti-neuronal cell antibody testing in CSF and serum. With serum testing positive for ANA, ds-DNA, antiphospholipid antibodies, and lupus anticoagulant (Table 30.1), a diagnosis of lupus/antiphospholipid antibody syndrome was established. Given this diagnosis, after completing plasmapheresis, she received intravenous immunoglobulin (2 g/kg divided over 3 days) and cyclophosphamide (750 mg/m² monthly for six doses). Electromyography/nerve conduction studies (EMG/NCS) at 3 weeks found absent motor unit potentials throughout bilateral lower extremities without abnormal spontaneous activity, absent bilateral peroneal and right tibial motor nerve responses, and normal upper extremity findings. Repeat EMG/NCV 6 weeks later was similar and further demonstrated profuse denervation potentials throughout all lower extremity muscles with a spinal level caudal to T8.

Due to continued fluctuating symptoms over 3 weeks after the start of therapy, she was treated with another course of intravenous immunoglobulin (2 g/kg divided over 3 days) and methylprednisolone (1 g daily for 5 days). After the diagnosis of lupus was established, she was started on aspirin (81 mg daily) and pentoxifylline (400 mg twice daily). Over the course of her 2-week inpatient treatment followed by 1-month rehabilitation stay, she reported improved sensation with a progressively improving spinal level and improved bladder control. Otherwise, she plateaued in symptom progression without ascending weakness but also without significant recovery of leg strength. With flaccid paralysis throughout both legs, she remained wheelchair-dependent for mobility but assisting in transfers and improving in wheelchair self-propelling at discharge. Over 3 years of follow-up, her deficits remained stable, and she did not present with any further episodes of demyelination (Fig. 30.1, Table 30.1).

## Clinical Reasoning Questions

1. What historical and/or examination features of this patient's initial presentation raise suspicion for demyelinating conditions other than transverse myelitis, e.g., Guillain-Barré syndrome (GBS)?
2. What is the association of transverse myelitis and other central demyelinating conditions with GBS? Is the presentation of overlapping central and peripheral demyelinating syndromes typically concurrent or sequential (i.e., relapsing)?
3. What serious or life-threatening systemic complications are common to both transverse myelitis and AIDP?
4. Are there specific prognostic indicators for outcomes in overlap syndromes? Is there evidence to support specific treatment regimens in overlap syndromes?

## Discussion

1. GBS, encompassing acute inflammatory demyelinating polyradiculopathy (AIDP) and acute motor axonal neuropathy (AMAN) and the variant Miller Fisher syndrome (MFS), represents the most frequent cause of acute flaccid paralysis in all age groups, with an incidence in Western countries of 1.1 per 100,000 person-years [1]. Recently proposed consensus diagnostic criteria (from the World Health Organization's Brighton collaboration) specify seven criteria whose presence converges to a high specificity (i.e., diagnostic certainty) for diagnosis of GBS. Validating these criteria in a large European adult cohort, sensitivity for a likely diagnosis (level 1 or 2 of certainty) was good at 96% [2]. Thus, in the appropriate clinical setting of a patient with acute flaccid paralysis and areflexia, without history or initial labs suggestive of classic infectious, autoimmune, or systemic mimicking conditions (e.g., poliomyelitis, botulism, myasthenia gravis, hypokalemia, or myopathy), a diagnosis of GBS is most likely given its prevalence.

   Acute transverse myelitis (TM), in contrast, is a relatively rare central demyelinating syndrome, with an estimated annual incidence of one to four cases per million person-years. With bimodal peaks in the second and fourth decades of life, ~20% of all cases occur in pediatric patients [3]. Consensus diagnostic criteria from the American Academy of Neurology (AAN) for TM include bilateral and progressive sensory, motor, or autonomic dysfunction attributable to the spinal cord, with evidence of inflammation and exclusion of compressive lesions in the spinal cord [4]. In up to 84% of cases of TM, a proximate cause or defined syndrome (e.g., multiple sclerosis, parainfectious myelitis, neuromyelitis optica, or systemic autoimmune disease) may be identified by history or initial work-up [5] which will guide further treatment to prevent recurrent attacks or other complications of the underlying disease. Therefore, after emergent contrast-enhanced spinal imaging to exclude compressive lesions, further work-up for transverse myelitis should include brain imaging and serum and CSF testing to identify typical findings of TM and to exclude alternative diagnoses. Isolated pediatric TM is discussed further in Chap. 28 [6].

Each of the aforementioned criteria was developed and proposed with explicit goals including establishing a uniform nosology and standardizing future research. They are best used clinically while keeping in mind their principal limitation, namely, a risk of low sensitivity for atypical or early presentations of disease. Such restrictive criteria are very useful in increasing specificity to differentiate similar conditions, as illustrated by their comparison in Table 30.2. Thus, while signs and symptoms of the conditions overlap, patterns of disease presentation for AIDP and TM contrast overall, making the exclusion of one or the other typically evident after appropriate investigation. CSF pleocytosis, significant asymmetry in weakness, and a clearly defined sensory level are uncommon in AIDP, whereas the absence of spinal reflexes and an ascending symmetric pattern of weakness or sensory loss would decrease suspicion for TM. Imaging and nerve conduction studies assist in further clarifying the diagnosis with typical patterns for each disease (Table 30.2).

2. TM and GBS have been rarely reported to co-occur, usually as single case reports either post-infection or postvaccination [7, 8] which give no clear indication of overall prevalence. Recently, by compiling and analyzing 66 previously published cases in the English literature, Mao and Hu published the largest case cohort yet available of overlapping GBS and acquired demyelinating syndromes (ADS) of the central nervous system [9]. Prodromal infection was common (up to 70%), and overlap syndromes typically presented concurrently (85% manifested both GBS and ADS within 4 weeks of initial symptoms). This pattern held for 21 cases of overlapping GBS/TM, which was the most common subtype (32%) of co-occurring ADS reported. TM diagnosis usually preceded or was simultaneous to diagnosis of GBS; only three patients (14%) were initially diagnosed with GBS, and only two patients (10%) had delay to secondary diagnosis of 10 days or more. In keeping with the common presenting symptoms of TM and GBS, paralysis or paresis was present in all 21 patients (100%), and sensory deficit and urinary disturbances were each present in 18 patients (86%).

GBS was further classified in the series to Miller Fisher syndrome (MFS) versus non-MFS. All 21 patients with TM/GBS were classified as non-MFS, though further classification (i.e., AIDP vs. AMAN) was not specified. The series also excluded all cases with evidence of vasculitis, granulomatous disease, and

**Table 30.2** Comparative features by history, examination, and diagnostic testing for the diagnosis of Guillain-Barré syndrome versus idiopathic acute transverse myelitis (adapted from the Brighton criteria [2] and AAN Transverse Myelitis Working Group [5])

|  | Guillain-Barré syndrome | Idiopathic acute transverse myelitis |
|---|---|---|
| History | Bilateral flaccid limb weakness (typically ascending) | Bilateral (not necessarily symmetric) sensory, motor, or autonomic dysfunction localizing to spinal cord |
|  | Symptom onset → nadir between 12H and 28D | Symptom onset → nadir between 4H and 21D |
| Exam | Diminished DTRs in weak limbs | Clearly defined sensory level DTRs can be increased or decreased in weak limbs |
| Laboratory/diagnostic studies | ± CSF pleocytosis, <50 cells/μL ↑ CSF protein (± cytoalbuminological dissociation) nerve conduction subtypes: Demyelinating polyneuropathy Axonal polyneuropathy Inexcitable | + CSF pleocytosis *or* + CSF elevated IgG index *or* MRI with spinal cord Gd enhancement (i.e., *inflammation within the spinal cord*) |
| Other/exclusion | Absence of alternative diagnosis | Exclusions: Radiation to the spine ≤10 years prior; arterial distribution clinical deficit; abnormal flow voids on spinal surface; evidence of connective tissue disease[a]; CNS viral manifestations (e.g., HIV, HTLV-1, HSV, VZV, EBV, etc.)[a]; brain MRI suggests multiple sclerosis[a]; history of optic neuritis[a] |

Refer to text for further discussion of the application of these criteria in establishing varying levels of diagnostic certainty

[a]Does not exclude disease-associated acute transverse myelitis

metabolic disorders and therefore may underrepresent disease-associated overlap syndromes, including GBS/TM. Thus, regardless of the actual incidence of post-infectious or "idiopathic" GBS/TM overlap, a high index of suspicion for disease-associated demyelination must be maintained in overlap syndrome cases, prompting investigation for infectious and systemic underlying causes. Regarding our patient, the association of systemic lupus erythematosus and demyelinating diseases is further explored here in Chap. 33.

3. Respiratory distress and autonomic dysfunction are common in both GBS and TM. Similarly, in Mao and Hu's cohort, 29% and 24% of patients with GBS/TM overlap had respiratory and autonomic dysfunction, respectively. Such high incidence of respiratory involvement and autonomic instability underscores the importance of vigilant monitoring and early intervention to prevent irreversible negative

outcomes. Both TM and GBS typically progress in a monophasic fashion, but the progression from onset to nadir of symptoms is variable, ranging from 4 h to 28 days [1, 2]. Frequent neurologic exams and cardiopulmonary monitoring in the initial treatment period of either condition are needed until it is established that there is no further clinical progression. Other complications such as urinary retention and constipation should be aggressively monitored and treated, and early individualized rehabilitation is essential to maximize functional outcomes [1].

4. Pharmacological treatment of GBS with intravenous immunoglobulin was demonstrated in adults to have similar outcomes to plasmapheresis. It is thus generally first recommended given its availability and favorable side effect profile. Steroids have not been found to effectively accelerate recovery or improve outcomes in GBS [1]. For TM, in contrast, class II evidence indicates the possible effectiveness of plasmapheresis for acute fulminating CNS demyelinating diseases unresponsive to high-dose corticosteroids; although only class IV studies have evaluated the effectiveness of steroids for TM specifically, they are typically offered initially for cases without a fulminant course [5, 6]. As there are no data from a standardized approach to treating patients with ADS/GBS overlap syndromes, a combination of treatments as indicated for the conditions independently, as used for our patient, is suggested as prudent at this time. Similarly, Mao and Hu [9] report that immunotherapy, "mostly prednisone and intravenous immunoglobulin," was prescribed in 85% of cases.

In their compiled series of overlap syndromes, Mao and Hu identified the presence of a sensory level as predictive of poor outcome [9]. However, with poor outcome defined as functional dependence and inability to ambulate independently, this is likely more reflective of the particular subtype of ADS than specifically related to sensory involvement; accordingly, patients with GBS/TM were among those most likely to have a sensory level (86%), and all manifested either paralysis or paresis. Overall, the functional outcome was good in 55% of patients with GBS/TM, with no patients dying from complications in the acute period.

## Clinical Pearls

- GBS and TM present with similar signs and symptoms; although careful examination and laboratory testing and imaging distinguish these clinical syndromes, overlapping central and peripheral demyelinating syndromes have been reported.
- The presentation of overlapping syndromes may represent disease-associated myelitis, and chronic diseases such as multiple sclerosis and lupus should be considered and investigated.
- The course of illness in GBS/TM overlap most often followed that of the independent syndromes, with early secondary diagnosis and progression to nadir within 30 days.

- Overlap syndromes should be regarded and treated with similar caution as their individual conditions, including close monitoring for and early treatment of respiratory compromise, autonomic instability, urinary retention, and bowel dysfunction.

# References

1. Sejvar JJ, Baughman AL, Wise M, Morgan OW. Population incidence of Guillain-Barré syndrome: a systematic review and meta-analysis. Neuroepidemiology. 2011;36:123–33.
2. Fokke C, van den Berg B, Drenthen J, Walgaard C, van Doorn PA, Jacobs BC. Diagnosis of Guillain-Barré syndrome and validation of Brighton criteria. Brain. 2014;137(1):33–43.
3. Berman M, Feldman S, Alter M, Zilber N, Kahana E. Acute transverse myelitis incidence and etiologic considerations. Neurology. 1981;31(8):966–71.
4. Group TMCW. Proposed diagnostic criteria and nosology of acute transverse myelitis. Neurology. 2002;59(4):499–505.
5. Scott TF, Frohman EM, Seze JD, Gronseth GS, Weinshenker BG. Evidence-based guideline: clinical evaluation and treatment of transverse myelitis report of the Therapeutics and Technology Assessment Subcommittee of the American Academy of Neurology. Neurology. 2011;77(24):2128–34.
6. Wolf VL, Lupo PJ, Lotze TE. Pediatric acute transverse myelitis overview and differential diagnosis. J Child Neurol. 2012;27(11):1426–36.
7. Sindern E, Schröder JM, Krismann M, Malin JP. Inflammatory polyradiculoneuropathy with spinal cord involvement and lethal [correction of letal] outcome after hepatitis B vaccination. J Neurol Sci. 2001;186(1–2):81–5.
8. Bajaj NP, Rose P, Clifford-Jones R, Hughes PJ. Acute transverse myelitis and Guillain-Barré overlap syndrome with serological evidence for mumps viraemia. Acta Neurol Scand. 2001;104(4):239–42.
9. Mao Z, Hu X. Clinical characteristics and outcomes of patients with Guillain-Barré and acquired CNS demyelinating overlap syndrome: a cohort study based on a literature review. Neurol Res. 2014;36(12):1106–13.

# Chapter 31
# Acute Flaccid Myelitis

Stephanie Morris, Young-Min Kim, Emmanuelle Waubant,
Keith Van Haren, and Soe S. Mar

## Case Presentation

**Case 1** A previously healthy 7-year-old girl presented to medical care after 5 days of progressive dysarthria, dysphagia, and weakness of her upper extremities. On the day of presentation, she developed a fever to 38.3 °C, posterior neck pain, and dyspnea. No bladder or bowel symptoms were noted. On physical exam, she was alert and attentive but had absent palatal rise, absent shoulder shrug, and asymmetric weakness in her proximal upper extremities. She had 0/5 strength in her proximal left arm and 1/5 strength in her proximal right arm while maintaining at least 3/5 strength distal to the elbow bilaterally with left hand strength more affected than the

S. Morris, M.D.
Department of Neurology, Washington University School of Medicine in St. Louis,
660 South Euclid Avenue, Campus Box 8111, St. Louis, MO, 63110, USA
e-mail: morris.s@wustl.edu

Y.-M. Kim, M.D.
Department of Pediatrics, Loma Linda University School of Medicine,
11175 Campus, St. Loma Linda, CA 92350, USA
e-mail: ymkim@llu.edu

E. Waubant, M.D., Ph.D.
Clinical Neurology and Pediatrics, Regional Pediatric MS Clinic at UCSF,
University of California San Francisco, 675 Nelson Rising Lane, Suite 221,
San Francisco, CA 94158, USA
e-mail: Emmanuelle.waubant@ucsf.edu

K. Van Haren, M.D.
Department of Neurology, Lucile Packard Children's Hospital and Stanford University
School of Medicine, 750 Welch Road, Suite 317, Palo Alto, CA 94304, USA
e-mail: kpv@stanford.edu

S.S. Mar, M.D. (✉)
Department of Neurology, Washington University School of Medicine, St. Louis, MO, USA
e-mail: mars@wustl.edu

© Springer International Publishing AG 2017
E. Waubant, T.E. Lotze (eds.), *Pediatric Demyelinating Diseases of the Central
Nervous System and Their Mimics*, DOI 10.1007/978-3-319-61407-6_31

right. She had normal power in her lower extremities. Sensation to all modalities was intact, and reflexes were absent at the biceps bilaterally, trace at the triceps bilaterally, and normal in the bilateral lower extremities with flexor plantar responses. She required endotracheal intubation for airway protection and required ventilation for respiratory failure due to diaphragmatic weakness.

The patient underwent magnetic resonance imaging (MRI) of her brain and spine that showed a longitudinally extensive, T2-hyperintense, non-enhancing lesion extending from the cervicomedullary junction to the level of C7 preferentially affecting the gray matter with expansion of the cervical cord (Fig. 31.1). Cerebrospinal fluid (CSF) analysis showed mixed pleocytosis, elevated protein, and normal glucose (Table 31.1). Rhino-/enterovirus was detected via polymerase chain reaction (PCR) from a nasopharyngeal specimen, but analysis of CSF, enteric, and serum samples did not detect a pathogenic organism or disease-specific antibodies. Electromyography and nerve conduction study (EMG-NCS) performed 1 week after initial symptoms showed very small median and ulnar compound muscle action potential (CMAP) amplitudes with normal distal latency and conduction velocities. There was decreased recruitment of the left vastus medialis and tibialis anterior and absent fibrillations and absent positive sharp waves (PSWs). Sensory nerve studies were normal.

The patient was treated with ten cycles of plasmapheresis and concomitant IV methylprednisolone (30 mg/kg/day for 5 days) followed by IV immunoglobulins

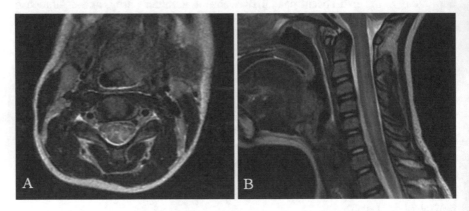

**Fig. 31.1** Cervical cord MRI from a 7-year-old girl with acute flaccid myelitis. (**a**) Axial T2-weighted image shows hyperintensity within the central gray matter of the spinal cord. (**b**) Sagittal T2-weighted image demonstrates longitudinally extensive lesion extending from the cervicomedullary junction to the level of C7 with expansion of the spinal cord

**Table 31.1** CSF results from the three cases

| Case | WBC (differential) | Protein (mg/dL) | Glucose (mg/dL) | IgG index | Oligoclonal bands |
|------|--------------------|------------------|------------------|-----------|-------------------|
| 1 | 179 (42% lymphocytes, 37% PMN, 21% monocytes) | 63 | 52 | Normal | Negative |
| 2 | 81 (55% lymphocytes, 33% PMN) | 31 | 53 | Normal | Negative |
| 3 | 3 (100% lymphocytes) | 35 | 63 | Normal | Negative |

(IVIG) (2 g/kg over 2 days) without notable improvement. After 2 months of intensive neuro-rehabilitation, she was weaned off of all respiratory support and had improvements in her head control (3/5 neck extension) and truncal stabilization via thoracolumbosacral orthosis (TLSO), which allowed her to ambulate, but she persisted to have hypernasal speech, swallowing dysfunction, and an elevated hemidiaphragm in addition to persistent flaccid weakness of her proximal upper extremities. She required a gastrostomy tube for chronic nutritional supplementation. Upon follow-up at 5 months after symptom onset, she had appreciable improvement in her elbow flexion bilaterally (both 3/5) via the use of her brachioradialis although deltoid and bicep activation was persistently absent.

**Case 2** A previously healthy 9-year-old boy presented to medical care after 4 days of fever, rhinorrhea, and pharyngitis with left arm weakness that progressed into flaccid paralysis within 48 h with a proximal predominance (proximally 1–2/5, distally 3/5). The day before the motor deficit, the patient had developed neck and left shoulder pain. Deep tendon reflexes were absent only in the left arm but normal otherwise. Sensation to all modalities was intact. The remainder of the neurologic exam was normal.

Blood test results were within normal range, except for the elevated neutrophils at 74% with a normal white blood cell (WBC) count. Spinal fluid analysis showed a lymphocytic pleocytosis (Table 31.1). An extensive evaluation for infection, including CSF PCR enterovirus, HSV1 and HSV2, serum qualitative *B. burgdorferi* antibodies, West Nile virus IgM, stool culture for enterovirus, and HTLV antibodies, was negative except for an elevated qualitative IgM titer for *Mycoplasma pneumoniae*. Mycoplasma infection was not confirmed. A rheumatologic evaluation and neuromyelitis optica (NMO) antibodies were also negative. The presence of polio antibodies suggested a lifelong immunity consistent with the patient's history of polio vaccination. Spine MRI showed a left-sided, longitudinally extensive T2 hyperintensity mainly affecting the gray matter between C4 and T1 without contrast enhancement (Fig. 31.2). Brain MRI was normal.

The patient was treated with methylprednisolone (20 mg/kg IV) for 7 days followed by IVIG (2 g/kg over 4 days). He was discharged on a 4-week oral steroid taper and started physiotherapy, occupational therapy, and electrical stimulations. After failing to mount a recovery at 2 months after symptom onset, the patient underwent a 7-day course of plasma exchange without appreciable benefit. Three months after symptom onset, he demonstrated marginal improvement in biceps (2–3/5) and hand (4–/5) function. Nine months after onset, electromyography (EMG) showed evidence of a motor neuronopathy affecting the left C5 > C6 > C7 myotomes with ongoing denervation. Ten months after onset, he still could not raise his left arm. Eighteen months after onset, the patient began to show improvement in proximal strength (3–4–/5).

**Case 3** A 16-year-old boy with a medical history notable only for asthma and eczema developed progressive numbness and tingling that began in his hands and traveled upward to include his arms and torso over the span of several days. Shortly after the onset of paresthesias, he developed progressive myalgias followed by progressive weakness in both arms. He also noted abrupt loss of bladder control. He denied preceding illnesses or sick contacts. Upon admission, he had a high thoracic sensory level, brisk reflexes at the left bicep, and diffuse weakness in all extremities.

**Fig. 31.2** Sagittal (**a**) and axial (**b**) T2-weighted images showing hyperintensity within the gray matter at C4–C5 with expansion of the cord

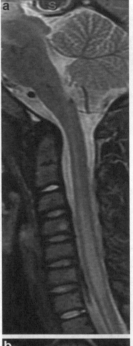

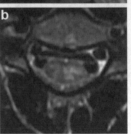

A cervical spine MRI revealed a cervical cord lesion affecting primarily the central gray matter but with involvement of adjacent white matter tracts (Fig. 31.3). CSF analysis showed normal WBC, glucose, and protein (Table 31.1). Infectious studies were unrevealing. Anti-aquaporin 4 antibody was negative. He was started on treatment presumptively for autoimmune myelitis with high-dose IV solumedrol (1000 mg IV daily), but after 3 days of treatment, his weakness progressed, he lost all spinal reflexes, his tone became flaccid, and he was intubated due to inability to protect his airway. Repeat imaging revealed enlargement and new enhancement of the cervical cord lesion. He was subsequently treated with plasmapheresis (1.5× volume exchange with 5% albumin over three sessions) followed by IVIG (2 g/kg divided over 3 days). His course was complicated by autonomic dysregulation, urinary retention, and prolonged intubation. After approximately 30 days of persistent, flaccid tetraparesis, he began mounting an abrupt motor recovery beginning in the distal extremities. Within 7 days, he was extubated, was able to stand, and was discharged to an acute rehab

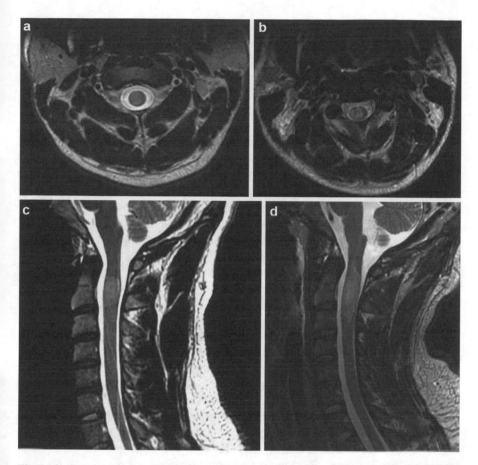

**Fig. 31.3** Both the initial (**a**, **c**) and follow-up (**b**, **d**) MRIs revealed mixed gray matter and white matter involvement

facility. Approximately 60 days after his initial onset of weakness, outpatient follow-up was notable for normal mental status and sensory exam with diminished reflexes and 4+/5 strength that was continuing to improve in all extremities.

## Clinical Questions

1. What are the clinical features of acute flaccid myelitis?
2. What ancillary studies can help differentiate anterior horn cell-specific myelitis?
3. What are the available treatment options?
4. What is known about the prognosis of acute flaccid myelitis?
5. What are potential etiologies of acute flaccid myelitis?

## *What Are the Clinical Features of Acute Flaccid Myelitis?*

Acute flaccid myelitis (AFM) is a poliomyelitis-like syndrome marked by manifestations of acute anterior horn cell disease. Poliomyelitis (*polio* meaning "gray" and *myelitis* referring to inflammation of the spinal cord) is an infectious disease of the spinal gray matter caused by the poliovirus, which preferentially affects the anterior horn cells of the spinal gray matter. It is caused by direct infection and replication of the poliovirus within the anterior horn cells leading to permanent destruction of lower motor neurons. Classically, as in poliomyelitis, AFM presents as an acute onset of painful asymmetric upper and/or lower extremity weakness with associated lower motor neuron signs including decreased tone and diminished (or absent) deep tendon reflexes. It typically presents without subsequent development of upper motor neuron signs such as increased tone and hyperreflexia. Motor deficits are typically proximal. Although sensory deficits may occur in AFM, they are typically minor in comparison to the motor deficits.

The extent of longitudinal cord involvement varies from one patient to the other, and the overall severity of the deficit is defined in the acute phase with a nadir typically reached within 48–72 h. Bulbar and cervical cord involvement can lead to dysarthria, swallowing dysfunction, and respiratory muscle weakness, which can be acutely life-threatening. Typically, neurological symptom onset is accompanied or preceded by a viral prodrome, which may include fever, headache, malaise, myalgias, nuchal rigidity, upper respiratory tract symptoms, and gastrointestinal symptoms. The frequency of encephalopathy, autonomic instability, and sphincter involvement in AFM have not yet been definitively established [1].

Due to the considerable overlap of presenting signs and symptoms, differentiating AFM from other causes of acute flaccid paralysis can be difficult during the early course of the illness. A broad differential diagnosis including acute idiopathic transverse myelitis, acute disseminated encephalomyelitis (ADEM), multiple sclerosis (MS), neuromyelitis optica (NMO), and acute inflammatory demyelinating polyradiculoneuropathy (AIDP) aka Guillain-Barre syndrome (GBS) should be considered, and attention should be given to arriving at an accurate and early diagnosis given the differences in acute treatment and long-term outcomes. In contrast to AFM, acute transverse myelitis typically presents with sensory loss below the affected spinal cord segment with the presence of a discrete spinal level; in addition, dysautonomia, bowel and bladder dysfunction, and eventual development of upper motor neuron signs characterize acute transverse myelitis. However, as Case 3 demonstrates, AFM may manifest upper motor neuron features that can appear more characteristic of transverse myelitis—although lower motor neuron signs should predominate. Furthermore, ADEM and NMO should be considered when the above signs and symptoms are accompanied by other neurologic signs including encephalopathy, cranial neuropathies, ataxia, and vision loss. AIDP/GBS is typified by a more subacute progression and an ascending pattern of weakness associated with sensory and autonomic disturbances.

## What Ancillary Studies Can Help Differentiate Anterior Horn Cell-Specific Myelitis?

In addition to obtaining a thorough history and performing a complete physical and neurologic examination, ancillary studies including CSF analysis, neuroimaging, and EMG-NCS can be useful in distinguishing AFM from other causes of acute flaccid paralysis. MRI with and without contrast of the brain and spine (cervical, thoracic, and lumbar) and EMG-NCS can provide localizing data pointing toward of anterior horn cell disease (Tables 31.2 and 31.3) [2, 3]. However, radiographic and electrophysiological findings can be non-specific in the early course. Therefore, a comprehensive evaluation should be pursued including further analysis of the CSF, serum, nasopharyngeal, and stool samples obtained at the time of presentation, some of which can be repeated at 6 weeks in coordination with the local Department of Health due to the time-dependent changes in antibody titers (Table 31.4).

## What Are the Available Treatment Options?

No effective treatment has been identified for AFM, and due to the relatively recent nature of the reemergence of pediatric cases in 2014, there is a dearth of evidence-based literature regarding optimal treatment. Therapies including high-dose IV corticosteroids, IVIG, interferon, and plasmapheresis have been tried empirically but have not demonstrated any consistent benefit in motor outcomes. This is likely due to irreversible anterior horn cell necrosis. Although case reports exist that document partial or complete recovery associated with immune-modulating therapies such as high-dose corticosteroids and IVIG, substantive evidence of treatment-related benefit is lacking [4, 5]. A consensus statement based on expert opinion released on November 7, 2014, from the Centers for Disease Control and Prevention (CDC) does not endorse the use of corticosteroids, IVIG, interferon, or plasmapheresis in the treatment of AFM due to the lack of data demonstrating efficacy. Corticosteroids may be helpful in treating cord edema, while it may also exacerbate an active viral infection by immunosuppression. Therefore, prompt and comprehensive evaluation to identify other possible etiologies including (but not limited to) acute transverse

**Table 31.2** Comparison of CSF findings

|  | CSF cell count (cells/mL) | CSF glucose | CSF protein | CSF oligoclonal bands |
|---|---|---|---|---|
| Acute flaccid myelitis | Moderately elevated (100–400) | Normal | Normal to mildly elevated | Negative |
| Acute transverse myelitis | Mildly elevated (<100) | Normal | Normal to mildly elevated | May be positive or negative |
| AIDP/GBS | Normal to mildly elevated (<50) | Normal | Moderately elevated | Negative |

**Table 31.3** Comparison of MRI and EMG-NCS findings

| | MRI | EMG-NCS |
|---|---|---|
| Acute flaccid myelitis | T2 hyperintensity affecting the central gray matter, typically non-enhancing, possibly isolated to anterior horns, commonly affecting brain stem and cervical spinal cord | 1–2 weeks: normal SNAPs, normal nerve conduction velocities, and small amplitude CMAPs<br>2–4 weeks: fibrillations and PSWs, reduced recruitment on EMG<br>>4 weeks: large duration and large amplitude CMAPs |
| Acute transverse myelitis | Poorly demarcated T2 hyperintensity, patchy enhancement, and cord thickening; may involve at least 2–3 spinal cord segments longitudinally or may be multifocal. Commonly affects cervicothoracic regions | Normal or reduced to absent recruitment on EMG |
| AIDP/GBS | Contrast enhancement and thickening of nerve roots within the cauda equina and surrounding the conus medullaris | <2 weeks: may be normal, earliest sign is reduced or absent H reflex<br>>2 weeks: prolonged F wave latency, reduced SNAPs, small CMAP amplitudes, delayed conduction velocities, temporal dispersion |

*SNAPs* sensory nerve action potentials, *CMAP* compound motor action potentials, *PSWs* positive sharp waves

**Table 31.4** Recommended investigations in suspected acute flaccid myelitis

| CSF | First tier: cell count, glucose, protein, culture; oligoclonal bands, IgG index, NMO (anti-aquaporin 4) Ab; PCR enterovirus, parechovirus, herpes simplex virus (HSV), cytomegalovirus (CMV), Epstein-Barr virus (EBV), human herpesvirus 6 (HHV-6), and human herpesvirus 7 (HHV-7); flow cytometry; cytology<br>Consider for second tier evaluation: arbovirus panel, mycoplasma Ab, paraneoplastic panel, anti-NMDA-receptor antibody, human T-lymphotropic virus 1 (HTLV-1) PCR |
|---|---|
| Serum | First tier: ANA, ENA, double-stranded DNA, ANCA, oligoclonal bands, IgG index, NMO (anti-aquaporin 4) Ab; mycoplasma antibodies (with convalescent titers after 4 weeks), arbovirus antibody panel, West Nile antibodies, Lyme testing<br>Consider for second tier evaluation: Aanti-NMDA receptor Ab, paraneoplastic panel |
| Nasopharyngeal | Viral multiplex swab |
| Stool | Enterovirus PCR |

myelitis, ADEM, MS, NMO, and AIDP/GBS is crucial given the proven efficacy of disease-specific immune-modulating therapies. At this time, supportive care and aggressive neuro-rehabilitation is the recommended treatment for AFM [6].

## What Is Known About the Prognosis of Acute Flaccid Myelitis?

Data describing the natural history and long-term prognosis of AFM are largely limited to case series and case reports that describe the long-term outcomes in acute flaccid myelitis cases associated with specific pathogens such as enterovirus 71 and West Nile virus. Even in these cases, the prognosis appears to be variable depending on the severity of the acute illness and ranges from complete motor recovery to substantial residual weakness with muscle atrophy, persistent bulbar dysfunction, and chronic respiratory failure [7]. The cases of AFM throughout the United States in 2014 without identified pathogens may represent a more heterogeneous group of anterior horn cell disease, and it remains unknown whether the available data regarding prognosis can be applied. Anecdotally, short-term motor recovery in these patients has been poor. The disease is thought to be monophasic.

## What Are Potential Etiologies of Acute Flaccid Myelitis?

Poliovirus is an enterovirus from the picornavirus family. Although the last case of wild poliomyelitis in the United States was documented to have occurred in 1979, four endemic locations (Afghanistan, India, Nigeria, and Pakistan) remain. Vaccine-associated paralytic poliomyelitis (VAPP) can occur (rate estimated at one case per 2.4 million doses administered) with administration of the oral polio vaccine (OPV), which is the vaccine of choice in endemic countries due to its ease of administration and superiority in conferring intestinal immunity. The inactivated polio vaccine (IPV) is routinely used alone in countries with high immunization coverage (>90%) and low risk of wild poliovirus importation and spread [8].

Since the eradication of poliovirus from the Western Hemisphere in 1991, several non-polio enteroviruses (such as types 68 and 71) and other viruses including West Nile virus, Japanese encephalitis virus, Epstein-Barr virus, echovirus type 4, and Coxsackie virus A and B have been linked to cases of acute flaccid paralysis. Although experts believe that AFM, like poliomyelitis, is due to active viral invasion and replication within the spinal cord, a specific pathogen has not been identified for the recent outbreak in the United States in 2014, which incidentally took place during an epidemic of enterovirus D68 [7].

## Clinical Pearls

1. Hallmark features of AFM include: rapid onset of asymmetric extremity weakness with a proximal predominance that typically nadirs in 2–3 days, decreased or flaccid tone, and absent deep tendon reflexes in affected extremities. Bulbar symptoms may occur, including dysphagia, dysarthria, and neurogenic respiratory failure.

2. Early comprehensive evaluation including CSF, serum, enteric, and nasopharyngeal specimen analysis, brain and spinal cord MRI, and EMG-NCS is critical for differentiating AFM from other treatable causes of acute flaccid paralysis.
3. There is no known effective treatment for AFM. Supportive treatment and aggressive neuro-rehabilitation are central to maximizing functional recovery.
4. Long-term outcomes are widely variable and range from complete motor recovery to permanent impairment.

# References

1. Ayscue P, Van Haren K, Sheriff H, et al. Acute flaccid paralysis with anterior myelitis—California, June 2012–June 2014. MMWR Morb Mortal Wkly Rep. 2014;63(40):903–6.
2. Sellner J, Luthi N, Schupbach WM, et al. Diagnostic workup of patients with acute transverse myelitis: spectrum of clinical presentation, neuroimaging, and laboratory findings. Spinal Cord. 2008;47:312–7.
3. Fokke C, Van Den Berg B, Drenthen J, et al. Diagnosis of Guillain-Barré syndrome and validation of brighton criteria. Brain. 2014;137(1):33–43.
4. Cohen HA, Ashkenasi A, Ring H, et al. Poliomyelitis-like syndrome following asthma attack (Hopkins' syndrome)—recovery associated with IV gamma globulin treatment. Infection. 1998;4:247–9.
5. Pyrgos V, Younus F. High-dose steroids in the management of acute flaccid paralysis due to West Nile virus infection. Scan J Infect Dis. 2004;36(6–7):509–12.
6. Acute flaccid myelitis: interim considerations for clinical management. Centers for Disease Control and Prevention Website. http://www.cdc.gov/ncird/investigation/viral/sep2014/hcp.html. Published November 7, 2014. Last Updated November 28, 2014. Accessed 5 Dec 2014.
7. Chang LY, Huang LM, Shur-Fen Gau S, et al. Neurodevelopment and cognition in children after enterovirus-71 infection. N Engl J Med. 2007;356:1226–34.
8. Poliomyelitis. World Health Organization Website. http://www.who.int/ith/vaccines/polio/en/. Accessed 4 Mar 2015.

# Chapter 32
# Neuromyelitis Optica Spectrum Disease with Transverse Myelitis Presentation

Wendy Vargas, Carlos Quintanilla Bordás, Carla Francisco, and Emmanuelle Waubant

## Case Presentations

**Case 1** A 9-year-old boy with a history of type 1 diabetes mellitus and Hashimoto's thyroiditis presented with acute onset of bilateral upper extremity and lower extremity numbness and weakness. On exam, he had proximal and distal weakness in bilateral upper and lower extremities as well as diminished sensation to light touch, pinprick, cold sensation, vibration, and proprioception. A C3 sensory level was present. He had clonus at the ankles and upgoing toes bilaterally. A contrast-enhanced MRI of the cervical spine showed hyperintense T2 signal from the cranio-cervical junction to the level of T1 with patchy gadolinium enhancement on T1 sequences (Fig. 32.1a, b). Brain MRI was normal. Lumbar puncture revealed a pleo-cytosis with 76 white cells (12% polymorphonuclear leukocytes). CSF protein and glucose were both within the normal range at 37 mg/dL and 67 mg/dL, respectively.

W. Vargas, M.D. (✉)
Department of Child Neurology, Morgan Stanley Children's Hospital of New York, Columbia University Medical Center, 180 Fort Washington Avenue, New York, NY 10032, USA
e-mail: wv2153@columbia.edu

C.Q. Bordás, M.D. (✉)
Department of Neurology, Servicio de Neurologia, Consorcio Hospital General Universitario de Valencia, Avenida Tres Cruces, 2, Valencia 46014, Spain
e-mail: carlosqb@gmail.com

C. Francisco, M.D.
Multiple Sclerosis and Neuroinflammation Center, University of California, San Francisco, San Francisco, CA, USA
e-mail: Carla.Francisco@ucsf.edu

E. Waubant, M.D., Ph.D.
Clinical Neurology and Pediatrics, Regional Pediatric MS Clinic at UCSF, University of California, San Francisco, 675 Nelson Rising Lane, Suite 221, San Francisco, CA 94158, USA
e-mail: Emmanuelle.waubant@ucsf.edu

© Springer International Publishing AG 2017
E. Waubant, T.E. Lotze (eds.), *Pediatric Demyelinating Diseases of the Central Nervous System and Their Mimics*, DOI 10.1007/978-3-319-61407-6_32

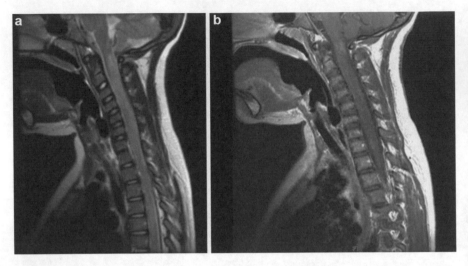

**Fig. 32.1** (a) T2-weighted MRI of the cervical spine demonstrating hyperintense T2 signal from the craniocervical junction to the level of T1; (b) T1-weighted MRI with contrast demonstrating patchy gadolinium enhancement

Oligoclonal bands were absent. Serum and CSF AQP4-IgG were negative. He was treated with IV methylprednisolone 30 mg/kg/day for 5 days followed by an oral prednisone taper over 4 weeks, and he gradually recovered completely without any residual neurologic deficits. He was diagnosed with idiopathic transverse myelitis.

Six months later, he again presented with acute quadriplegia, urinary retention, and complete sensory loss in the upper and lower extremities. A C5 sensory level was present on exam. MRI of the spine demonstrated a longitudinally extensive hyperintense T2 lesion with corresponding enhancement on T1 sequences extending from C4 to T1. Within a week of this presentation, he developed bilateral optic neuritis with bilateral optic nerve pallor noted on direct fundoscopy. Serum and CSF AQP4-IgG were again negative and brain MRI was normal. Dedicated orbital MRI was not performed. He was again treated with IV methylprednisolone 30 mg/kg/day for 5 days followed by an oral prednisone taper over 4 weeks. His vision, sensory, and urinary functions recovered to normal, but he had mild residual left lower extremity weakness. He was lost to follow up after this attack.

Five months later, he presented with recurrent quadriplegia secondary to another episode of acute transverse myelitis, with an associated longitudinally enhancing lesion from T4 to T10. His vision was not affected with this event. Serum and CSF AQP4-IgG remained negative. Additional testing for serum double-stranded DNA antibodies, Smith antibodies, ssA and ssB antibodies, and rheumatoid factor antibodies was negative, and angiotensin-converting enzyme levels were normal. Serum antithyroid peroxidase (TPO) antibodies and anti-glutamic acid decarboxylase (GAD) 65 antibodies were positive prior to the development of neurologic symptoms but were never identified in the CSF on testing at the time of his attacks.

He was diagnosed with an NMO spectrum disorder (NMOSD) after this third attack. He was initially treated with rituximab 750 mg/m$^2$ at weeks 0 and 2 and then every 6 months as an immunomodulatory treatment, but he developed anaphylaxis after the second dose of the initial infusion. He was subsequently treated with mycophenolate mofetil 1000 mg twice daily and has remained on this medication for 4 years. He has not had a relapse since going on immunomodulatory medication.

**Case 2** A 16-year-old previously healthy Caucasian female presented with approximately 2 weeks of fluctuating perineal and abdominal numbness, asymmetric bilateral leg numbness and paresthesias, urinary incontinence, and constipation. She went on to have severe weakness and gait difficulty and was admitted to the hospital. On admission she had left more than right leg weakness, with strength rated 1–3/5 bilaterally in the lower extremities. Her legs and ankles were cool to touch, and she had hyperreflexia in her lower extremities and positive Babinski signs bilaterally. MRI of the thoracic spine showed a lesion from T2 to T8 that was partially enhancing (Fig. 32.2a, b). A repeat MRI cervical/thoracic/lumbar spine 5 weeks later showed persistent T2–T8 hyperintensity that had not appreciably changed but much more avid T3–T7 dorsal cord enhancement (Fig. 32.2c, d). The lesion was initially suspected to be tumor. MRI of the brain was normal. The patient had a lumbar puncture with normal cell count, protein, and cytology and no oligoclonal bands (OCB). Aquaporin-4-immunoglobulin (AQP4-IgG) was positive at >1/160 titer, and she was then diagnosed with NMO. She was treated with intravenous methylprednisolone (IVMP) 1000 mg daily over 3 days, and then she underwent therapeutic plasma exchange (PE) four times every other day for 7 days. She was concomitantly started on mycophenolate mofetil that was titrated to a goal dose of 1000 mg twice a day. During the first day after plasma exchange, some improvement was noted; however, 3 weeks later, she developed increasing lower extremity weakness, urinary retention, and incontinence of stool. She had been on mycophenolate mofetil for only 1 week; thus, it was continued. She was given a further round of high-dose IVMP followed by another four rounds of PE every other day for 7 days. Three months later her examination showed decreased appreciation of light touch, vibration, and proprioception in toes of both feet. She had moderate to severe spasticity in the legs, right worse than left, with 3–4/5 grade weakness in lower extremities. She had normal upper limb reflexes but hyperreflexia in the lower limbs. Babinski sign was positive bilaterally. She could ambulate with a four-wheeled walker while dragging her right leg and was easily fatigued. Twenty-five-foot timed walk was performed in 53 s with the use of a four-wheeled walker. She had normal bladder function and daily bowel movements with the use of polyethylene glycol.

# Clinical Questions

1. In patients presenting with acute transverse myelitis, what ancillary studies are beneficial in prognosticating as to which children are more likely to have a recurrent course?
2. How do the current diagnostic criteria for NMOSD apply to these cases?
3. What acute and chronic treatment options are available for these patients?

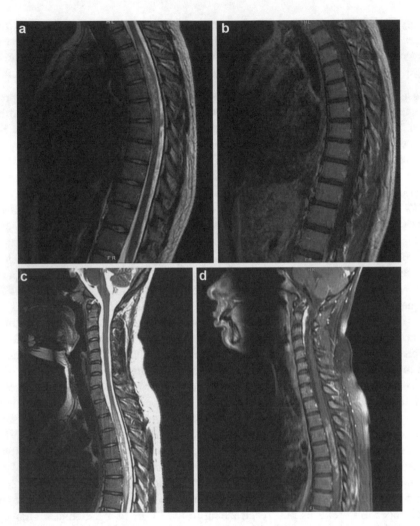

**Fig. 32.2** (**a**) T2-weighted MRI of the thoracic spine demonstrating a hyperintense lesion from T2 to T8; (**b**) T1-weighted MRI with contrast of thoracic spine at onset of symptoms demonstrating patchy enhancement from T2 to T8; (**c**) T2-weighted MRI of the lower cervical and upper thoracic spine approximately 5 weeks later showing persistent T2–T8 hyperintensity; (**d**) T1-weighted MRI with contrast of lower cervical and upper thoracic spine approximately 5 weeks later with more avid T3–T7 dorsal cord enhancement

4. What is the prognosis and what factors affect NMO with spinal cord involvement?

## Diagnostic Discussion

1. Children presenting with acute transverse myelitis can represent a diagnostic dilemma. It can be challenging to find a cause for their presentation and to prognosticate as to whether the initial event heralds the development of a relapsing disorder. In addition to the MRI of the total spine with and without gadolinium, which will be used to make the diagnosis of transverse myelitis, an MRI of the brain with and without gadolinium should be obtained. Imaging of the orbits should also be performed if there are historical or clinical findings suggestive of optic neuritis. This can help determine whether the child meets criteria for pediatric multiple sclerosis or if there are features more indicative of NMOSD. Imaging has become a principal method by which distinguishing patterns of disease can be used to differentiate between MS and NMOSD.

Brain lesions seen in pediatric MS are typically ovoid and perpendicular to the long axis of the corpus callosum and associated with T1 hypointensity [1]. Lesions of the optic pathway and spinal cord tend to be short and segmental, as opposed to the longer tracks of inflammation encountered in NMOSD.

In contrast to pediatric multiple sclerosis, hyperintense T2 lesions seen on brain MRI in pediatric NMOSD are most commonly located in aquaporin-4-rich areas of the brain. These include the periventricular region of the third ventricle (including hypothalamic and thalamic lesions), periventricular region of the fourth ventricle (including the medulla, midbrain, pons, and area postrema), periaqueductal gray matter, and parahippocampal regions. Periventricular lesions in NMOSD tend to have a broader base than those encountered in MS. In addition, lesions can be found in the corpus callosum, cerebral white matter, and juxtacortical white matter.

The characteristic spine MRI finding of longitudinally extensive transverse myelitis may be less specific for NMOSD in children. In a study investigating 87 children with inflammatory demyelination, longitudinally extensive transverse myelitis was found in 14% of the children with relapsing remitting multiple sclerosis [2]. Thus, a longitudinally extensive spinal cord lesion does not exclude the diagnosis of MS in children and is less predictive for NMOSD than in adult patients [3].

Cerebrospinal fluid findings in NMOSD include a pleocytosis often with a polymorphonuclear predominance in addition to elevated protein. In distinction from MS, the pleocytosis seen in the CSF of patients with NMOSD can sometimes be markedly high (>100 white cells) [4]. In contrast to pediatric multiple sclerosis where oligoclonal bands are seen in the cerebrospinal fluid of approximately 60% of children, only 6% of pediatric NMOSD patients have oligoclonal bands [5].

The astrocytic water channel, aquaporin-4 (AQP4), is the antigenic target of the pathogenic IgG autoantibody found in many patients with NMOSD [6]. Children presenting with acute transverse myelitis should undergo serum and CSF evaluation for AQP4-IgG. The detection of this antibody in serum or spinal fluid of children presenting with CNS inflammation is specific to NMOSD. In a study of 87 children with inflammatory demyelination, none of the 41 children with relapsing remitting multiple sclerosis were seropositive for AQP4-IgG, nor has it been identified in other acquired demyelinating syndromes [2]. However, this antibody may be negative in up to 30% of cases of children with NMOSD [7]. In addition, the use of steroids or other immunotherapies may mask the presence of the antibody. Therefore, the absence of the AQP4-IgG does not exclude an NMO spectrum disorder. In cases where there is strong clinical suspicion with initial negative testing, the antibody should be tested again in 6 months. Seropositivity for AQP4-IgG is not required to make a diagnosis of NMOSD, provided other criteria are met [8].

Other serum antibodies should be measured to evaluate for comorbid systemic autoimmune disease. In contrast to multiple sclerosis, autoimmune disorders and related antibodies are commonly found in patients with NMOSD. In one series of pediatric AQP4-IgG seropositive patients, coexisting autoimmune disorders were found in 42% of patients [5]. Among the identified disorders were systemic lupus erythematosus, Sjögren's syndrome, Graves disease, and juvenile rheumatoid arthritis. In addition, other serum autoantibodies suggestive (but not diagnostic) of coexisting autoimmunity were detected in 76% of patients. These antibody findings included antinuclear antibodies, extractable nuclear antigen antibodies, neural specific antibodies, and thyroid antibodies [5]. As noted in Case 1, the patient had comorbid diabetes mellitus and autoimmune thyroid disease with associated seropositive antibody titers. AQP4-IgG has not been identified in patients with systemic lupus erythematosus or Sjögren's syndrome except for those meeting diagnostic criteria for NMOSD. This finding is consistent with NMOSD being a distinct disorder rather than a complication of systemic autoimmune disease [9].

2. The 2015 international consensus diagnostic criteria for NMOSD can be used for evaluating pediatric cases [10]. In considering these criteria, Case 1 illustrates the difficulty of diagnosing seronegative disease upon initial presentation. With this patient's first manifestation of transverse myelitis, he did not meet criteria for NMO spectrum disorder [10]. However, despite having a negative AQP4-IgG titer, he presented with recurrent episodes of longitudinally extensive acute transverse myelitis, bilateral optic neuritis, and a brain MRI that was not diagnostic for multiple sclerosis. Thus, upon his subsequent attacks, he was diagnosed with NMO spectrum disorder and began immunomodulatory treatment. In contrast, Case 2 tested positive for the NMO antibody at the time of her initial presentation, meeting diagnostic criteria for NMOSD at the time of the first clinical event.

Of note, Case 1 had the finding of optic nerve pallor at the time of his second attack, which could be suggestive of a prior history of subclinical optic neuritis. This finding might prompt earlier initiation of immunomodulatory treatment in suspected NMOSD patients presenting with seemingly isolated transverse myelitis. In fact, this patient would have been offered immunomodulatory treatment after his second attack when he met clinical criteria for NMOSD, but he was unfortunately lost to follow up. In the absence of a positive aquaporin-4 antibody test, a child having an initial presentation or subsequent relapses consistent with NMO spectrum disorder should be offered treatment with a preventative therapy to reduce the chance of further potentially disabling attacks. Children with a single attack consistent with NMOSD who are AQP4-IgG positive should also be offered preventative treatment given that the antibody is predictive of a relapsing course [2].

3. Patients with an acute demyelinating attack, irrespective of the cause, should be treated without delay. The mainstay of treatment for an attack includes high-dose intravenous corticosteroids and plasmapheresis. Plasmapheresis may be particularly useful in the setting of an antibody-mediated disease, such as NMOSD. However, there are no randomized trials for treatment, and information is based on limited uncontrolled retrospective studies and expert opinions. Typical practice includes methylprednisolone 30 mg/kg/dose given intravenously daily for 3–5 days, with a maximum dose of 1 g/day. If response is poor over the course of this treatment or if symptoms progress in the midst of this treatment, then plasmapheresis should be initiated. Typically, pheresis of one plasma volume is performed every other day for a total of five to six exchanges. This number of treatments allows for near complete filtration of pathogenic antibodies from the serum.

Given the severity of residual disability produced by the neuroinflammation in NMOSD attack, long-term immunomodulatory treatment is indicated. Though there are no specific guidelines, rituximab, azathioprine, and mycophenolate mofetil have been used with success. Daily oral prednisone (1 mg/kg/day) is usually initiated with a transition to a steroid-sparing agent. Before starting azathioprine, patients should be tested for thiopurine methyltransferase deficiency, as lower levels of this enzyme may potentiate toxicity. The usual target dosage is 2.5–3 mg/kg/day. Mycophenolate mofetil is typically dosed at 600 mg/m$^2$/dose or 15 mg/kg/dose twice daily to a maximum of 1000 mg twice daily. Rituximab can be given at 375 mg/m$^2$/dose (maximum of 1000 mg) weekly for 4 weeks or 750 mg/m$^2$/dose (maximum of 1000 mg) for two doses separated by 2 weeks, with booster dosing given every 6 months or depending on recovering CD19/20 B cell counts. When side effects, medication failure, or compliance issues arise, an alternative medication from the list of three should be initiated. Adequate dosing should be ensured to prevent treatment failure. Parents should be counseled on the long-term side effects of corticosteroids and immunosuppressants.

4. NMO has a relapsing course in over 90% of patients, typically presenting with severe recurrent attacks of LETM, ON, or both [11]. Recovery from attacks is variable, and disability usually accumulates with recurrent attacks, leading to a stepwise decline in visual, motor, sensory, and bladder function. Children have been reported to have better outcome than adults. However, outcomes in children with NMOSD can be more severe than in children with multiple sclerosis [5]. In

a study of 48 children with NMOSD with a median of 12 months of follow-up, 54% had visual impairment, 54% had motor impairment, and 12% had urinary difficulties [5]. Antibody status seems to influence rate of relapses. In the UK national cohort of pediatric patients, time to relapse for antibody-positive patients was 0.76 years vs. 2.4 years in antibody-negative cases [12]. Younger age also seems to set a higher risk for optic neuritis and visual disability. On the other hand, motor outcomes are worse in older-onset patients, suggesting a diminished capability of spinal cord repair in these patients. Conversely, monophasic courses in seronegative patients appear to have excellent outcomes. These prognostic data underline the importance of starting disease-modifying therapy in patients who are likely to have a recurrent course. In a recent French multicenter retrospective study with long-term data available on 12 pediatric patients with a median follow-up of 19 years, the median times to reach expanded disability status scores of 4 and 6 were 20.7 and 26 years, respectively, which were significantly longer when compared to adults [13].

## Clinical Pearls

1. The presence of the AQP4-IgG is predictive of a relapsing course, and long-term treatment should be started to prevent further disabling attacks.
2. The absence of AQP4-IgG does not rule out an NMO spectrum disorder, and children who meet diagnostic criteria for NMOSD should be offered long-term preventative treatment.
3. Systemic autoimmune disorders are commonly seen in pediatric patients with NMO spectrum disorders. These include systemic lupus erythematosus, Sjögren's disease, juvenile rheumatoid arthritis, and thyroid disorders.
4. Rituximab, azathioprine, and mycophenolate mofetil have been used with success in the prevention of relapses for pediatric NMO and NMO spectrum disorder.

## References

1. Verhey LH, Branson HM, Shroff MM, Callen DJ, Sled JG, Narayanan S, et al. MRI parameters for prediction of multiple sclerosis diagnosis in children with acute CNS demyelination: a prospective national cohort study. Lancet Neurol. 2011;10(12):1065–73.
2. Banwell B, Tenembaum S, Lennon VA, Ursell E, Kennedy J, Bar-Or A, et al. Neuromyelitis optica-IgG in childhood inflammatory demyelinating CNS disorders. Neurology. 2008;70(5):344–52.
3. Wingerchuk DM, Lennon VA, Pittock SJ, Lucchinetti CF, Weinshenker BG. Revised diagnostic criteria for neuromyelitis optica. Neurology. 2006;66(10):1485–9.

4. Jarius S, Paul F, Franciotta D, Ruprecht K, Ringelstein M, Bergamaschi R, et al. Cerebrospinal fluid findings in aquaporin-4 antibody positive neuromyelitis optica: results from 211 lumbar punctures. J Neurol Sci. 2011;306(1–2):82–90.
5. McKeon A, Lennon VA, Lotze T, Tenenbaum S, Ness JM, Rensel M, et al. CNS aquaporin-4 autoimmunity in children. Neurology. 2008;71(2):93–100.
6. Lennon VA, Wingerchuk DM, Kryzer TJ, Pittock SJ, Lucchinetti CF, Fujihara K, et al. A serum autoantibody marker of neuromyelitis optica: distinction from multiple sclerosis. Lancet. 2004;364(9451):2106–12.
7. Tillema JM, McKeon A. The spectrum of neuromyelitis optica (NMO) in childhood. J Child Neurol. 2012;27(11):1437–47.
8. Wingerchuk DM, Banwell B, Bennett JL, Cabre P, Carroll W, Chitnis T, et al. International consensus diagnostic criteria for neuromyelitis optica spectrum disorders. Neurology. 2015;85(2):177–89.
9. Pittock SJ, Lennon VA, de Seze J, Vermersch P, Homburger HA, Wingerchuk DM, et al. Neuromyelitis optica and non organ-specific autoimmunity. Arch Neurol. 2008;65(1):78–83.
10. Krupp LB, Tardieu M, Amato MP, Banwell B, Chitnis T, Dale RC, et al. International Pediatric Multiple Sclerosis Study Group criteria for pediatric multiple sclerosis and immune-mediated central nervous system demyelinating disorders: revisions to the 2007 definitions. Mult Scler. 2013;19(10):1261–7.
11. Mealy MA, Wingerchuk DM, Greenberg BM, Levy M. Epidemiology of neuromyelitis optica in the United States: a multicenter analysis. Arch Neurol. 2012 Sep 1;69(9):1176–80.
12. Kitley J, Leite MI, Nakashima I, Waters P, McNeillis B, Brown R, et al. Prognostic factors and disease course in aquaporin-4 antibody-positive patients with neuromyclitis optica spectrum disorder from the United Kingdom and Japan. Brain. 2012;135(6):1834–49.
13. Collongues N, Marignier R, Zephir H, Papeix C, Fontaine B, Blanc F, et al. Long-term follow-up of neuromyelitis optica with a pediatric onset. Neurology. 2010;75(12):1084–8.

# Chapter 33
# Transverse Myelitis in Lupus

Maryam Nabavi Nouri and E. Ann Yeh

## Case Presentation

A 15-year-old girl with a known diagnosis of systemic lupus erythematosus (SLE) presented with difficulty walking and urinary incontinence. She was diagnosed with SLE at age 10 based on the following features: malar rash, photosensitivity, arthritis and hypocomplementemia. Her autoantibody profile was positive for anti-dsDNA, ANA, anti-RNP, and anti-Sm. She was maintained on 500 mg of hydroxychloroquine and 7.5 mg of prednisone daily and had achieved adequate disease control. At current presentation, she reported a self-limited gastrointestinal illness followed 2 weeks later by difficulty voiding and stooling. This progressed quickly to bilateral lower extremity weakness and total anesthesia of her legs up to her umbilicus. She also reported diplopia. Physical examination revealed nystagmus in all fields of gaze with left eye exotropia. She was found to have flaccid paralysis and areflexia of lower extremities with a T10 sensory level. She was incontinent of stool and urine.

Her MRI spine showed T2 hyperintensity extending from T1 to conus with marked swelling of the conus and nerve root enhancement (Fig. 33.1). MRI of the brain showed T2 hyperintensity of the dorsal pons and cerebellar peduncles bilaterally (Fig. 33.1).

Her autoantibody workup was positive for the following: anti-dsDNA (190), anti-Sm (>100), anti-RNP (28), and anti-neutrophil cytoplasmic antibody (1/320). Anti-NMO IgG (IFA) was negative. CSF analysis was as follows: WBC 693 (neutrophils 76%, lymphocytes 12%), RBC 0, protein 0.58, and normal glucose. CSF

M.N. Nouri, M.D. • E.A. Yeh, M.D., F.R.C.P.C. (✉)
Department of Pediatrics, Division of Neurology, The Hospital for Sick Children, University of Toronto, 555 University Avenue, Toronto, ON, Canada, M5G 1X8
e-mail: Maryam.nabavinouri@mail.utoronto.ca; ann.yeh@sickkids.ca

© Springer International Publishing AG 2017                                    261
E. Waubant, T.E. Lotze (eds.), *Pediatric Demyelinating Diseases of the Central Nervous System and Their Mimics*, DOI 10.1007/978-3-319-61407-6_33

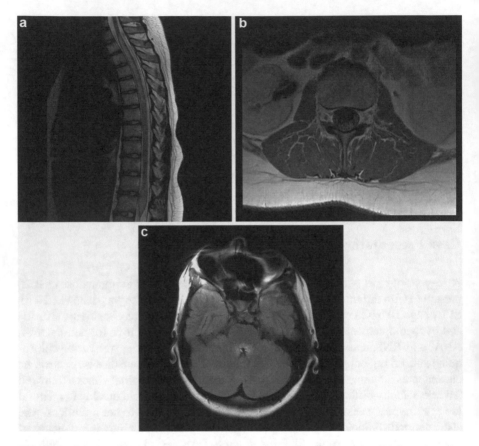

**Fig. 33.1** Spinal MRI: sagittal T2 (**a**) showing a longitudinally extensive T2 hyperintensity extending from T1 to the conus. Axial T1 with gadolinium (**b**) showing nerve root enhancement. Brain MRI: axial T2 (**c**) showing dorsal pons T2 hyperintensity

IgG index was normal. CSF Oligoclonal bands were negative. An extensive infectious workup was unremarkable for serum herpes simplex virus (HSV), varicella zoster virus (VZV), cytomegalovirus (CMV), Epstein–Barr virus (EBV), parvovirus B19, *Borrelia burgdorferi*, West Nile, *Bartonella henselae*, and VDRL. CSF studies were negative for HSV, enterovirus, *Mycoplasma pneumoniae*, and bacterial culture. Stool was negative for enterovirus. Nasopharyngeal swab was negative for enterovirus and *Mycoplasma pneumoniae*.

She was treated empirically with antibiotics. Immunotherapy was initiated with IV methylprednisolone (MP) (30 mg/kg/dose) for 7 days with an oral prednisone (starting with 1 mg/kg/day) wean thereafter. She was started on plasmapheresis within 4 days of her presentation to the hospital (total of 7 exchanges. IVIG replacement of 0.1 g/kg/exchange also administered). Following this, she received two doses of rituximab (500 mg/m²/dose, separated by 2 weeks). Clinically, her diplopia improved within 3 days of starting IV MP. While receiving plasmapheresis, she regained sensation in a patchy distribution at T6. Follow-up MRI within 3 weeks showed interval improvement of the brainstem and upper thoracic T2 hyperintensities, with ongoing nerve root enhancement. Subsequently, she received monthly cyclophosphamide (750–1000 mg/m²/dose) for 6 months. No further disease progression was noted.

## Clinical Questions

1 How do the presenting signs and symptoms relate to patient's underlying diagnosis?
2. What is the differential diagnosis of the patient's presentation?
3. Which laboratory investigations can aid with diagnosis in this case?
4. Based on the diagnosis, how can we proceed with the treatment plan?
5. What do we know about the anticipated course and prognosis?

## Diagnostic Discussion

### How Do the Presenting Signs and Symptoms Relate to Patient's Underlying Diagnosis?

In this case, the patient presented with a sensory level and flaccid paraparesis in the context of an underlying diagnosis of SLE. SLE is a multisystem, inflammatory, and autoimmune disorder affecting between 5000 and 10,000 children in the United States [1]. Adult studies have shown that up to 60% of SLE patients develop neurological symptoms, including seizures, aseptic lymphocytic meningitis, and migraine. Acute transverse myelitis (ATM) occurs in 1–2% of SLE cases, primarily in the form of longitudinally extensive transverse myelitis (LETM) [2]. Little is known about the frequency of ATM in cases of pediatric SLE; 11 pediatric cases have been described in the literature (Table 33.1).

The pathogenesis of ATM in SLE may be related to immune complex-mediated vasculitis causing ischemic necrosis or an antiphospholipid antibody (APLA)-related mechanism associated with vascular thrombosis. In some cases, neuromyelitis optica spectrum disorders (NMOSDs) [12] have been described; in one case series, NMO-IgG positivity was reported in 35.7% of patients with NMOSDs with SLE and Sjögren's syndrome [13]. In a separate review, prevalence of antiphospholipid antibody (APLA) ranged from 18 to 60% [14]. SLE-associated ATM (SLE-ATM) occurs most commonly as a monophasic illness that tends to occur within the first 5 years of SLE diagnosis, with at least one recurrence in 21–55% of patients [2]. In adult series, systemic symptoms commonly precede those of SLE-ATM, but 23–39% of SLE patients present initially with ATM [15]. Females account for three-fourths of cases (mean age at ATM diagnosis 29.3 ± 9.4 years). The rate of recovery

**Table 33.1** Literature review of pediatric patients with SLE-ATM

| Patient number (Refs.) | Age (years) | Sex | Duration of SLE | Systemic SLE Features | Duration of myelitis-related symptoms | Clinical features | Treatment | MRI | Follow-up duration | Improvement | Exam |
|---|---|---|---|---|---|---|---|---|---|---|---|
| 1 [3] | 12 | M | Onset | None | 4 months | Fever, paraplegia, hyporeflexia, sensory level (T1), urinary sphincter dysfunction | CS | LETM-C2-conus | NA | Partial recovery | Spastic paraplegia |
| 2 [4] | 16 | F | 8 months | Alopecia, arthritis | 2 months | Paraplegia, sensory level (T7) | CS 2 mg/kg/day | LETM | NA | Poor recovery | NA |
| 3 [4] | 17 | F | 3 months | Fever, rash, arthralgia | NA | NA | MP 500 mg + CP 0.8 g/m², q4w, RTX 500 mg, q1w, twice | 8 focal speckle-like lesions | NA | Poor recovery | NA |
| 4 [4] | 15 | F | 3 months | Fever, low complements | NA | Lower extremity paraparesis | | Focal cervical lesions | MP 500 mg | Good | NA |
| 5 [5] | 19 | F | Onset | None | Acute onset | Fever, neck stiffness, tetraplegia, sensory level (T6), urinary sphincter dysfunction | CS IVIG | LETM | 13 months | Complete improvement | Normal exam |
| 6 [6] | 13 | F | 3 years | Fever, weight loss, arthralgia, chorea | Few days | Sensory level, brisk reflexes, and positive Babinski sign | MP for 3 days CP (0.5 g/m²) over 2 days | LETM | 1 month | Complete | Normal |
| 7 [7] | 13 | F | Onset | None | 2 weeks | Bilateral LE weakness, areflexia, T7 sensory level | 7 cycles of CP, 3 cycles of PE | LETM-C5 down to the conus | 16 months | Partial recovery | Spastic paraplegia |

| | | | | | | | | | | | |
|---|---|---|---|---|---|---|---|---|---|---|---|
| 8 [8]ᵃ | 10 | F | Onset | None | 3 months | Hypertonic paraparesis and right UE weakness | NA | NA | NA | NA | NA |
| 9 [9] | 5 | F | 7 months | Fever, anorexia, weight loss, cutaneous erythematous eruption | Acute onset | Flaccid paraplegia, para-anesthesia, D10 level, urinary retention | 3 weeks pulses of MP and CP | LETM-c2-conus | 12 months | Partial recovery of motor and sensory function | NA |
| 10 [10] | 12 | F | Onset | None | 1 week | Thrombocytopenia, fever, weight loss, followed by urinary retention and flaccid paralysis | CS for 3 days. CP (500 mg/m² in 2 days and 750 mg/m² monthly for the following 6 months) | LETM-T1-T9 | 2 years | Partial recovery | NA |
| 10 [11]ᵃ | NA | NA | NA | NA | NA | NA | CS + CP | NA | NA | NA | NA |

CS corticosteroids, MP methylprednisolone, CP cyclophosphamide, RTX rituximab, PE plasma exchange
ᵃUnable to access articles

in the 11 reported pediatric cases was variable (3/11 had good recovery and the remainder had poor/partial recovery) (Table 33.1).

Suspicion of undiagnosed SLE in a patient with ATM should be increased when the patient is African American and has a high ANA titer, inflammatory CNS lesions on MRI, a high IgG index on CSF analysis, and a high sedimentation rate [2].

## What Is the Differential Diagnosis of the Patient's Presentation?

Various clinical entities can be responsible for longitudinally extensive spinal cord lesions. Given this patient's clinical presentation, autoimmune or inflammatory etiologies are most likely (a and b below). Given the history of immunosuppression, infectious etiologies (c below) should also be considered [16]:

(a) Autoimmune: NMO, Sjögren's syndrome, antiphospholipid antibody syndrome (APAS), rheumatoid arthritis, immune thrombocytopenic purpura, and inflammatory bowel disease
(b) Inflammatory: MS, neuro-sarcoidosis, and neuro-Behçet
(c) Infectious: viruses (HSV, VZV, CMV, EBV, HTLV-1, HIV), bacteria (*Treponema pallidum*, *Mycobacterium tuberculosis* and *Mycobacterium bovis*, *Borrelia burgdorferi*), and parasitic (Schistosomiasis, *Toxocara canis*, *Ascaris suum*)
(d) Neoplastic: B-cell lymphoma, ependymoma and astrocytoma
(e) Paraneoplastic syndromes
(f) Spinal cord infarction
(g) Traumatic injuries
(h) Nutritional deficiencies: B12 and copper deficiency

## Which Laboratory Investigations Can Aid with Diagnosis in This Case?

MRI of the spine is an essential diagnostic step. In LETM, MRI shows a holocord zone of high signal on T2 images extending along greater than 3 vertebral segments. In addition, serum testing for systemic inflammatory processes together with lumbar puncture, including cells, protein, glucose, IgG index, oligoclonal bands, and evaluation for infectious etiologies, should be performed. In a review of 22 patients with SLE-ATM [15], 94% had increased white blood cell count, with polymorphonuclear predominance in 73%. Infectious evaluations including viral PCR and culture were negative in this series. Positive anti-dsDNA antibodies and low levels of complement were detected in 60% of the patients. Half the patients tested were positive for APLA. Given the MRI findings in this case, diagnostic testing should include serologies for NMO-IgG, APA, and rheumatological serologies, namely,

ANA, anti-dsDNA, and ESR. Infectious processes should be ruled out by specific viral PCR testing of the cerebrospinal fluid and serum.

## Based on the Diagnosis, How Can We Proceed with the Treatment Plan?

Therapeutic strategies for treatment of SLE-ATM include the use of immunosuppressive therapies when the underlying pathogenesis is considered primarily inflammatory. As ATM in SLE is a rare manifestation, treatment guidelines for this entity have not been developed. The combination of intravenous methylprednisolone and intravenous cyclophosphamide can be effective if used promptly. Plasmapheresis and intravenous immunoglobulin are recommended in severe cases [12]. In a review of 22 adult patients [15], a combination of corticosteroids and cyclophosphamide was used, but only 14% had complete resolution of symptoms and 59% had a partial recovery. Rituximab was associated with reduced disease activity related to SLE-ATM and prevention of disability in two observational studies [16].

In 2010, the European League Against Rheumatism (EULAR) issued recommendations for neuropsychiatric involvement of SLE [12]. In SLE-ATM, based on these recommendations, prompt induction therapy with high-dose glucocorticosteroids (1000 mg/day × 3–5 days) was suggested followed by monthly intravenous cyclophosphamide (750–1000 mg/m² or 500 mg/m² over 2 days) for 6 months (strength of statement A). Maintenance therapy with less intensive immunosuppressive regimens such as 1 mg/kg/day of oral corticosteroids with a standard progressive dose decrease for at least 12 months may be considered to prevent recurrence (strength of statement D). In severe myelitis not responding to standard immunosuppressive therapy, rituximab (anti-CD20Ab) could be considered (500 mg/m² rituximab once a week, 2 weeks apart alternatively 375 mg/m² weekly for 4 weeks) (strength of statement D). Anticoagulation/antiplatelet therapy has been suggested in APLA-positive or APAS patients not responding to immunosuppressive therapy (strength of statement D).

## What Do We Know About the Anticipated Course and Prognosis?

In SLE-ATM, the rule of thirds typically applies: one-third recover with minimal sequelae, one-third retain a moderate degree of disability, and the final third has severe residual disability. Patients with NMO-IgG antibody are likely to experience recurrence and can be classified as having NMOSDs if they satisfy diagnostic criteria.

# Clinical Pearls

1. ATM is a rare neurological condition characterized by local inflammation within the spinal cord resulting in motor, sensory, and autonomic dysfunction. Mechanical injury, infections, and neoplastic and paraneoplastic syndromes must be ruled out before autoimmune etiologies are considered.
2. In SLE, ATM tends to occur within the first 5 years of diagnosis, and in nearly half the cases, it is the first clinical manifestation of SLE. A recurrence of myelitis is seen within several months of the first event, and at least one recurrence occurs in 21–55% of patients.
3. Longitudinally extensive transverse myelitis is a rare, but serious, complication of SLE, leading to a variable degree of disability in the majority of patients. In SLE-ATM, one-third of patients will recover with little or no sequelae, one-third is left with a moderate degree of permanent disability, and one-third has severe residual disability.
4. In SLE, myelitis may be associated with NMO and APS (20% and 45%, respectively). Anti-aquaporin-4 antibody and APLA testing in patients with SLE-associated extensive ATM are suggested as part of initial investigations.
5. No clinical trials have been performed on this disorder. However, high-dose glucocorticoids and cyclophosphamide are the standard of care for SLE-ATM, while in more severe steroid-resistant cases, plasmapheresis is also recommended.

# References

1. Pineles D, Valente A, Warren B, Peterson MG, Lehman TJ, Moorthy LN. Worldwide incidence and prevalence of pediatric onset systemic lupus erythematosus. Lupus. 2011;20(11):1187–92.
2. Schulz SW, Shenin M, Mehta A, et al. Initial presentation of acute transverse myelitis in systemic lupus erythematosus: demographics, diagnosis, management and comparison to idiopathic cases. Rheumatol Int. 2012;32:2623–7.
3. Katramados AM, Rabah R, Adams MD, Huq AH, Mitsias PD. Longitudinal myelitis, aseptic meningitis, and conus medullaris infarction as presenting manifestations of pediatric systemic lupus erythematosus. Lupus. 2008;17:332–6.
4. Lu X, Gu Y, Wang Y, Chen S, Ye S. Prognostic factors of lupus myelopathy. Lupus. 2008;17:323–8.
5. Lehnhardt FG, Scheid C, Holtik U, Burghaus L, Neveling M, Impekoven P, et al. Autologous blood stem cell transplantation in refractory systemic lupus erythematosus with recurrent longitudinal myelitis and cerebral infarction. Lupus. 2006;15:240–3.
6. Baca V, Sanchez-Vaca G, Martinez-Muniz I, Ramirez-Lacayo M, Lavalle C. Successful treatment of transverse myelitis in a child with systemic lupus erythematosus. Neuropediatrics. 1996;27(1):42–4.
7. Shivamurthy VM, Ganesan S, Khan A, Hussain N, Sridhar AV. Acute longitudinal myelitis as the first presentation in child with systemic lupus erythematosus. J Pediatr Neurosci. 2013;8(2):150–3.

8. Linssen WHJP, Fiselier TJW, Gabreëls TJW, Wevers RA, Cuppen MPMJ, Rotteveel JJ. Acute transverse myelopathy as the initial manifestation of probable systemic lupus erythematosus in a child. Neuropediatrics. 1988;19(4):212–5.
9. Vieira JP, Ortet O, Barata D, Abranches M, Gomes JM. Lupus myelopathy in a child. Pediatr Neurol. 2002;27:303–6.
10. Campana A, Buonuomo PS, Insalaco A, Bracaglia C, Di Capua M, Cortis E, Ugazio AG. Longitudinal myelitis in systemic lupus erythematosus: a paediatric case. Rheumatol Int. 2012;32(8):2587–8.
11. Al-Mayouf SM, Bahabri S. Spinal cord involvement in pediatric systemic lupus erythematosus: case report and literature review. Clin Exp Rheumatol. 1999;17(4):505–8.
12. Bertsias GK, Ioannidis JP, Aringer M, Bollen E, Bombardieri S, Bruce IN, Cervera R, Dalakas M, Doria A, Hanly JG, Huizinga TW, Isenberg D, Kallenberg C, Piette JC, Schneider M, Scolding N, Smolen J, Stara A, Tassiulas I, Tektonidou M, Tincani A, van Buchem MA, van Vollenhoven R, Ward M, Gordon C, Boumpas DT. EULAR recommendations for the management of systemic lupus erythematosus with neuropsychiatric manifestations: report of a task force of the EULAR standing committee for clinical affairs. Ann Rheum Dis. 2010;69(12):2074–82.
13. Pittock SJ, Lennon VA, de Seze J, Vermersch P, Homburger HA, Wingerchuk DM, Lucchinetti CF, Zéphir H, Moder K, Weinshenker BG. Neuromyelitis optica and non organ-specific autoimmunity. Arch Neurol. 2008;65(1):78–83.
14. Saison J, Costedoat-Chalumeau N, Maucort-Boulch D, et al. Systemic lupus erythematosus-associated acute transverse myelitis: manifestations, treatments, outcomes, and prognostic factors in 20 patients. Lupus. 2015;24:74–81.
15. Espinosa G, Mendizábal A, Mínguez S, et al. Transverse myelitis affecting more than 4 spinal segments associated with systemic lupus erythematosus: clinical, immunological, and radiological characteristics of 22 patients. Semin Arthritis Rheum. 2010;39:246–56.
16. Nardone R, Fitzgerald RT, Bailey A, et al. Longitudinally extensive transverse myelitis in systemic lupus erythematosus: case report and review of the literature. Clin Neurol Neurosurg. 2015;129:57–61.

# Chapter 34
# Acute Demyelination Associated with TNF-Alpha Inhibiting Biologic Therapy

Ian Ferguson, Gulay Alper, Sara Vila Bedmar, Jennifer S. Graves, and Emmanuelle Waubant

**Case 1** A 14-year-old girl presented to an ophthalmologist with a history of bilateral eye pain and blurred vision. On examination, she was noted to have bilateral non-granulomatous anterior and posterior uveitis. She otherwise had normal visual acuity, no afferent pupillary defect, and normal visual fields. She began treatment with topical prednisolone acetate, subconjunctival hydrocortisone injections, and cycloplegic eye drops. She was subsequently evaluated by a rheumatologist for joint pain and swelling in the knees and ankles. Laboratory investigations were notable only for a positive antinuclear antibody (1:320). She otherwise had negative markers for HLA-B27 and had a normal ESR and CRP. Given her constellation of symptoms,

I. Ferguson, M.D.
Division of Pediatric Rheumatology, Department of Pediatrics, Yale University School of Medicine, 789 Howard Avenue, New Haven, CT 06519, USA
e-mail: ian.ferguson@yale.edu

G. Alper, M.D. (✉)
Division of Child Neurology, Department of Pediatrics, Children's Hospital of Pittsburgh, University of Pittsburgh School of Medicine, 4401 Penn Avenue, Pittsburgh, PA 15224, USA
e-mail: Gulay.Alper@chp.edu

S.V. Bedmar, M.D.
Department of Neurology, Hospital Universitario 12 de Octubre,
Córdoba Ave, s/n, Acuerdo St., 35, 6°B, Madrid 28041, Spain
e-mail: vilabed@gmail.com

J.S. Graves, M.D., Ph.D., M.A.S. • E. Waubant, M.D., Ph.D.
Clinical Neurology and Pediatrics, Regional Pediatric MS Clinic at UCSF,
University of California San Francisco, 675 Nelson Rising Lane, Suite 221,
San Francisco, CA 94158, USA
e-mail: jennifer.graves@ucsf.edu; Emmanuelle.Waubant@ucsf.edu

© Springer International Publishing AG 2017      271
E. Waubant, T.E. Lotze (eds.), *Pediatric Demyelinating Diseases of the Central Nervous System and Their Mimics*, DOI 10.1007/978-3-319-61407-6_34

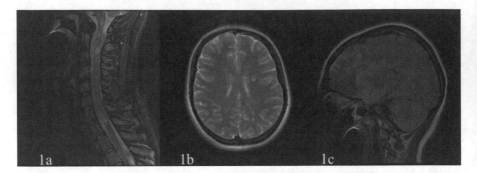

**Fig. 34.1** (**a**) Sagittal T2-FLAIR image demonstrates multiple short segment cervical and thoracic spinal cord lesions. (**b**) Axial T2 image demonstrates multiple periventricular lesions. (**c**) Sagittal T2-FLAIR image with "Dawson's fingers" (periventricular lesions perpendicular to ventricular edge)

juvenile idiopathic arthritis (JIA) and uveitis were diagnosed, and treatment was initiated with an anti-inflammatory TNF-alpha inhibiting (TNFi) medication. She initially received subcutaneous adalimumab (40 mg) every other week for 6 months but was nonadherent to the regimen. She was subsequently changed to monthly intravenous infliximab (5 mg/kg/dose) and completed two doses of this treatment. Seven months after the start of therapy with TNFi and 17 days after her last dose of TNFi, she presented with numbness in the left upper and right lower extremity, difficulty with her balance, trouble walking, and lower extremity weakness.

A brain MRI at that that time showed multifocal well-circumscribed hyperintense T2 lesions throughout the supratentorial white matter and corpus callosum as well as in the cervical and thoracic cord. Many of these lesions enhanced on T1-weighted imaging with gadolinium contrast (Fig. 34.1a). CSF analysis showed 0 WBC, 0 RBC, protein of 40 mg/dL, glucose of 45 mg/dL, positive oligoclonal bands by isoelectric focusing, and an elevated IgG index of 1.28. ANA titer remained positive at 1:1280.

TNFi treatment was immediately stopped, and she was started on methylprednisolone 1000 mg IV daily for 3 days with a subsequent oral taper of prednisone over 12 weeks. Three months after this event, and 2 days after cessation of steroids, she again developed bilateral leg weakness and gait instability. On examination, she was noted to have patchy sensory loss below the waist and loss of taste sensation over the right side of the tongue. Repeat imaging at this time showed multiple new T1-weighted gadolinium-enhancing white matter lesions in the brain as well as in the mid-cervical and upper thoracic spinal cord. She was again treated with methylprednisolone 1000 mg IV daily for 5 days followed by an oral taper over 12 weeks. In addition, she received IVIg (1 g/kg/dose) once monthly intervals for 3 months.

During the course of her oral steroid taper, she developed severe arthritis of the right hip. A repeat laboratory panel at that time showed persistent positive ANA, high positive anti-double stranded DNA, and low complement values. Her clinical syndrome was felt to be most consistent with systemic lupus erythematosus (SLE) at that time. She was placed on mycophenolate mofetil and hydroxychloroquine with improved control of her arthritis, and she subsequently did not develop any further flares of neurological disease. While her signs and symptoms of weakness and numbness resolved, she continued to have ophthalmological problems to include the development of glaucoma and cataracts in association with uveitis.

As there was a temporal relationship between the onset of her acquired demyelinating syndrome and the start of anti-TNF treatment, the drug was thought to have a causative role in the demyelinating disorder.

**Case 2** A 15-year-old girl with a 6-year history of polyarticular juvenile idiopathic arthritis on oral methotrexate (10 mg weekly) developed breakthrough activity and started intravenous infliximab (10 mg/kg every 6 weeks). One year into this new therapy, she woke up with blurred vision in her right eye. She had retro-orbital pain, worsened by eye movements. She had no other neurological symptoms. She had no preceding illness or fever, and her arthritis was under good control. Her examination confirmed right optic neuritis with severely impaired visual acuity (20/200–2), dyschromatopsia, and a right afferent pupillary defect. The rest of her neurological examination was normal.

She was admitted to the hospital for further evaluation and management. Blood test results were within normal range (including complete blood count, creatinine, transaminases, C-reactive protein, and sedimentation rate), except for low levels of 25(OH) vitamin D (17 ng/mL, range 30–100 ng/mL). Extensive infectious workup and aquaporin 4 antibody were negative. A brain MRI performed 1 week after the onset of symptoms revealed asymmetric T2 hyperintensity and enlargement of the right prechiasmatic optic nerve, compatible with optic neuritis without gadolinium enhancement. The remainder of the brain parenchyma appeared unremarkable (Fig. 34.2). She and her family declined to have a lumbar puncture, which had been proposed for routine studies (cell count, protein, glucose, cultures) and IgG index and oligoclonal bands.

She was treated with corticosteroids (methylprednisolone 1000 mg IV daily for 3 days followed by an oral prednisone taper) for 1 week and experienced rapid improvement. Infliximab was discontinued and oral methotrexate was increased to 25 mg weekly. She was started on vitamin D3 supplementation. After 3 years of follow-up, her central acuity is 20/20 in the right eye. She has had no clinical or MRI evidence of additional demyelinating lesions.

## Clinical Questions

1. In Case 1, how does the differential diagnosis evolve through the disease course with the development of new neurological symptoms and imaging findings?
2. What is the pharmacology of TNFi medications?
3. What is the hypothesis for development of demyelination with these medications?

**Fig. 34.2** On axial
T2-weighted FLAIR
image, the cisternal and
canalicular segments of the
right prechiasmatic optic
nerve appear
asymmetrically
hyperintense and enlarged
compatible with given
history of optic neuritis

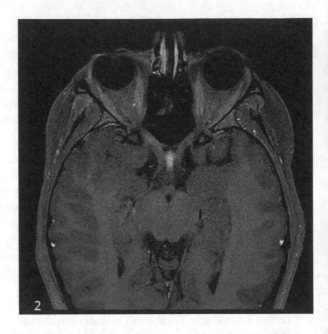

4. What is the experience with TNFi medications and CNS demyelinating disease? Is the association of TNFi with CNS demyelinating disease a causal relationship or is the link between CNS demyelination and the underlying disease the cause?

## Diagnostic Discussion

1. The first patient presented had a long clinical course prior to the ultimate diagnosis of systemic lupus erythematosus. At her initial presentation of bilateral uveitis and a positive ANA, the differential diagnosis included inflammatory disorders such as SLE, sarcoidosis, juvenile idiopathic arthritis, Behcet's disease, and infectious disorders such as herpetic uveitis, tuberculosis, or toxoplasmosis. With the development of focal paresthesia, she was subsequently diagnosed with transverse myelitis. The differential was then further expanded to include multiple sclerosis (MS), sarcoidosis, SLE, and TNFi-related demyelination.

   Review of the initial imaging shows a picture that is more classically associated with multiple sclerosis than other etiologies such as SLE. This includes short segments of demyelination involving the cervical cord. SLE is more typically noted to have longitudinally extensive disease. In addition, the prominence of the lesions in the corpus callosum and periventricular areas (Dawson's fingers) is more linked to MS. While the final diagnosis of SLE was made based on the autoantibody panel and associated arthritis, other potential etiologies were also treated to include cessation of the TNFi medication, which has been associated with acute demyelinating disease.

2. TNF-alpha is synthesized as a monomeric type-2 transmembrane precursor protein (tmTNF) which is active as either the transmembrane form or the soluble form, when cleaved through the action of the TNF-alpha cleaving enzyme [1]. TNF-alpha is produced by many cell types, including macrophages, lymphocytes, dendritic cells, and natural killer cells in the periphery. In the CNS, it is produced by microglia and astrocytes [2]. These transmembrane or soluble forms of TNF-alpha form trimers, which are biologically active and bind to one of two receptors: TNFR1 and TNFR2 [2]. It is here that the biological effects differ. TNFR1, which is preferentially activated through soluble TNF-alpha, triggers the production of pro-inflammatory mediators or caspases, which trigger cell death. TNFR2, activated by transmembrane TNF-alpha, lacks the ability to generate apoptosis and functions to propagate the inflammatory cascade through NfkB, an intracellular transcription factor key in regulating the immune response [1, 3].

   There are currently five approved medications with important variations in the formulation (one soluble TNF receptor and four monoclonal antibodies against TNF) and dosing schedule that is beyond the scope of this discussion. They all function to bind both sTNF and tmTNF and reduce the subsequent signaling cascade.

3. Speculation as to the pathophysiology of TNFi-related demyelinating disease was proposed by Kaltsonoudis [4]. These theories are largely based on the CNS as an immunologically privileged site. Demyelinating lesions in multiple sclerosis patients have shown elevations of TNF-alpha. The molecule is localized to the lesions and produced in the central nervous system by microglia and CNS macrophages. It is not produced in the periphery, as serum levels in these patients are routinely normal. TNFi medications cannot reach past the blood-brain barrier to affect this production.

   In considering the role of TNF-alpha in diseases of the peripheral immune system, the signaling protein serves a joint role to stimulate both pathologic effector T-cells and regulatory T-cells. TNFi medications would be expected to be effective by a balanced inhibition or activity biased against the pathologic effector T-cells. However, in some patients, the administration of TNF-inhibiting medication appears to have a greater inhibiting effect on the regulatory cells over pathogenic effector T-cells, resulting in a paradoxical inflammatory response in the periphery. The inflammatory cytokines subsequently produced pass freely into the CNS, stimulating an inflammatory response in microglia and macrophages. While the peripheral inflammation is negated by the activity of the TNF-inhibiting medication, the drug does not cross the blood-brain barrier, resulting in unchecked paradoxical CNS inflammation.

4. There are conflicting studies regarding the relationship between TNFi medications and acquired demyelinating syndromes. One study of 10,000 patients with rheumatoid arthritis exposed to TNFi showed that up to 30% of the cohort developed demyelinating disease [7], whereas other studies suggest that the incidence of demyelination with TNFi does not differ from the general incidence of multiple sclerosis [8, 9]. A phase 1 study investigating infliximab as a potential

treatment for multiple sclerosis paradoxically found an increased number of CNS lesions and elevated inflammatory laboratory markers in two patients with progressive MS [5]. A multicenter review of patients on the TNF-inhibiting medications infliximab, etanercept, and adalimumab suggested that the prevalence of developing demyelinating lesions with these treatments was 0.05–0.2% per patient. Reported CNS demyelinating syndromes included isolated optic neuritis (60%), multiple sclerosis (15%), and transverse myelitis (3%). In addition, demyelinating disease of the peripheral nervous system also occurred to include Guillain-Barre syndrome (7%), mononeuritis multiplex (1.5%), and small fiber neuropathy (2.5%) [6]. This study also stratified according to the medication used and found that etanercept had the lowest prevalence of demyelinating disease (0.02%), while adalimumab had the highest (0.1%) with infliximab in the middle (0.05%).

The causative role of TNFi medications in demyelinating disease remains unclear. While there does not appear to be a clear association, the data suggests a risk for the development of demyelinating disease with TNFi usage, whether the etiology is from the drug itself or from genetic predisposition for autoimmunity. Patients seem to develop symptoms after the start of the medication and there is some relief with cessation of the drug.

Consensus opinion seems to be that TNFi should not be used in patients with MS or other acquired demyelinating syndromes. Any patient under TNFi therapy should be well informed that the development of neurological symptoms should not be taken lightly and the medication should be stopped if such symptoms occur. While there is no consensus on the use of these medications in patients with a family history of MS, caution and close follow-up may be warranted. In general, clinicians should evaluate the choice of medication and monitor all patients closely for the development of even seemingly benign concerns.

## Clinical Pearls

Side effects related to dosing with TNFi include acquired demyelinating disorders of the central nervous system. After starting any immune modulating therapy, there should be close evaluation to determine side effects or new disease symptoms.

## References

1. Caminero A, Comabella M, Montalban X. Tumor necrosis factor alpha (TNF-α), anti-TNF-α and demyelination revisited: an ongoing story. J Neuroimmunol. 2011;234:1–6.
2. McCoy MK, Tansey MG. TNF signaling inhibition in the CNS: implications for normal brain function and neurodegenerative disease. J Neuroinflammation. 2008;5:45–57.

3. Tracey D, Klareskog L, Sasso EH, Salfeld JG, Tak PP. Tumor necrosis factor antagonist mechanisms of action: a comprehensive review. Pharmacol Ther. 2008;117:244–79.
4. Kaltsonoudis E, Voulgari PV, Konitsiotis S, Drosos AA. Demyelination and other neurological adverse events after anti-TNF therapy. Autoimmun Rev. 2014;13:54–8.
5. van Oosten BW, Barkhof F, Truyen L, Boringa JB, Bertelsmann FW, von Blomberg BM, Woody JN, Hartung HP, Polman CP. Increased MRI activity and immune activation in two multiple sclerosis patients treated with the monoclonal anti-tumor necrosis factor antibody cA2. Neurology. 1996;47:1531–4.
6. Bosch X, Saiz A, Ramos-Casals M, BIOGEAS Study Group. Monoclonal antibody therapy-associated neurological disorders. Nat Rev Neurol. 2011;7(3):165–72.
7. Bernatsky S, Renoux C, Suissa S. Demyelinating events in rheumatoid arthritis after drug exposures. Ann Rheum Dis. 2010;69:1691–3.
8. Fernández-Espartero MC, Pérez-Zafrilla B, Naranjo A, Esteban C, Ortiz AM, Gómez-Reino JJ, Carmona L, BIOBADASER Study Group. Demyelinating disease in patients treated with TNF antagonists in rheumatology: data from BIOBADASER, a pharmacovigilance database, and a systematic review. Semin Arthritis Rheum. 2011;40:330–7.
9. Magnano MD, Robinson WH, Genovese MC. Demyelination and inhibition of tumor necrosis factor (TNF). Clin Exp Rheumatol. 2004;22(5 Suppl. 35):S134–40.

# Chapter 35
# Myelopathy Due to Occult Trauma Mimicking Transverse Myelitis

Carlos Quintanilla Bordás, Bardia Nourbakhsh, and Emmanuelle Waubant

## Case Presentation

A previously healthy 16-year-old girl presented over a 2-month period with numbness and tingling in her lower limbs that spread to her upper limbs with concomitant stiffness. Two weeks prior to presentation, she noticed increasing weakness in all four limbs, to the point of needing help for getting dressed and support for walking. She denied bladder or bowel problems or any systemic symptoms. During the previous year, she had experienced on and off right predominant shooting pain and tingling in the arms that lasted 30 min at a time. She had a positive family history of autoimmune disorders in two sisters and three second-degree relatives. Neurological examination at the time of presentation revealed upper limb predominant quadriparesis. She had increased tone throughout, and strength was 4/5 proximally and 3/5 distally in upper limbs and 4+/5 in lower limbs. Sensation was reduced multimodally in all four limbs without any clear level. Deep tendon reflexes (DTR) were 3+ throughout, and both

C.Q. Bordás, M.D. (✉)
Department of Neurology, Servicio de Neurologia, Consorcio Hospital General Universitario de Valencia, Avenida Tres Cruces, 2, Valencia 46014, Spain
e-mail: carlosqb@gmail.com

B. Nourbakhsh, M.D., M.A.S.
University of California San Francisco, 675 Nelson Rising Lane, Suite 221, San Francisco, CA 94158, USA

Department of Neurology, Johns Hopkins University,
600, N Wolfe Street, Pathology 627, Baltimore, MD 21287, USA
e-mail: bnourba1@jhmi.edu

E. Waubant, M.D., Ph.D.
Clinical Neurology and Pediatrics, Regional Pediatric MS Clinic at UCSF,
University of California San Francisco, 675 Nelson Rising Lane, Suite 221, San Francisco, CA 94158, USA
e-mail: Emmanuelle.waubant@ucsf.edu

© Springer International Publishing AG 2017
E. Waubant, T.E. Lotze (eds.), *Pediatric Demyelinating Diseases of the Central Nervous System and Their Mimics*, DOI 10.1007/978-3-319-61407-6_35

Hoffmann's sign and extensor plantar responses were present bilaterally. Cognition and cranial nerves were intact. MRI of her neuraxis revealed intramedullary T2 signal change from C3 to C5 with patchy enhancement and degenerative changes in discs and vertebrae but no sign of compression (Fig. 35.1a–c). Brain MRI was normal. CSF analysis was normal (total protein of 33 mg/dL, glucose of 49 mg/dL, 1 lymphocyte, no oligoclonal bands, IgG index of 0.5, no bacteria on Gram staining, and negative cultures). Extensive workup included PCR for other herpesviruses and enterovirus in CSF, infectious serologies, and autoimmunity panel that returned negative except for positive antinuclear antibodies (ANA) at a 1:320 titer. She was first diagnosed with a myelitis of uncertain origin (infectious vs. inflammatory) and received high-dose steroids plus acyclovir IV but did not recover.

Two months after being discharged, she developed increasing weakness, and repeat MRI revealed persistence of the previously seen cord lesion and ongoing enhancement (Fig. 35.1d–f). HSV-1 serology was negative (IgG and IgM). Since the patient had a positive ANA titer, ongoing enhancement, clinical worsening, and a family history of autoimmune disease, an inflammatory transverse myelitis was suspected, and plasma exchange was performed for four cycles without clinical improvement.

Reexamination of imaging focused on disc and vertebral body changes raised additional consideration for the possibility of a past trauma. The patient had not had any major cervical trauma but had a motor tic involving her neck for the past 11 years with increasing frequency in the past months, up to several times per hour.

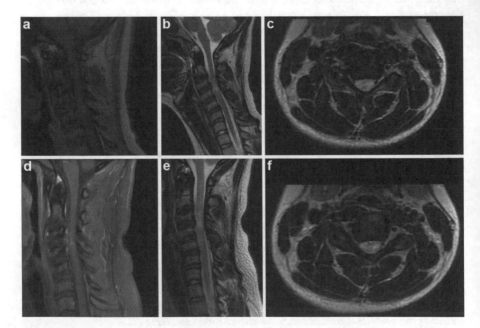

**Fig. 35.1** MRI sagittal T1 post-contrast (*left*) and T2 sequences (*middle and right*) of cervical spine at presentation (**a–c**) and 5 months later (**d–f**). The T2 signal hyperintensity extending from C3 to C4 persists, while enhancement is slightly increased on follow-up. Note also mild disc protrusion at C3–C4, mild disc desiccation, and cervical canal narrowing, which are surprising findings for a 16-year-old girl

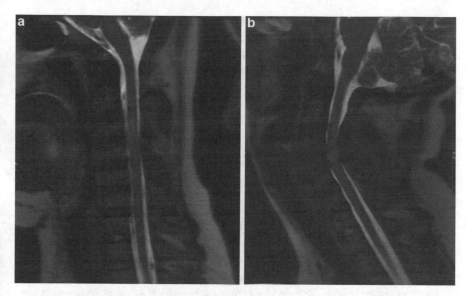

**Fig. 35.2** MRI T2 sequence dynamic sagittal images of the spine demonstrate progressive spinal canal narrowing at C3–C4 in neck extension compared to neutral flexion position, related to combination of progressive disc bulge and ligamentum flavum buckling

The tic involved "cracking" her neck by pulling her head laterally to each side with the help of her hands. Dynamic plain radiographs of her neck did not show signs of spine instability. However, dynamic MRI demonstrated cervical spinal canal narrowing at the level of the lesion in neck extension due to disc protrusion and ligamentum flavum buckling (Fig. 35.2). The patient underwent multilevel laminoplasty, and upon clinical follow-up 8 months later, neurological deficits had stabilized and neuropathic pain had improved.

## Clinical Questions

1. Where is the lesion based on her symptoms and physical exam?
2. What can cause an enhancing lesion in the spinal cord?
3. How can a spondylotic myelopathy present on MRI?
4. What may cause a spondylotic myelopathy in a teenager?

## Discussion

1. Where is the lesion based on her symptoms and physical exam?
   The patient presented with a 10-week history of weakness and multimodal sensory loss involving both lower and upper limbs with increased DTR and plantar extensor responses. This presentation is consistent with cervical myelopathy.

A peripheral origin such of the Guillain-Barré spectrum can be ruled out because of very prominent upper motor neuron signs. Also, a higher than cervical lesion is unlikely due to sparing of cognitive function and cranial nerves. MRI of her neuraxis revealed a partially enhancing intramedullary lesion that spanned from C3 to C5 as well as some degenerative changes in discs and vertebra (see Fig. 35.1a–c)

2. What can cause an enhancing lesion in the spinal cord?

The differential diagnosis for an enhancing lesion in the spinal cord is broad and includes vascular, inflammatory, infectious, neoplastic, paraneoplastic, and compressive etiologies. Chronology of symptoms is crucial to narrow down the differential diagnosis. Myelopathies are acute when nadir of maximum disability is reached between 4 h and 21 days [1]. Hyperacute presentations (below 4 h) will usually have a vascular etiology. The differential diagnosis of acute myelopathy is discussed further in Chap. 32, "Neuromyelitis optica spectrum disease with transverse myelitis presentation."

Since presentation was consistent with a subacute process, causes for both acute and progressive myelopathies had to be considered. CSF analysis can help to further narrow down the differential diagnoses. Brain imaging can also help to detect accompanying abnormalities in inflammatory diseases (i.e., multiple sclerosis) and certain tumors (i.e., multifocal hemangioblastoma, multiple cavernomas).

- An infectious myelopathy was ruled out because of CSF parameters within normal range and negative PCR and serologies for common infectious agents. Transverse myelitis can be isolated (i.e., idiopathic) or part of an inflammatory disease. CSF can exhibit oligoclonal band (OCB) or increased IgG index but may be normal.

  - Multiple sclerosis (MS) lesions in the spinal cord tend to be asymmetrical and short (<3 vertebral segments). Approximately, 90% of cases will have OCB in CSF at disease onset. Brain imaging will show typical lesions, although about 10% of isolated TM without brain abnormalities will convert to MS later in life.
  - Neuromyelitis optica spectrum disorders (NMOSD) lesions tend to be symmetrical and longitudinally extensive (>3 vertebral segments). In the absence of other typical findings, serum positivity for AQP4-IgG is required for diagnosis. CSF is usually abnormal with elevated WBC.
  - Serum autoimmunity panel (e.g., antinuclear antibodies) and other systemic findings are important to exclude rheumatological diseases or associated cancer when suspected.
  - Persistence of enhancement beyond 2 months should question an inflammatory origin [2]. One exception to this rule is sarcoidosis, where enhancement may persist chronically. Meningeal enhancement and other systemic findings (i.e., hilar lymphadenopathy) may help with the diagnosis [3].

- Vascular malformation can present in many forms. Fluctuating symptoms due to vascular steal phenomenon are typical. MRI T2-weighted images may show hyperintense intramedullary signal changes due to edema. Post-contrast T1 images may show enhancement and mimic transverse myelitis. CSF may show elevated protein without pleocytosis. The presence of abnormal vascular flow voids and serpentine enhancement along the surface of the cord are suggestive. Digital subtraction arteriography is the gold standard to confirm the diagnosis.

- Intramedullary tumors may be difficult to distinguish from transverse myelitis. The most frequent tumors in childhood include astrocytoma and ependymoma. A nearby syrinx may be present when the tumor obstructs the central canal. In contrast to inflammatory lesions, tumors will usually enlarge cord diameter. A lesion that continues to worsen beyond the acute time frame despite medical treatment should raise suspicion for a tumor.
- Compressive myelopathy is an uncommon cause for an enhancing lesion. See next question for further details.

3. How does a spondylotic myelopathy present on MRI?

Spondylotic myelopathy presents with intramedullary hyperintense T2 signal that can be accompanied by gadolinium enhancement. In addition, cervical spondylosis is a common finding in the adult population and may coexist with other spinal pathology. Therefore, the combination of hyperintense T2 signal with post-contrast enhancement may first suggest transverse myelitis or intramedullary tumor [4]. Recognizing spondylotic myelopathy is important as it can be treated, while misdiagnosis may expose patients to hazardous treatments and procedures (i.e., biopsy). The lesion appears on T2 sequence as a nonspecific fusiform area that may extend longitudinally for a variable number of segments away from the site of compression. Gadolinium enhancement when present will show characteristic transverse band, often referred as "pancake like," just below the site of maximum stenosis. This band may be complete or partial. Interestingly, this pattern of enhancement may persist from several months to years despite successful decompression and clinical recovery [5]. However, our case presented with a more longitudinal and patchy enhancement pattern that may reflect dynamic factors contributing to the myelopathy.

4. What may cause a spondylotic myelopathy in a teenager?

Children and teenagers are not expected to have degenerative spondylotic changes in their spine and, when present, should always raise suspicion for a secondary process. Our patient was discovered to have a motor tic, a potential cause for continuous, repetitive low-grade trauma to the spinal cord. The association between cervical tic and myelopathy has been previously reported. An association with other movement disorders such cervical dystonia has also been described [6]. In one case, the spinal cord lesion preceded spondylotic changes, suggesting that initial cord injury may arise from mechanical stretch or other dynamic factors [7]. In our case, dynamic MRI showed cervical canal narrowing on neck extension (Fig. 35.2) which may further explain the dynamic nature of the myelopathy.

# Clinical Pearls

1. MRI for a suspected lesion to the cervical spine should also include brain imaging with and without contrast. Many etiologies causing a cervical lesion share concomitant brain abnormalities which may be clinically silent.
2. The presence of MRI enhancement or elevated protein in CSF does not necessarily indicate an inflammatory origin.
3. Clinical worsening beyond 3 weeks is unusual for an inflammatory lesion and should question alternative diagnosis. An exception to the rule is sarcoidosis.

Spondylotic myelopathy may cause intramedullary T2-bright changes and pancake-like gadolinium enhancement immediately caudal to the site of maximum stenosis.

# References

1. Transverse Myelitis Consortium Working Group. Proposed diagnostic criteria and nosology of acute transverse myelitis. Neurology. 2002;59:499–505.
2. Cotton F, Weiner HL, Jolesz FA, Guttmann CRG. MRI contrast uptake in new lesions in relapsing-remitting MS followed at weekly intervals. Neurology. 2003;60:640–6.
3. Flanagan EP, Kaufmann TJ, Krecke KN, et al. Discriminating long myelitis of neuromyelitis optica from sarcoidosis. Ann Neurol. 2016;79:437–47. doi:10.1002/ana.24582.
4. Cabraja M, Abbushi A, Costa-Blechschmidt C, et al. Atypical cervical spondylotic myelopathy mimicking intramedullary tumor. Spine (Phila Pa 1976). 2008;33:E183–7. doi:10.1097/BRS.0b013e318166f5a6.
5. Ozawa H, Sato T, Hyodo H, et al. Clinical significance of intramedullary Gd-DTPA enhancement in cervical myelopathy. Spinal Cord. 2010;48:415–22. doi:10.1038/sc.2009.152.
6. Fung GPG, Chan KY. Cervical myelopathy in an adolescent with Hallervorden-Spatz disease. Pediatr Neurol. 2003;29:337–40.
7. Dobbs M, Berger JR. Cervical myelopathy secondary to violent tics of Tourette's syndrome. Neurology. 2003;60:1862–4.

# Chapter 36
# Hypomyelination with Brainstem and Spinal Cord Abnormalities and Leg Spasticity (HBSL)

Nicole Ulrick and Adeline Vanderver

## Case Presentation

A 15-year-old girl came to the attention of neurologists after experiencing weakness and gait abnormalities while playing softball. Symptoms initially presented as weakness in the lower extremities accompanied by decreased sensitivity to temperature and vibration below the knee. This patient reportedly felt a sense of coldness in her feet, particularly on the right side. She also experienced a notable increase in her urinary and bowel urgency, as well as a "shocking" feeling radiating down her legs subsequent to physical activity. Until this time, her medical history was relatively uneventful. At the age of 2, she experienced a possible episode of transient neurologic dysfunction of unknown origin that resolved 1 week later. At the age of 10, a series of headaches ensued following a trivial fall. A magnetic resonance imaging study (MRI) at that time demonstrated bilateral multifocal white matter disease, but the headaches resolved after a month and never recurred.

In response to the subacute onset of symptoms, an MRI of the brain was ordered. When compared to previous imaging, an assessment revealed stable periventricular multifocal white matter abnormalities. The patient's symptoms progressed rapidly over several months with worsening gait dysfunction and falls. A 5-day course of IV steroids was administered with a positive response with improved bowel control, subjective sensory improvement, decreased frequency of falls, and improved gait abnormalities. Episodic declines were seen, with a return of gait abnormalities approximately 3 months after treatment with IV methylprednisolone. She thus

N. Ulrick, B.A.
Department of Neurology and Center for Genetic Medicine Research, Children's National Medical Center, 111 Michigan Avenue NW, Washington, DC 20010, USA
e-mail: nulrick@childrensnational.org

A. Vanderver, M.D. (✉)
Children Hospital of Pennsylvania, Philadelphia, PA 19104, USA
e-mail: Avanderv@childrensnational.org

© Springer International Publishing AG 2017
E. Waubant, T.E. Lotze (eds.), *Pediatric Demyelinating Diseases of the Central Nervous System and Their Mimics*, DOI 10.1007/978-3-319-61407-6_36

received several courses of pulse steroid therapy every few months to manage her symptoms. Taking into account the gait abnormalities, imaging studies, and steroid responsiveness, multiple sclerosis (MS) was initially considered.

This patient underwent extensive genetic and laboratory testing that ultimately eliminated a neuroinflammatory process and suggested a possible leukoencephalopathy. A follow-up MRI of the brain and spine exhibited dorsal spinal cord lesions and T2-weighted abnormalities in the anterior pons and middle cerebellar peduncles. These findings, complimented by an amplified lactate peak on a magnetic resonance spectrometry study (MRS), suggested the possibility of a transfer RNA (tRNA) synthetase disorder, such as leukoencephalopathy with brainstem and spinal cord involvement and lactate elevation (LBSL) or hypomyelination with brainstem and spinal cord abnormalities and leg spasticity (HBSL). LBSL is an autosomal recessive condition attributable to a mutation in the *DARS2* gene coding for mitochondrial aspartyl-tRNA synthase (mt-AspRS) [1, 2]. HBSL is an autosomal recessive condition attributable to a mutation in the *DARS* gene coding for cytoplasmic aspartyl-tRNA synthase (AspRS). The patient was found to be heterozygous for p.His280Lys and p.Asp367His variants on the *DARS* gene.

The patient has continued to be stable over a period of 7 years. She attends a regular college education, ambulates independently, and plays college-level sports.

## Clinical Questions

1. What are the clinical features of HBSL?
2. Which studies can be performed to diagnose HBSL?
3. What is the mechanism of disease in HBSL?
4. What other neurologic diseases should be considered when making a differential diagnosis of HBSL?
5. What are current treatment options?
6. What is the prognosis for an individual with HBSL?

## Diagnostic Discussion

### *What Are the Clinical Features of HBSL?*

HBSL is a rare hereditary leukoencephalopathy resulting from an autosomal recessive mutation in the *DARS* gene, which affects the production of essential enzymes used in protein translation [3]. These mutations cause non-synonymous changes to highly conserved amino acids [4]. Most patients identified with HBSL have an infantile onset and appear to grow normally until 6–18 months of age [3, 4].

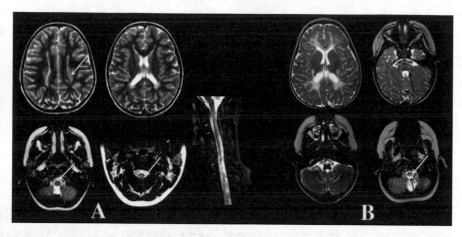

**Fig. 36.1** HBSL imaging features. T2-weighted images in a 15-year-old female (**a**) and a 3-year-old female (**b**) with HBSL. Note the selective tract involvement including pyramidal tracts through their entire length (*white arrows*), sensory tracts including medial lemniscus (*red arrows*), superior and inferior cerebellar peduncles (*blue arrow*), and the intraparenchymal trajectory of the trigeminal nerve (*black arrow*). Note the longitudinal cord involvement (**a**) as well as the multifocal supratentorial white matter changes in the adolescent patient (**a**) versus the diffuse white matter changes in the childhood onset case (**b**)

Neurological care is frequently sought after the patient experiences an acute regression of motor skills, often following an infection or vaccination. Hypotonia and lower limb spasticity contribute to progressive motor dysfunction that results in a delay or regression in motor abilities. Nystagmus in the first year of life is also a common occurrence for patients with an infantile onset [4]. Over time, patients continue to have severe motor abnormalities predominating in the lower extremities, and many never achieve independent ambulation or are wheelchair bound. Symptoms suggestive of peripheral nerve dysfunction such as paresthesias and loss of vibration and position sense are common, but nerve conduction velocities are normal. Many patients experience mild epilepsy, with infrequent, easily controlled seizures.

Patients with a subacute disease presentation in late adolescence have been recently identified, broadening the clinical spectrum associated with this disease [3]. Patients with a later onset tend to have a less severe clinical picture, which seems to correlate with less severe brain abnormalities.

In both clinical variants, MRI studies reveal distinct abnormalities (Fig. 36.1) in the supratentorial white matter as well as signal changes in the lateral corticospinal tracts and the dorsal columns of the spinal cord [3]. In the infantile variants, supratentorial white matter changes are confluent, initially appearing consistent with hypomyelination but over time often developing increasing T2 signal intensity. In the later-onset variants, MRI features of HBSL more closely mimic LBSL, with multifocal periventricular white matter changes.

## Which Studies Can Be Performed to Diagnose HBSL?

Because hyperintense T2 white matter changes and steroid responsiveness may mimic the presence of a neuroinflammatory disease such as multiple sclerosis, careful attention should be given to exclude this possibility. CSF should be analyzed for the presence of oligoclonal bands and other inflammatory markers. Involvement of selective tracts in the brainstem and spinal cord is suggestive of the diagnosis [3]. Although an MRI is informative in diagnosing HBSL (Fig. 36.1), the neuroradiological features are conspicuously similar to those present in LBSL. MRS studies to rule out elevated lactate levels may help differentiate LBSL from HBSL. Typically lactate elevations are seen in LBSL, although LBSL can exist even if elevated lactate is absent [2] and elevated lactate may be seen in HBSL. Definitive diagnosis is obtained by sequencing of the *DARS* gene and identifying pathogenic mutations inherited in an autosomal recessive manner. Because of the close clinical and radiologic overlap with LBSL, consideration may be given to concomitant screening of *DARS2*.

## What Is the Mechanism of Disease in HBSL?

Aminoacyl tRNA synthetases (ARS) are a class of enzymes that play an essential role in protein translation. ARS are responsible for the aminoacylation of tRNA, the first step in protein translation. During this process, tRNA becomes "charged" when it is covalently attached to its cognate amino acid in the cytoplasm, mitochondria, or ribosomes of a cell [5, 6]. Each ARS is specifically assigned to at least one amino acid. The *DARS* gene encodes for AspRS, the cytoplasmic ARS that attaches aspartate to its cognate tRNA [3, 5, 6]. Accurate translation of genetic material is necessary for the survival and physiology of all cells. Patients with HBSL have a *DARS* mutation that affects the production of AspRS, an essential enzyme used in the first step of protein translation.

## What Other Neurologic Diseases Should Be Considered When Making a Differential Diagnosis of HBSL?

LBSL is remarkably similar to HBSL. Clinically, both patient populations present with profound spasticity that is greater in the lower limbs. Moreover, both disorders demonstrate selective spinal pathway involvement with abnormalities evident along entire tracts [1, 3]. Genetic testing is one way in which these leukoencephalopathies can be distinguished, as HBSL is caused by mutations in the *DARS* gene and LBSL is a result of mutations in the *DARS2* gene.

HBSL mimics neuroinflammatory diseases, such as multiple sclerosis (MS), because of its responsiveness to steroids and sometimes multifocal or spine T2 white matter changes [3]. However, in HBSL, oligoclonal bands are not present in the CSF as they may be in a neuroinflammatory disease. Moreover, MRIs in HBSL reveal stagnant or very slowly progressing patterns of white matter changes, as opposed to the new foci of demyelination typically seen in MS.

## What Are Current Treatment Options?

Although there is no current treatment option to slow or stop the progression of the disease, therapeutic options are available for symptom management. Careful attention should be given to rehabilitative care to avoid orthopedic complications such as hip dislocation and scoliosis. Patients should be aware of decreased lower extremity sensation and the potential for injury. Chemodenervation in the flexor muscles and pharmacologic management of lower limb spasticity may be useful. A history of seizures should be sought and treated with standard anticonvulsant regimens. Developmental evaluations and educational support depending on the child's cognitive level should be considered.

At this time, despite anecdotal response to IV methylprednisolone, insufficient evidence exists to recommend steroid treatment to all patients with HBSL [3]. Additional studies are needed to assess mechanisms by which steroids may be beneficial.

## What Is the Prognosis for an Individual with HBSL?

Although longitudinal data is limited, the disease course of known patients suggests that prognosis could be linked to age of onset, with more severe forms of the disease presenting earlier in life. Symptom severity ranges from profound cognitive difficulties and the inability to independently ambulate to normal intellectual ability and full functional mobility into the third decade of life. The diagnostic criteria for HBSL have recently been redefined, broadening the clinical spectrum of the disease [3]. As more patients are accurately diagnosed and carefully tracked, greater insight will be gained about the prognosis of HBSL.

## Clinical Pearls

1. Presentation in late adolescence may mimic a neuroinflammatory disease. CSF studies should be analyzed for inflammatory markers, and MRI patterns should be reviewed to determine if white matter changes are static or progressive.

2. HBSL and LBSL share a similar neuroradiologic pattern characterized by signal changes in the lateral corticospinal tracts and the dorsal columns of the spinal cord. Concomitantly screening *DARS* and *DARS2* genes for known pathogenic variants will facilitate a definitive differentiation between these closely related leukoencephalopathies.
3. A number of patients have shown responsiveness to IV methylprednisolone, but not all HBSL patients should be recommended steroid therapy. Symptom management is the current standard of care for HBSL, and treatment considerations should be made with a patient's specific presentation in mind.

# References

1. van der Knaap MS, van der Voorn P, Barkhof F, Van Coster R, Krageloh-Mann I, Feigenbaum A, et al. A new leukoencephalopathy with brainstem and spinal cord involvement and high lactate. Ann Neurol. 2003;53(2):252–8. Epub 2003/01/31.
2. Lin J, Chiconelli Faria E, Da Rocha AJ, Rodrigues Masruha M, Pereira Vilanova LC, Scheper GC, et al. Leukoencephalopathy with brainstem and spinal cord involvement and normal lactate: a new mutation in the DARS2 gene. J Child Neurol. 2010;25(11):1425–8. Epub 2010/05/27.
3. Wolf NI, Toro C, Kister I, Latif KA, Leventer R, Pizzino A, et al. DARS-associated leuko-encephalopathy can mimic a steroid-responsive neuroinflammatory disorder. Neurology. 2015;84(3):226–30. Epub 2014/12/21.
4. Taft R. Mutations in DARS cause hypomyelination with brain stem and spinal cord involvement and leg spasticity. Am J Hum Genet. 2013;92(5):774–80.
5. Antonellis A, Green ED. The role of aminoacyl-tRNA synthetases in genetic diseases. Annu Rev Genomics Hum Genet. 2008;9:87–107. Epub 2008/09/05.
6. Wallen RC, Antonellis A. To charge or not to charge: mechanistic insights into neuropathy-associated tRNA synthetase mutations. Curr Opin Genet Dev. 2013;23(3):302–9. Epub 2013/03/08.

# Part IV
# Diseases That Affect the Optic Nerve

# Chapter 37
# Acute Disseminated Encephalomyelitis Followed by Recurrent or Monophasic Optic Neuritis

Amy T. Waldman

## Case Presentation

A 5-year-old female presented with 2 weeks of intermittent emesis, headache, and fatigue. There were no recent or intercurrent illnesses. She awoke one day with left-sided weakness and incontinence. She was taken to an emergency department where her examination was notable for decreased visual acuity (20/50) in the left eye, disc swelling OS, nystagmus, left-sided weakness, a positive Romberg sign, ataxic gait, and extensor plantar responses bilaterally. An MRI revealed multiple nonenhancing lesions in the brain (see Fig. 37.1a) and three extensive lesions in cord (C4–C7, T2–T5, conus; Fig. 37.1b). A lumbar puncture revealed 57 white blood cells in the cerebrospinal fluid (CSF) with 21% neutrophils, 15% monocytes, and 64% lymphocytes. The CSF red blood cell count was 8, protein was 32, and glucose was 62. Testing for oligoclonal bands was not sent from the emergency department. Based on her clinical presentation of encephalopathy with polyfocal neurologic signs and diffuse, poorly demarcated lesions on MRI, she was diagnosed with acute disseminated encephalomyelitis (ADEM) and treated with intravenous methylprednisolone (30 mg/kg/day) for 5 days and a a 16-day oral taper with resolution of her symptoms.

She had two recurrences in the 3 months following her diagnosis with symptoms similar to her initial presentation. Both of these relapses were treated with IV methylprednisolone for 3 days, followed by a prednisone taper. During the third attack, which occurred 3 months after her disease onset and 1 month after completion of her steroid taper, a repeat MRI revealed several new lesions in the bilateral cerebral

A.T. Waldman, M.D., M.S.C.E. (✉)
Division of Neurology, The Children's Hospital of Philadelphia,
Philadelphia, PA 19104, USA
e-mail: WALDMAN@email.chop.edu

© Springer International Publishing AG 2017
E. Waubant, T.E. Lotze (eds.), *Pediatric Demyelinating Diseases of the Central Nervous System and Their Mimics*, DOI 10.1007/978-3-319-61407-6_37

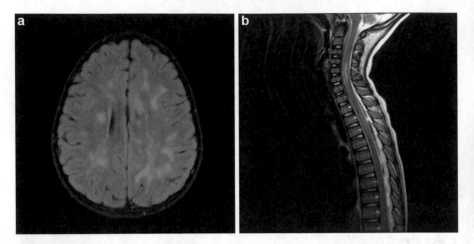

**Fig. 37.1** MRI scans revealing diffuse T2 and FLAIR hyperintensities throughout the brain, optic nerves, and spinal cord, with subsequent resolution of brain abnormalities. Initial presentation: (**a**) Diffuse nonenhancing FLAIR hyperintensities throughout the brain and (**b**) additional T2 hyperintensities in the spinal cord (C4–C7, T2–T5, conus—not visualized)

peduncles, posterior limb of the right internal capsule, right hippocampus, and left thalamus. A routine follow-up MRI of the brain 6 months after symptom onset also revealed new asymptomatic lesions with enhancement after gadolinium administration (see Fig. 37.2a, b).

She had a fourth clinical relapse 7 months after initial presentation with lethargy, blurry vision in the left eye, facial weakness, and an abnormal gait. MRI revealed a new enhancing lesion in the left optic nerve, with additional new nonenhancing lesions in the brainstem (see Fig. 37.3a, b). A repeat lumbar puncture was unrevealing (CSF WBC 0, RBC 0, protein 18, glucose 60, oligoclonal bands negative, IgG index, and myelin basic protein normal). She was treated with high-dose methylprednisolone for 5 days, followed by a 3-month taper.

One year after symptom onset, a routine MRI showed near-complete resolution of supra- and infratentorial lesions (see Fig. 37.4a–c); however, she was noted to have enlargement and subtle FLAIR signal abnormality with subtle enhancement of the intraorbital left optic nerve. Two weeks later, she was noted to have left eye pain and blurry vision. Her visual acuity was 20/80 OS with a left afferent pupillary defect and decreased color vision in that eye. She was treated with a 3-day methylprednisolone pulse (30 mg/kg/day) followed by an oral taper.

Over the next 6 years, she had 7 additional relapses of unilateral optic neuritis, sometimes affecting the left eye and other times affecting the right eye. Her visual acuities during these relapses ranged from 20/40 to 20/200, with pain as a prominent symptom accompanying vision loss. During the relapses, the MRI of the optic nerves at times showed T2 hyperintensities with enhancement; however, the MRI of the brain and C- and T-spine remained normal. Serum and CSF aquaporin-4 antibodies were negative. Over the years, she was treated with glatiramer acetate, then interferon-beta; however, neither prevented optic neuritis recurrence. She was

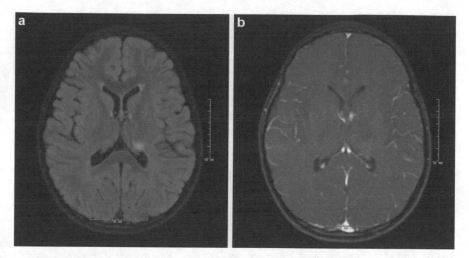

**Fig. 37.2** Routine surveillance MRI performed 6 months after initial presentation: (**a**) new left thalamic lesion is visualized on FLAIR images with (**b**) mild enhancement on post-contrast images

treated with high-dose methylprednisolone and prolonged prednisone tapers for relapses and improved. Chronic prednisone use (for 3-month intervals after an acute episode) helped decrease new attacks, and she was ultimately switched to a steroid-sparing agent (mycophenolate mofetil). However, after being on mycophenolate mofetil for over a year, she continued to relapse and was started on rituximab (750 mg/m² given 2 weeks apart). Her vision has been stable on rituximab with the exception of a single relapse during a gap in therapy. At the time of her last neuro-ophthalmologic evaluation 6 years after her initial presentation, her visual acuity was 20/150 in the right eye with moderate pallor of the right optic nerve and 20/20 distance acuity in the left eye with temporal pallor of the left optic nerve, with a 2+ relative afferent pupillary defect on the right.

## Clinical Questions

1. What are the clinical features and proposed diagnostic criteria for ADEM followed by recurrent or monophasic optic neuritis?
2. What distinguishes ADEM followed by recurrent or monophasic optic neuritis from multiphasic ADEM, NMO, MS, and other relapsing demyelinating diseases?
3. What is the treatment and prognosis for ADEM followed by optic neuritis?
4. What is the role of anti-myelin oligodendrocyte glycoprotein (MOG) antibodies in ADEM followed by recurrent or monophasic optic neuritis?
5. Should this disorder be considered as a separate entity from other relapsing diseases?

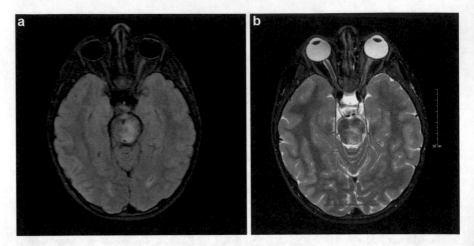

**Fig. 37.3** MRI performed 7 months after symptom onset (with recurrence of similar symptoms): (**a**) new lesions in the deep gray structures and (**b**) brainstem on FLAIR and T2 images. The left optic nerve (also pictured) is hyperintense and expanded, with enhancement (not shown)

## Discussion

Acute disseminated encephalomyelitis followed by recurrent or monophasic optic neuritis (ADEM followed by ON) was described in 2012 by Huppke et al. who recognized the unique features of this recurrent disease in seven children [1]. As the name implies, children present with signs and symptoms of diffuse central nervous system inflammation and encephalopathy meeting diagnostic criteria for acute disseminated encephalomyelitis [2]; however, they later relapse with attacks only involving the optic nerves. The clinical features are highlighted by the present case, and the rationale for distinguishing this disorder from other demyelinating syndromes is discussed.

In Huppke's original cohort of children with ADEM followed by ON [1], the median age at presentation was 6 years of age (range 4–8), a common age group for ADEM. All children have encephalopathy (as is required for an ADEM diagnosis) and polyfocal neurologic symptoms localizing to the brain, optic nerve, and spinal cord (such as paraparesis, tetraparesis, ataxia, bladder dysfunction). Other reported features include fever, meningismus, headaches, recurrent vomiting, hallucinations, and seizures. Isolated optic neuritis (characterized by visual acuity loss, pain with eye movements, abnormal color vision, and/or visual field deficits) presents weeks to several years later. Typically, the ON attack is unilateral but can be bilateral, and the vision loss may not fully recover even with treatment (discussed below). As in the present case, multiple ADEM and ON attacks can occur, with the original paper describing 1–4 attacks of ADEM followed by 1–9 attacks of ON [1].

The differential diagnosis for relapsing demyelinating diseases includes multiple sclerosis (MS), neuromyelitis optica spectrum disorders (NMOSD), multiphasic ADEM, chronic relapsing inflammatory optic neuropathy (CRION), relapsing

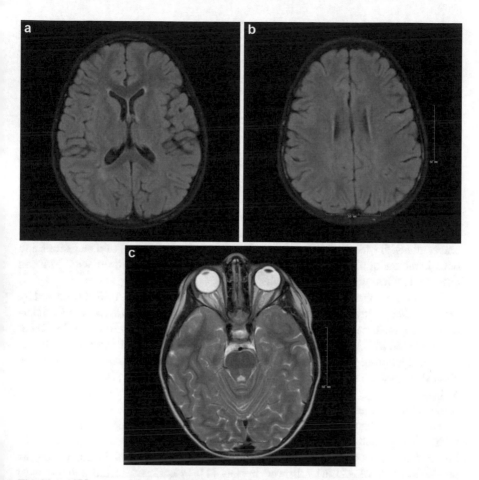

**Fig. 37.4** MRI performed 1 year after the initial presentation: (**a–c**) substantial resolution of the supratentorial lesions

transverse myelitis, and relapsing ON. However, the clinical, radiographic, and laboratory features of ADEM followed by ON (Table 37.1) help distinguish this disorder from the others. For example, multiphasic ADEM requires encephalopathy with each relapse; however, encephalopathy is absent in the recurrent ON portion of this disease. Similarly, CRION is isolated to the optic nerves, and diffuse CNS involvement is absent [3]. In ADEM followed by ON, the initial MRI reveals hyperintense T2 lesions affecting white and gray matter, including the deep gray structures (such as the basal ganglia or thalamus), and possibly the spinal cord, as typical of ADEM. In ADEM followed by ON, contrast enhancement of the brain lesions was not reported in the initial cohort [1], and only faint enhancement was seen during an ADEM relapse in the present case. New lesions may appear on subsequent MRI scans (with clinical symptoms). However, with time, there is resolution or substantial improvement of MRI abnormalities outside of the optic nerves. Although

**Table 37.1** Proposed diagnostic criteria for ADEM followed by recurrent or monophasic optic neuritis (derived from Huppke et al. [1])

| |
|---|
| 1. Initial presentation fulfills criteria for ADEM |
| 2. ON diagnosed after ADEM with objective evidence of loss of visual function |
| 3. The ON occurs after a symptom-free interval of 4 weeks and not as part of the ADEM or recurrent ADEM |
| 4. Diagnostic criteria for pediatric MS are not fulfilled |
| 5. Oligoclonal bands are not detected in the CSF (a pleocytosis may be present) |
| 6. MRI reveals typical brain or spinal cord T2 lesions consistent with ADEM initially; however, subsequent imaging shows resolution or near-complete resolution of lesions, and new brain or spinal cord lesions do not appear during the ON attacks |

in teenagers and adults, most MS lesions do not resolve with time, in children younger than 11, T2-bright foci frequently resolve substantially [4]. In teenagers and adults with MS, the MRI remains abnormal with the accrual of new lesions and occasional gadolinium-enhancing lesions, while younger children with MS can develop new lesions that may later resolve.

The cerebrospinal fluid may also be helpful in distinguishing ADEM followed by ON from MS. While a cerebrospinal fluid pleocytosis may be present in both disorders, oligoclonal bands are often absent in children with ADEM followed by ON at onset, as well as NMOSD. For those children in the original cohort whose CSF was retested, including our patient, oligoclonal bands remained absent throughout the clinical disease course [1]. The absence of oligoclonal bands also argues against MS, although in pediatric MS under the age of 11 the presence of oligoclonal bands is much less frequent than in teenagers and adults with the disease.

The clinical features of ADEM followed by ON are perhaps most similar to NMOSD, especially in cases featuring a longitudinally extensive myelitis in addition to ON. However, aquaporin-4 antibodies were not present in our patient or published cases of ADEM followed by ON [1]. In contrast, serum antibodies to myelin oligodendrocyte glycoprotein (MOG), a protein expressed only on the outer portion of the myelin sheath in the CNS (discussed below), were identified in all children with ADEM followed by ON (including 3 during an ADEM attack, and all 7 during an ON event) [1]. Follow-up serologic testing revealed persistently elevated high anti-MOG antibodies between and during ON episodes in 4 of 7 patients. Of note, testing for anti-MOG antibodies is not currently clinically available, and such testing is considered "experimental and investigational" in pediatric demyelinating diseases by a major insurance carrier in the United States [5].

The neurologic deficits and visual impairment in ADEM followed by ON in children improve with high-dose intravenous corticosteroids. As demonstrated by the present case and two other cases reported by Huppke [1], interferon-beta or glatiramer acetate has not been successful in preventing relapses in ADEM followed by ON. Treatment with azathioprine by Huppke was beneficial in one of two patients. The decision to begin immunosuppression in the present case was due to the concern for further visual loss with subsequent relapses of ON; however, the prognosis of ADEM followed by ON is unclear. To date, a few of the reported cases had residual deficits from myelitis (mild spastic paraparesis, bladder dysfunction) or mild vision loss (20/30 to 20/40) as in the present case.

An area of active research, anti-MOG antibodies have been increasingly implicated in pediatric but also adult inflammatory diseases of the central nervous system, especially with improved methods for detection [6]. Original assays (ELISA, Western blot) measured antibodies to the linear epitope of denatured protein, whereas cell-based assays use the conformational epitope. In addition, newer cell-based assays [7] use the full-length protein, rather than the extracellular and transmembrane domains, further increasing the sensitivity of the test. Anti-MOG antibodies have been identified in research studies of pediatric inflammatory diseases, such as ADEM, ON, and ADEM followed by ON, TM, and NMOSD without aquaroin-4 antibodies and occasionally pediatric MS [1, 6–10]. Anti-MOG antibodies are also rarely seen in adult MS [7, 9, 10] but may be more common in NMOSD patients negative for aquaporin-4 antibodies [11, 12], and as such its significance remains to be determined.

ADEM followed by ON is a demyelinating disorder with a distinct phenotype with multiple relapses over time. While the prevalence is unknown, the number of patients with this disorder was similar to NMOSD in one cohort [1], and ADEM followed by ON is likely under-recognized. The long-term course is not unclear, and it is possible that some of these patients will meet MS or NMOSD criteria in the future. Corticosteroids may improve acute clinical symptoms; however, it is unclear whether chronic immunosuppression alters the disease course or severity of attacks. Given the rarity of the phenotype, collaborative research is needed to determine treatment algorithms and prognostic implications for children with these clinical features. Whether elevated serum or CSF anti-MOG IgG antibodies are a distinct marker for specific demyelinating diseases requires further study, and additional research into the presence of anti-MOG antibodies and persistence of these antibodies throughout ADEM followed by ON, as well as long-term follow-up, will inform the pathophysiology of this disorder.

## Clinical Pearls

- Acute disseminated encephalomyelitis followed by recurrent or monophasic optic neuritis may be a distinct relapsing syndrome in children characterized by single or multiple attacks of encephalopathy and polyfocal neurologic symptoms with diffuse, poorly demarcated MRI T2 hyperintensities followed by resolution of these symptoms and MRI lesions; however, children subsequently develop isolated recurrences of optic neuritis.
- The absence of oligoclonal bands, aquaporin-4 antibodies, and contrast-enhancing brain lesions in acute disseminated encephalomyelitis followed by recurrent or monophasic optic neuritis may help distinguish this disorder from multiple sclerosis and neuromyelitis optica.

- Acute clinical symptoms improve with corticosteroids, although there is insufficient evidence for preventative treatment recommendations.
- Antibodies to myelin oligodendrocyte glycoprotein during relapses of ADEM followed by ON have been detected in research studies and may play a role in the pathophysiology of this disorder.
- Given the rarity of this disorder, collaborative investigations are needed to determine the long-term neurologic and visual prognosis for children with ADEM followed by ON and confirm if this phenotype is clearly distinct from MS and NMOSD.

# References

1. Huppke P, Rostasy K, Karenfort M, et al. Acute disseminated encephalomyelitis followed by recurrent or monophasic optic neuritis in pediatric patients. Mult Scler. 2013;19(7):941–6. doi:10.1177/1352458512466317.
2. Krupp LB, Tardieu M, Amato MP, et al. International Pediatric Multiple Sclerosis Study Group criteria for pediatric multiple sclerosis and immune-mediated central nervous system demyelinating disorders: revisions to the 2007 definitions. Mult Scler. 2013;19(10):1261–7. doi:10.1177/1352458513484547.
3. Petzold A, Plant GT. Chronic relapsing inflammatory optic neuropathy: a systematic review of 122 cases reported. J Neurol. 2014;261(1):17–26. doi:10.1007/s00415-013-6957-4.
4. Chabas D, Castillo-Trivino T, Mowry EM, Strober JB, Glenn OA, Waubant E. Vanishing MS T2-bright lesions before puberty: a distinct MRI phenotype? Neurology. 2008;71(14):1090–3. doi:10.1212/01.wnl.0000326896.66714.ae.
5. Antibody tests for neurologic diseases. Aetna policy 0340. http://www.aetna.com/cpb/medical/data/300_399/0340.html.
6. Reindl M, Di Pauli F, Rostásy K, Berger T. The spectrum of MOG autoantibody-associated demyelinating diseases. Nat Rev Neurol. 2013;9(8):455–61. doi:10.1038/nrneurol.2013.118.
7. Hacohen Y, Absoud M, Deiva K, et al. Myelin oligodendrocyte glycoprotein antibodies are associated with a non-MS course in children. Neurol Neuroimmunol Neuroinflamm. 2015;2(2):e81. doi:10.1212/NXI.0000000000000081.
8. Baumann M, Sahin K, Lechner C, et al. Clinical and neuroradiological differences of paediatric acute disseminating encephalomyelitis with and without antibodies to the myelin oligodendrocyte glycoprotein. J Neurol Neurosurg Psychiatry. 2015;86(3):265–72. doi:10.1136/jnnp-2014-308346.
9. Pröbstel AK, Dornmair K, Bittner R, et al. Antibodies to MOG are transient in childhood acute disseminated encephalomyelitis. Neurology. 2011;77(6):580–8. doi:10.1212/WNL.0b013e318228c0b1.
10. Brilot F, Dale RC, Selter RC, et al. Antibodies to native myelin oligodendrocyte glycoprotein in children with inflammatory demyelinating central nervous system disease. Ann Neurol. 2009;66(6):833–42. doi:10.1002/ana.21916.
11. Rostásy K, Mader S, Hennes EM, et al. Persisting myelin oligodendrocyte glycoprotein antibodies in aquaporin-4 antibody negative pediatric neuromyelitis optica. Mult Scler. 2013;19(8):1052–9. doi:10.1177/1352458512470310.
12. Sato DK, Callegaro D, Lana-Peixoto MA, et al. Distinction between MOG antibody-positive and AQP4 antibody-positive NMO spectrum disorders. Neurology. 2014;82(6):474–81. doi:10.1212/WNL.0000000000000101.

# Chapter 38
# Chronic Relapsing Inflammatory Optic Neuropathy (CRION)

Seanna Grob, Gena Heidary, and Leslie Benson

## Case Presentation

A 10-year-old girl presented with 2 weeks of headache, photophobia, nausea, and vomiting. Initial ophthalmic examination revealed visual acuities of 20/20 in each eye with mild bilateral optic disc edema. A lumbar puncture showed an elevated opening pressure of 34 cmH$_2$O, and cerebrospinal fluid (CSF) analysis was suggestive of viral meningitis (207 white blood cells/mm$^3$, 44% polymorphonuclear cells, 50% lymphocytes, 4 red blood cells/mm$^3$ with total protein of 73.5 mg/kL and glucose of 45 mg/dL). CSF analysis and all other pertinent infectious studies were

S. Grob, M.D., M.A.S. (✉)
Department of Ophthalmology, Harvard Medical School,
243 Charles St., Boston, MA 02114, USA

Department of Ophthalmology, Massachusetts Eye and Ear Infirmary, Boston, MA, USA
e-mail: Seanna_Grob@meei.harvard.edu; seannagrob@gmail.com

G. Heidary, M.D., Ph.D.
Department of Ophthalmology, Harvard Medical School, Boston Children's Hospital,
243 Charles St., Boston, MA 02114, USA
e-mail: gena.heidary@childrens.harvard.edu

L. Benson, M.D.
Department of Pediatric Neurology, Harvard Medical School, Boston Children's Hospital,
Boston, MA, USA
e-mail: Leslie.Benson@childrens.harvard.edu

© Springer International Publishing AG 2017
E. Waubant, T.E. Lotze (eds.), *Pediatric Demyelinating Diseases of the Central Nervous System and Their Mimics*, DOI 10.1007/978-3-319-61407-6_38

negative. She was started on oral acetazolamide. Over the following week, she developed worsening pain with eye movements and progressive left eye visual dysfunction with visual acuity of 20/200, a relative afferent pupillary defect (rAPD), color vision loss, and increased optic disc edema on exam. Formal visual field testing demonstrated a normal visual field in the right eye and generalized constriction in the left eye (Fig. 38.1). The remaining neurological exam was unremarkable. Magnetic resonance imaging (MRI) showed enhancement of the left optic nerve without evidence of any intracranial lesions (Fig. 38.1). MRI of the spine was negative for spinal cord disease. Repeat lumbar puncture was consistent with aseptic meningitis without oligoclonal bands. An extensive infectious and rheumatological workup was negative. A chest x-ray and angiotensin-converting enzyme (ACE) were normal. Neuromyelitis optica (NMO) antibody was negative. Treatment included intravenous Solu-Medrol (1 mg/kg for 3–5 days) followed by an oral prednisone taper for post-infectious optic neuritis with complete recovery of her vision and near complete recovery of her visual field in the left eye.

Subsequently, the patient had four similar recurrent episodes of isolated optic neuritis (one left eye, three right eye). Each episode began with periorbital eye pain exacerbated by eye movements and visual loss over 1–5 days with an interval range of 1–19 months between episodes. Visual acuity varied from 20/20 to 20/200 during the attacks. Each episode resolved with systemic corticosteroids. The first two recurrences were temporally related to corticosteroid taper, and the first occurred 1 month after the initial episode. The third recurrence occurred 4 months after tapering off a year-long course of monthly intravenous immunoglobulin (IVIG) therapy (1 g/kg for 2 days for initial dosing, then 1 g/kg for subsequent monthly doses) and the fourth 6 months after stopping IVIG again (over 2 years after her initial presentation). Current treatment includes mycophenolate mofetil with low-dose oral corticosteroids. Current visual acuity is best corrected to 20/20 in the right eye and 20/20-1 in the left eye. Clinical exam shows a trace relative afferent pupillary defect on the left and mild optic nerve pallor. This clinical course is consistent with chronic relapsing inflammatory optic neuropathy (Figs. 38.1 and 38.2).

## Clinical Questions

1. What are the clinical features that distinguish CRION from other forms of optic neuritis?
2. How is the diagnosis of CRION established?
3. What is known about the pathophysiology of CRION?
4. In what ways does the management of CRION differ from other forms of optic neuritis?
5. How do you approach acute management of CRION and what are the long-term management options in cases of CRION?

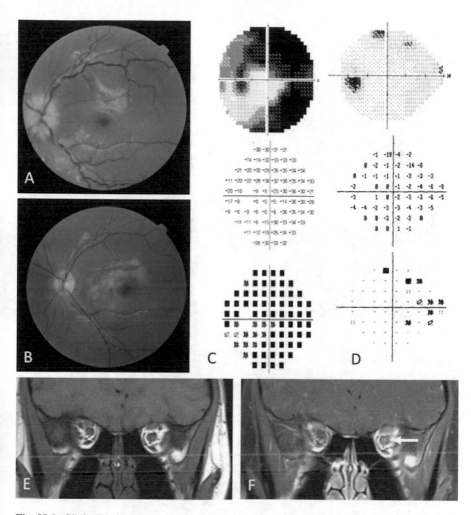

**Fig. 38.1** Clinical and Radiographic Images. (**a**) Fundus photograph of first episode of optic neuritis of the left eye showing optic disc edema. (**b**) Fundus photograph after resolution of first episode of optic neuritis showing resolution of optic disc edema. (**c**) Humphrey automated visual field 30-2 from the first episode of optic neuritis in the left eye showing a superior altitudinal defect and an inferior arcuate defect. The *gray scale* and pattern deviation plots are featured. The mean deviation was −23.89 DB. (**d**) Humphrey automated visual field 24-2 after resolution of the first episode of optic neuritis showing significant improvement in her visual field exam with mild decreased sensitivity primarily superonasally. The *gray scale* and pattern deviation plots are featured. The mean deviation was −3.59 DB. (**e**) Pre-contrast coronal magnetic resonance image during the first episode of optic neuritis. (**f**) Post contrast coronal magnetic resonance image during the first episode of optic neuritis showing enhancement of the left optic nerve (*arrow*)

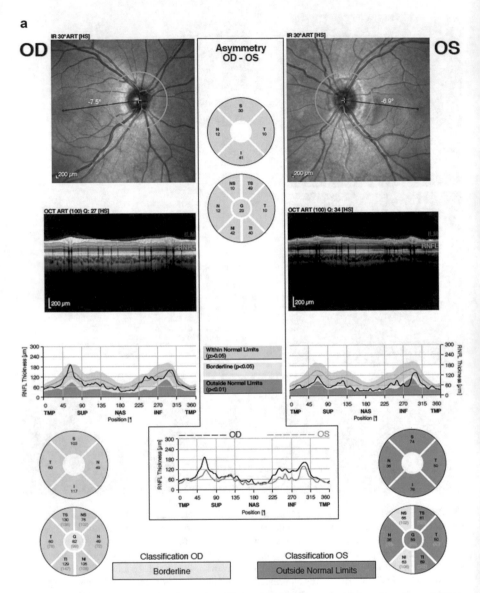

**Fig. 38.2** Optical coherence tomography (OCT) assessment of retinal nerve fiber layer (rNFL). (**a, b**) These are circle scans centered on the optic nerve head measuring rNFL thickness using the Heidelberg Spectralis (Heidelberg Engineering, Germany). (**a**) OCT showing rNFL thinning of the left eye after the patient's initial episode of optic neuritis on the left. (**b**) OCT taken approximately three and a half years later showing bilateral rNFL thinning after the right eye had also been affected

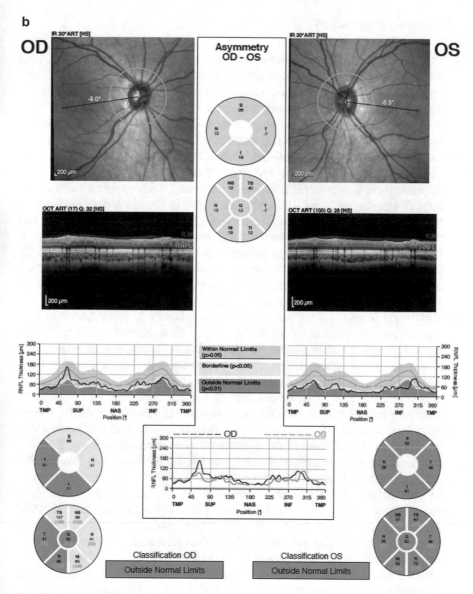

**Fig. 38.2** (continued)

# Diagnostic Discussion

1. CRION is a recurrent, corticosteroid-sensitive, isolated optic neuritis without evidence of any other neurological, infectious, inflammatory, or systemic autoimmune disease. In the acute setting, presenting findings are similar to demyelinating optic neuritis (pain increased with eye movement, relative afferent pupillary defect, decreased color vision, visual field defect, optic disc edema); however, it is the negative workup and multiple relapses and remissions of isolated optic neuritis that distinguish this condition from other demyelinating optic neuropathies [1, 2]. Kidd et al. described 15 cases of CRION and found that in the majority of the cases, the pain was severe and persistent even after development of visual symptoms. In addition, the degree of visual loss was more severe than in demyelinating optic neuritis, and peripheral visual field constriction was more common than a central scotoma [1]. Involvement of both optic nerves is common and often happens sequentially, as in the case of our patient [1, 2]. Latency between episodes varies widely between each case and between each episode within the same case [1, 2]. These patients classically respond promptly to systemic corticosteroids and relapse upon steroid withdrawal [1, 2].

2. CRION is a diagnosis of exclusion and is established by the clinical course of the disease and the absence of another systemic disease process. An extensive workup to rule out other causes of optic neuritis is necessary. MRI is important to evaluate enhancement of the affected optic nerve and the absence of brain lesions suggestive of multiple sclerosis (MS) or neuromyelitis optica (NMO). Demyelinating optic neuropathies can also occur following viral infections, especially in pediatric patients. The optic neuritis which ensues is different from infectious neuroretinitis associated with Bartonella infection (cat scratch disease); this is characterized by the appearance of optic nerve edema with perifoveal exudates or a "macular star" and was not a consideration in this specific case. A viral infection may have been the inciting factor for the primary episode of optic neuritis in our patient; however, post-viral optic neuritis would most commonly be monophasic rather than recurrent. Testing should include NMO immunoglobulin (NMO-IgG), CSF oligoclonal bands, evaluation for sarcoidosis, and further workup based on the individual presentation to rule out alternative etiologies. Proposed diagnostic criteria include (1) history of optic neuritis with at least one relapse, (2) loss of visual function, (3) NMO antibody negative, (4) contrast enhancement of the affected optic nerve, and (5) response to immunosuppressive treatment and relapse on withdrawal [2].

3. The pathophysiology of CRION is largely unknown [1, 2]. The robust response to immunosuppressive treatment suggests the etiology is at least in part immune-mediated. The clinical syndrome resembles other inflammatory optic neuropathies, including sarcoidosis. Nerve biopsies in granulomatous optic neuropathy have shown nerve swelling to be due to infiltration of inflammatory cells (lymphocytes, plasma cells, epithelioid and giant cells) and granuloma formation. Vision loss is likely from inflammation within the nerve [1]. There is a suggestion

that anti-myelin oligodendrocyte glycoprotein (MOG) antibodies may be linked to recurrent optic neuritis and other non-MS demyelinating diseases, including CRION, antibody negative NMO, and acute disseminated encephalomyelitis (ADEM) with optic neuritis [3–5]. MOG antibodies remain a research test at this time with unclear implications. Further research may reveal details regarding the etiology of this recurrent disease.

4. Patients with CRION are corticosteroid dependent and may suffer significant vision loss without treatment, distinguishing this condition from several forms of optic neuritis in which corticosteroids may not affect final visual outcomes [6]. With treatment, often complete restoration of normal visual acuity and color vision is achieved in between episodes, but relapses may occur upon cessation of corticosteroid [1, 2]. Some of these patients require a low dose of systemic steroids indefinitely, either alone or in combination with other immunomodulatory agents. There are reports of remission off treatment, as well.

5. Treatment of CRION consists of three phases: restoring vision in the acute phase, stabilizing vision in the interim period, and preserving vision over the long term with minimal side effects [2]. The acute phase is often treated with intravenous corticosteroids for 3–5 days or plasmapheresis (five exchanges is typical for neuro-inflammatory disease but can range from three to seven exchanges). Oral steroids are most often used in the interim period and can be very slowly tapered with rigorous follow-up for evaluation of visual function. Even with a slow taper, patients can relapse. Long-term therapy often involves the addition of steroid-sparing medications to minimize the potentially significant systemic side effects of steroids. Many different steroid-sparing medications have been described in CRION, including azathioprine, methotrexate, cyclophosphamide, mycophenolate mofetil, IVIG, cyclosporine, plasma exchange, and infliximab [2, 7, 8]. The decision on which medication to use often depends on the patients age and comorbidities. The patient should establish care with a specialist who can manage these medications and their side effects. At this time, there are no standardized methods for following this disease overtime. We have chosen to follow the patient with serial OCTs and MRIs to monitor for changes.

## Clinical Pearls

1. CRION is a recurrent, corticosteroid-dependent, isolated optic neuritis without evidence of other neurological, infectious, inflammatory, or systemic autoimmune diseases.
2. Diagnosis is one of exclusion, and a thorough evaluation to identify other systemic and demyelinating diseases is important for establishing the diagnosis.
3. Patients with CRION are corticosteroid dependent and may suffer significant and permanent vision loss without treatment, distinguishing this condition from several forms of optic neuritis in which corticosteroids may not affect final visual outcomes.

4. Steroids sparing immunomodulatory agents may be necessary for long-term management of patients with CRION with multiple or frequent recurrences to avoid the systemic side effects of chronic steroid use. There is not a well-established consensus on treatment for CRION, and comparative data are not available. Current knowledge is based on case reports and small case series.

# References

1. Kidd D, Burton B, Plant GT, Graham EM. Chronic relapsing inflammatory optic neuropathy (CRION). Brain. 2003;126:276–84.
2. Petzold A, Plant G. Chronic relapsing inflammatory optic neuropathy: a systemic review of 122 cases reported. J Neurol. 2014;261:17–26; Epub 2013 May 23.
3. Rostasy D, Mader S, Schanda K, et al. Anti-myelin oligodendrocyte glycoprotein antibodies in pediatric patients with optic neuritis. Arch Neurol. 2012;69:752–6.
4. Huppke B, Seidi R, Leiz S, et al. Acute disseminated encephalomyelitis followed by recurrent or monophasic optic neuritis in pediatric patients. Mult Scler. 2013;19(7):941–6.
5. Hacohen Y, Absoud M, Deiva K, et al. Myelin oligodendrocyte glycoprotein antibodies are associated with a non-MS course. Neurol Meuroimmunol Neuroinflamm. 2015;2(2):e81.
6. Beck RW. The optic neuritis treatment trial: three year follow-up results. Arch Ophthalmol. 1995;113:136–7.
7. Stiebel-Kalish H. Intravenous immunoglobulin in recurrent-relapsing inflammatory optic neuropathy. Can J Ophthal. 2010;45:71–5.
8. Myers TD, Smith JR, Wertheim MS, Egan RA, Shutts WT, Rosenbaum JT. Use of corticosteroid sparing systemic immunosuppressives for the treatment of corticosteroid dependent optic neuritis not associated with demyelinating diseases. Br J Ophthal. 2004;88:673–80.

# Chapter 39
# Optic Neuritis as the Presenting Symptom for MS

Dorlyne M. Brchan and Teri L. Schreiner

## Case Presentation

A 15-year-old right-handed Caucasian girl with history of migraine and ADHD presented to the hospital with a 3-day history of central visual loss from the right eye. She had no prior history of visual complaints and had recently been healthy. Family history was notable for mother with rheumatoid arthritis and maternal aunt with hypothyroidism. She was in the tenth grade with no learning difficulties and active in school athletics. She denied any recent trauma.

When covering the left eye, she could only see gray shadows of bright moving objects in the periphery of the vision of the right eye. She was unable to differentiate the color red from dark gray. She had pain with eye movement on the right. She denied concurrent weakness, sensory changes, or coordination problems. She was evaluated by an ophthalmologist who noted a relative afferent pupillary defect in the right eye but no optic nerve swelling nor retinal pathology. MRI brain and orbits with and without contrast were performed and notable for enlargement of the right optic nerve compared to the left and enhancement of the right optic nerve (Fig. 39.1). There were several foci of increased T2 and FLAIR signal in the subcortical white matter and periventricular region of the bilateral frontal and occipitoparietal lobes, as well as a small focus of abnormal signal in the juxtacortical white matter and the right optic radiation. There was no evidence of enhancement of brain lesions.

D.M. Brchan, M.D.
Tanana Valley Clinic, Foundation Health Partners, 1432 102nd Street, Unit 4,
Fort Wainwright, AK 99703, USA
e-mail: Dorlyne585@gmail.com

T.L. Schreiner, M.D., M.P.H. (✉)
Department of Neurology and Pediatrics, Children's Hospital Colorado, University of
Colorado-Denver, 13123 E. 16th Avenue., B155, Aurora, CO 80045, USA
e-mail: Teri.schreiner@ucdenver.edu

© Springer International Publishing AG 2017      309
E. Waubant, T.E. Lotze (eds.), *Pediatric Demyelinating Diseases of the Central Nervous System and Their Mimics*, DOI 10.1007/978-3-319-61407-6_39

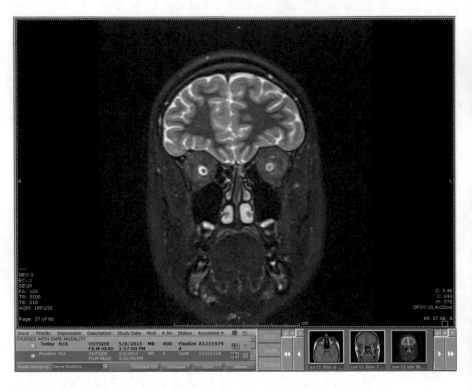

**Fig. 39.1** MRI orbits. This coronal STIR image shows edema of the right optic nerve

Laboratory workup included a lumbar puncture with 1 WBC, 0 RBC, normal glucose, and elevated protein of 61 mg/dL (The upper limit of normal was 25 mg/dL). She had positive oligoclonal bands in the CSF. NMO aquaporin-4 IgG antibody was negative in the CSF. Serum studies included a negative ANA titer and normal glucose, thyroid function, B12, and normal 25-OH-Vitamin D.

## Clinical Questions

1. What is the differential diagnosis of vision loss in children?
2. What features of our clinical scenario suggest optic neuritis?
3. What does the age of the patient as well as MRI findings and presence of unilateral or bilateral optic neuritis portend for prognosis?
4. What treatment is recommended for optic neuritis in children?
5. What is the likelihood of complete visual recovery of optic neuritis in children?

# Diagnostic Discussion

## *Answer #1*

Optic neuritis is a common cause of vision loss in children. This may occur as part of acute disseminated encephalomyelitis, as the result of a chronic, relapsing condition such as multiple sclerosis and neuromyelitis optica, or it may be idiopathic. Prior to attributing the cause as idiopathic, alternative diagnoses should be considered. While the differential diagnosis for vision loss is broad, the clinician must consider the probability of a given disease in the pediatric age group. For example, syphilis and ischemic optic neuropathy are extraordinarily rare in children, whereas cat-scratch disease and inherited disorders are more common. Along with childhood onset, the associated constitutional signs and symptoms can help to further narrow differential considerations. A detailed history should include complaints of dry eyes and dry mouth (sicca symptoms) related to Sjögren's syndrome. A detailed exam should evaluate for cutaneous stigmata of neurofibromatosis and optic pathway gliomas. Inflammation of the cavernous sinus associated with Tolosa-Hunt syndrome classically presents with a painful ophthalmoplegia and proptosis in association with optic neuropathy. Some conditions may also be distinguished by their propensity to more commonly produce either unilateral or bilateral disease as well as demonstrate disease-related fundoscopic findings (Table 39.1)

Evaluation of acute vision loss in children should begin with identification of whether vision loss is monocular or binocular. Adolescents are typically aware of unilateral vision changes, but younger children can accommodate with the healthy eye and may not come to attention until a visual field defect is suspected during regular play activities. Monocular vision loss is suggestive of retinal or optic nerve pathology. Binocular vision loss is more suggestive of a lesion involving the optic chiasm and posterior optic pathways. The presence of a relative afferent pupillary defect helps to narrow the localization to either retina or optic nerve. Subsequent evaluation should establish the extent of visual field deficit.The classic triad of symptoms in optic neuritis is subacute unilateral vision loss, periocular pain, and decreased color vision. Symptoms usually progress over a period of days to 2 weeks. A history of a more chronic progressive vision loss might prompt consideration for an alternate diagnosis from optic neuritis. It is not unusual for the funduscopic examination to show a normal optic nerve head with no signs of inflammation.

## *Answer #2*

The presented patient's history and examination findings are consistent with the features of optic neuritis: monocular vision loss, painful eye movement, and decreased color vision. Moreover, the presence of a swollen, enhancing optic nerve on MRI as well as lymphocyte predominance and elevated protein in CSF is supportive. The presence of oligoclonal bands is supportive of intrathecal inflammation which portends a chronic condition.

**Table 39.1** Differential diagnosis for acute/subacute vision loss

| Disease category | Disease name | Presenting exam findings | Ancillary tests |
|---|---|---|---|
| Infectious | Cat-scratch disease | Unilateral, macular star sign, neuroretinitis | CSF CBC +/− *Borrelia* IgM +/− PPD or quantiferonTB |
| | Lyme disease or syphilis | Uveitis/retinitis | |
| | Tuberculosis | Uveitis/choroiditis, herpes zoster | |
| Rheumatologic | Behçet's disease or Wegener's granulomatosis | Papillitis, uveitis, retinal vasculitis, possible systemic symptoms | ANA ESR/CRP +/− ACE |
| | Sarcoidosis | Painful vision loss, possible systemic symptoms | |
| | Systemic lupus erythematosus (SLE) | Unilateral vision loss, possible systemic symptoms | |
| | Sjögren's syndrome | Bilateral vision loss, possible systemic symptoms | |
| Neoplastic | Optic glioma | Painless and progressive vision loss; +/− protrusion of one or both globes | CBC CSF |
| Ischemic | Retinal artery occlusion | Painless, severe vision loss | MRI brain Vessel imaging (CTA/MRA) |
| Toxic/ nutritional | B12 deficiency Methanol toxicity | Painless, bilateral, symmetric vision loss | B12 testing, CBC, methanol screening |
| Inherited | Leber's hereditary optic neuropathy | Painless, progressive, bilateral vision loss | Family history Genetic testing |
| Ocular | Posterior scleritis | Eye pain, minimal vision loss | Ultrasound ESR/CRP |
| | Retinopathies/ maculopathies | Painless vision loss, retained color vision | |

## *Answer #3*

Age has been identified as one of the key factors in the relationship between presentation and the development of multiple sclerosis. Optic neuritis in young children (<10 years of age) is more likely to be bilateral than unilateral and less likely to lead to multiple sclerosis. In one study, children with optic neuritis were noted to have at least a 36% risk of developing multiple sclerosis within 2 years. Although children with bilateral optic neuritis were noted to have a 71% likelihood of an abnormal MRI versus 33% with unilateral optic neuritis, patients with normal MRI's in the setting of unilateral or bilateral optic neuritis were less likely to go on to develop multiple sclerosis. Overall, a negative MRI at the time of presentation of optic neuritis is prognostically favorable [1–4].

The patient described has a high risk of subsequent demyelinating attacks given the presence of brain lesions on MRI. She meets criteria for dissemination in space with the presence of at least one lesion in 2 of 4 locations: periventricular, juxtacortical, infratentorial, and spinal cord. Our patient has both periventricular and juxtacortical lesions. However, she does not meet McDonald criteria for dissemination in time as she has only had one clinical event and one MRI scan and does not have an asymptomatic, enhancing lesion. If she had had an asymptomatic, enhancing brain lesion in addition to the enhancing optic nerve lesion, she would have met criteria for dissemination in time per McDonald criteria. Our patient was diagnosed with a clinically isolated syndrome. She subsequently developed new T2 lesions on MRI and was diagnosed with relapsing and remitting multiple sclerosis.

Treatment for acute optic neuritis includes high-dose steroids followed by oral prednisone taper. Appropriate follow-up would occur within a few weeks of presentation.

## Answer #4

No clinical trials of treatment of optic neuritis in a pediatric population have been done. Thus, our knowledge of the treatment of pediatric-onset optic neuritis is extrapolated from studies in adult patients. For example, the Optic Neuritis Treatment Trial [5, 7] found that adult patients who received intravenous methylprednisolone (250 mg IV every 6 h for 3 days followed by an oral prednisone taper) had accelerated visual recovery; however, compared to placebo, this treatment did not improve visual outcomes at 6 months or 1 year after the event. As with adults, steroids are the mainstay of treatment in pediatric-onset optic neuritis, as well. Intravenous methylprednisolone (20–30 mg/kg/day) may be considered for a 3–5-day course to hasten the return of vision. This high-dose course of steroids may be followed by a 2–4-week course of oral prednisone, starting at 1–2 mg/kg/day and tapered over a 2–4-week period.

## Answer #5

Complete visual recovery is more likely in children than adults. In one study [4], >80% of children had full visual recovery after optic neuritis with a mean follow-up period being 2.4 years (0.3–8.3 years). In another study [6], >90% of patients had complete recovery of visual symptoms within 2–3 weeks, regardless of treatment. Through the course of recovery, accommodations should be made for school, and caution should be exercised in sports activities to prevent a collision injury from residual field deficits.

Consultation with an ophthalmologist experienced in pediatric optic neuritis is important during the acute presentation and during follow-up. Specific studies can be used to better assess deficits to include direct fundoscopy evaluating for optic nerve pallor, formal visual field testing, Ishihara color-plate testing, and visual acuity to include low-contrast visual acuity, which is often more significantly affected. More advanced evaluations, which are becoming common, include the use of optical coherence tomography (OCT) to measure ganglion cell layer (GCL) and the retinal nerve fiber layer (RNFL) thickness. This technology can be used to determine the degree of permanent injury from a case of optic neuritis, although patients are not typically visually impaired by minor thinning of the retina. In one study [8], the mean RNFL thickness was about 25% lower in patients with demyelinating disease, suggesting that there may be permanent damage to the retina over time even if not clinically evident.

## Clinical Pearls

1. Painful eye movements with vision loss developing over days should trigger consideration of optic neuritis.
2. Children less than 10 years of age with a normal MRI brain at the time of presentation of unilateral or bilateral optic neuritis have a low likelihood of progressing to multiple sclerosis. Children with optic neuritis in association with other brain lesions and not having ADEM should be evaluated for multiple sclerosis using current diagnostic criteria.
3. The majority of pediatric patients with optic neuritis have recovery within 2–3 weeks, regardless of treatment.
4. Current standard treatment for optic neuritis is a 3-5 day course of intravenous methylprednisolone followed by oral steroids.

## References

1. Bonhomme GR, Waldman AT, Balcer LJ, Daniels AB, Tennekoon GI, Forman S, Galetta SL, Liu GT. Pediatric optic neuritis: brain MRI abnormalities and risk of multiple sclerosis. Neurology. 2009;72:881–5.
2. Waldman AT, Stull LB, Galetta SL, Balcer LJ, Liu GT. Pediatric optic neuritis and risk of multiple sclerosis: meta-analysis of observational studies. J AAPOS. 2011;15:441–6.
3. Subramanian PS. Pediatric optic neuritis and multiple sclerosis: who is at risk for progression? J AAPOS. 2011;15(5):419–20.
4. Wilejto M, Shroff M, Buncic JR, Kennedy J, Goia C, Banwell B. The clinical features, MRI findings, and outcome of optic neuritis in children. Neurology. 2006;67:258–62.
5. Voss E, Raab P, Trebst C, Stangel M. Clinical approach to optic neuritis: pitfalls, red flags, and differential diagnosis. Ther Adv Neurol Disord. 2011;4(2):123–34.
6. Beck RW, Gal RL. Treatment of acute optic neuritis: a summary of findings from the optic neuritis treatment trial. Arch Ophthalmol. 2008;126(7):994–5.
7. Optic Neuritis Study Group. Multiple sclerosis risk after optic neuritis: final optic neuritis treatment trial follow-up. Arch Neurol. 2008;65(6):727–32.
8. Yeh EA, Marrie RA, Reginald YA, Buncic JR, Noguera AE, O'Mahony J, Mah JK, Banwell B, Costello F. Functional-structural correlations in the afferent visual pathway in pediatric demyelination. Neurology. 2014;83(23):2147–52.

# Chapter 40
# Steroid-Dependent Recurrent Optic Neuritis in Pediatric Multiple Sclerosis

Hardeep Chohan, Emmanuelle Waubant, and Jennifer S. Graves

## Case Presentation

A 15-year-old previously healthy female of Chinese descent first presented with a 1-week history of bilateral eye pain and subsequent blurred vision. She had moved to the United States 2 years prior, was up-to-date with her immunizations, and had no family history of neurological disease. She had tested positive for tuberculosis exposure upon arrival to the United States and had previously been treated with a 9-month course of isoniazid. She had no precipitating signs or symptoms of illness identified, but she did develop upper respiratory symptoms after her visual symptoms began. She denied any diplopia or external redness or swelling of her eyes.

On examination her visual acuity was counting fingers at 1 ft in each eye, and there was no relative afferent pupillary defect (RAPD). On dilated fundus exam, she had bilateral optic nerve head edema (ONHE). Her MRI showed bilateral optic nerve T2 prolongation and gadolinium enhancement anterior to the chiasm (L > R), one small, isolated T2 non-enhancing 2 mm lesion in the right cerebellum and no cord lesions. Lumbar puncture (LP) showed normal opening pressure and WBC and protein levels, no oligoclonal bands, and a normal IgG index. Extensive laboratory workups, which included infectious, rheumatic, and inflammatory panels, were all unremarkable. She was admitted and received IV methylprednisolone 1000 mg/day for 3 days. She had significant improvement after initiation of steroids with resolution of eye pain,

H. Chohan, M.D. (✉)
Department of Neurology, University of California San Francisco,
350 Parnassus Avenue, Suite 304 A, San Francisco, CA 94117, USA
e-mail: Hardeep.k.chohan@gmail.com

E. Waubant, M.D., Ph.D. • J.S. Graves, M.D., Ph.D., M.A.S.
Clinical Neurology and Pediatrics, Regional Pediatric MS Clinic at UCSF,
University of California San Francisco, 675 Nelson Rising Lane, Suite 221,
San Francisco, CA 94158, USA
e-mail: Emmanuelle.waubant@ucsf.edu; Jennifer.graves@ucsf.edu

© Springer International Publishing AG 2017                                          315
E. Waubant, T.E. Lotze (eds.), *Pediatric Demyelinating Diseases of the Central Nervous System and Their Mimics*, DOI 10.1007/978-3-319-61407-6_40

improved ONHE and visual acuity of 20/25 in the left eye and 20/20 in the right after the third day of pulse steroids. She was discharged on a 3-week prednisone taper starting with 50 mg per day.

She had a follow-up visit at the ophthalmology clinic 2 days after discharge and was found to have 20/20 vision in each eye and was instructed to stop the steroid taper. Within a week of stopping steroids, blurred vision returned, worse on the left side, and she was restarted on oral steroids starting at 40 mg daily with a prolonged taper. Six weeks later, she self-discontinued her steroids and within the week had an episode of dizziness, vomiting, fever, and vision loss. At the visual nadir, her acuity was reduced to finger counting on the left but maintained 20/20 on the right. She had a left RAPD, bilateral optic disc pallor, and significant visual field deficits bilaterally (left > right). At this point she was diagnosed with a steroid-dependent optic neuropathy suggestive of chronic relapsing inflammatory optic neuropathy (CRION).

Repeat CSF analyses showed the presence of two oligoclonal bands and an elevated IgG index of 0.7 (normal range = 0.3–0.6). MRI at the time demonstrated left optic nerve enhancement, along with a new enhancing left paravermian cerebellar white matter lesion in conjunction with multiple new punctate supratentorial lesions. While these MRI findings met 2010 McDonald criteria for multiple sclerosis (MS) with dissemination in space and time, she had no signs or symptoms of disease outside the visual pathway. Also, her steroid-dependent course of disease was atypical for MS and for those reasons raised concern for CRION.

She was restarted on prednisone 20 mg/day, and 1 month later, her vision was 20/40 in the left eye. Ocular coherence tomography (OCT) at that time demonstrated retinal nerve fiber layer (RNFL) thinning bilaterally. Repeat OCT 3 months later showed further loss with global mean peripapillary RNFL of 53 μm in right and 43 μm in left eye. Given the severity of her visual deficits, she was tested for aquaporin-4 antibodies but these were not present. Repeat testing for these antibodies 1 year later was also negative.

With new baseline Snellen acuity of 20/20 in the right and 20/25 in the left side, mycophenolate mofetil was introduced progressively up to 1000 mg twice daily as a steroid-sparing agent along with a prednisone taper that was completed after 4 months. Within days of being off steroids, blurred vision in her left eye returned with a visual nadir of only being able to count fingers at 2 ft. She remained 20/20 on the right. She received 5 days of IV methylprednisolone 1000 mg/day, and left eye vision again improved to 20/50 at the end of the course. A prolonged prednisone taper was restarted at 60 mg/day along with an increase in mycophenolate mofetil to 1500 mg twice daily.

A brain MRI obtained toward the end of the 6-month prolonged steroid taper demonstrated two new asymptomatic brain parenchymal lesions and atrophied optic nerves. A few weeks later and after stopping prednisone, she had another severe relapse of painful left ON. Her acuity in the left eye was 20/800 and right remained 20/20. Repeat brain MRI demonstrated 13 new clinically silent enhancing brain lesions plus enhancement of the left optic nerve. Once again IV methylprednisolone 1000 mg daily improved the visual loss, but recovery was more gradual, and new baseline acuity for the left eye after the episode was 20/30. Her OCT demonstrated extensive axonal loss with mean global RNFL of 39 μm in the left eye. Given numerous enhancing brain lesions suggestive of MS (although asymptomatic) and negative anti-aquaporin-4 antibodies, mycophenolate mofetil was discontinued, and natalizumab was initiated along with prolonged steroid taper.

After five monthly infusions of natalizumab and completion of the steroid taper, she had recurrence of left ON with visual nadir of 20/200. There was no change in her brain parenchymal lesion burden. Repeat testing for aquaporin-4 antibodies (for a total of three assays) was negative. She was not found to have anti-natalizumab antibodies. After additional pulse steroid and resumption of prolonged taper to 20 mg daily prednisone, she returned to her baseline of 20/30 in the left eye.

Rituximab 1000 mg per dose given in two doses 2 weeks apart was infused after a 1-month washout from natalizumab. She remained stable until prednisone was tapered to less than 10 mg daily. She had recurrence of left ON with visual nadir of 20/50 but, with higher doses of steroids, returned to 20/30 in the left eye. Further attempt to maintain her on rituximab and 10 mg daily prednisone was insufficient to prevent ON relapse, but there was no change in brain parenchymal lesion burden. Throughout her disease course, she had a normal neurological exam except for her visual findings. She developed steroid side effects of acne, moon facies, and bone mineral loss. As a final attempt with a steroid-sparing agent, methotrexate was initiated, but when steroids were tapered below 20 mg daily, she experienced another episode of left ON. After careful consultation with the family and an endocrinologist, a decision was made to continue on monotherapy with daily prednisone 20 mg with careful monitoring and management of steroid side effects. She has been without further relapse and is performing well in college without any evidence of symptoms or clinical findings outside the visual system for over 1-year follow-up.

## Clinical Reasoning Questions

1. What is the differential diagnosis for optic neuritis in patients NOT meeting MS criteria?
2. What is chronic relapsing inflammatory optic neuropathy (CRION)?
3. What are treatment options and considerations for relapsing optic neuritis that is not associated with MS or NMO?
4. What are the long-term visual outcomes for non-MS- and non-NMO-related forms of optic neuritis?

## Discussion

1. Optic neuritis (ON) is a subacute loss of vision usually accompanied by retro-orbital pain and pain with eye movements. Both viral and bacterial infections can cause ON. Viral agents include herpes simplex, hepatitis A, and enteroviruses [1]. Bacterial infections involve organisms such as streptococcus, meningococcus,

brucella, pertussis, salmonella, *Treponema pallidum*, borrelia, and *Mycobacterium tuberculosis* [1]. After infectious etiologies have been ruled out, the differential for autoimmune inflammatory optic neuropathies must be considered. Acute demyelinating ON is primarily associated with MS. More severe cases of ON, often with less responsiveness to corticosteroids, raise concern for neuromyelitis optica spectrum disorders (NMOSD), diseases now known to be associated with an astrocytopathy but with secondary demyelination [1, 2]. Besides these two, many less common forms of autoimmune ON exist that may be associated with systemic autoimmune diseases, such as lupus erythematosus, vasculitis, rheumatoid arthritis, and inflammatory bowel diseases; some recurrent forms of autoimmune ON, however, are not yet clearly understood. These latter syndromes have acquired descriptive labels including the moniker's single isolated ON (SION) for an idiopathic monophasic syndrome, recurrent isolated ON (RION), and chronic relapsing inflammatory optic neuropathy (CRION). CRION, defined further below, is by definition a steroid-dependent syndrome, whereas the term RION has largely been used to describe less severe isolated, idiopathic recurring ON events [3]. The underlying pathophysiology of these descriptive syndromes are not yet known, yet neuroimmunology specialists are still often asked to aid neuro-ophthalmologists in designing the most appropriate treatment plans. Sarcoidosis may also manifest as ON or perineuritis [1–3]. Lastly, compressive or infiltrative lesions, such as metastatic carcinoma, meningioma and glioma, and fungal disease, must be considered as alternative diagnoses as appropriate in atypical presentations of acute optic neuritis or chronic optic neuropathy [2].

2. CRION was first described by Kidd et al. in 2003 [1]. Since then there have been various case reports of patients with similar presentations, including one comprehensive global review of the literature published between 2003 and 2013 which identified 122 cases [2, 4]. CRION is a clinical syndrome characterized by >1 episode of ON, strong corticosteroid dependence, and normal brain imaging [1, 2]. However, rarely brain imaging abnormalities might be seen. Petzold et al. identified abnormal brain MRI findings outside of the optic nerve in 3 out of 122 cases, though none of them met MS criteria [2]. In our patient, MS criteria was met, but the atypical steroid-dependent disease course as well as a lack of response to MS therapy raised concern for CRION. Other common features of CRION include severe pain at onset and overall worse outcome than multiple sclerosis optic neuritis (MSON). In fact 68% of all reported CRION cases presented with visual acuity (VA) of 0.1 (IQR 0–0.25) or less compared to 36% in the optic neuritis treatment trial (ONTT), the largest trial of acute demyelinating optic neuritis [2]. Recurrence of pain and visual loss shortly after reducing or stopping a steroid taper is a red flag, and a non-MSON such as NMOSD, sarcoidosis, or CRION should be suspected. One concern regarding the initial description of CRION was that anti-aquaporin-4 antibodies were not available at the time and some cases could have been NMOSD. In later reports of CRION, this has been less of an issue. Anti-aquaporin-4 antibodies should be checked more than once in cases of suspected CRION given similarities in the optic neuritis phenotype in the two diseases.

3. Treatment for an atypical, recurrent autoimmune ON such as CRION consists of three phases: restoring visual function in the acute phase, stabilizing the vision in the interim, and preserving vision in the long term with minimal side effects from treatments [2]. For the acute phase, intravenous glucocorticosteroids (methylprednisolone, 30 mg/kg/dose; maximum 1000 mg) for 3–5 days. If there is no response to glucocorticoids, plasmapheresis may be considered. For steroid-dependent optic neuritis, a prolonged prednisone taper over several months should be considered, often starting at a dose of 1 mg/kg/day which is then weaned down to a minimal effective dose that may vary between patients. During the oral steroid taper, stringent follow-up should be implemented to not go below the minimal effective dose associated with a risk of relapse. For the final phase, emphasis is on minimizing side effects of long-term steroid use by adding a steroid-sparing medication. Commonly used agents are azathioprine, methotrexate, cyclophosphamide, or mycophenolate mofetil. There are reports of patients benefitting from monthly intravenous immunoglobulin (IVIG) treatment [5]. The response to treatment is very much case dependent; some patients might not respond to any of these steroid-sparing agents, as in our patient, and require long-term steroid treatment. Long-term steroid use is a particularly challenging situation in pediatric patients due possible effect on bone growth. Simultaneous osteoporosis prophylaxis is recommended.

4. Overall, steroid-dependent forms of ON including CRION and NMOSD have more severe and potentially blinding loss of vision over time when compared to MSON. Petzold et al. noted that 33% of patients with CRION had residual VA of less that 0.1 (IQR 0.1–1.0) compared to only 1% in the ONTT [2]. It is pertinent that ON patients are critically examined and followed up so that steroid-dependent cases can be identified early and treated appropriately to decrease the risk of further visual loss. A typical short glucocorticosteroid taper as used in MS can be detrimental for a CRION patient due to ON recurrence upon treatment discontinuation. Prompt and long-term glucocorticosteroid use and/or broad-spectrum immunosuppression is essential to decrease the rate of ON relapses in CRION.

## Clinical Pearls

- Optic neuritis commonly occurs in the context of multiple sclerosis and neuromyelitis optica spectrum disorders, but many other rare etiologies exist.
- Chronic relapsing inflammatory optic neuropathy is a syndrome characterized by isolated recurrent optic neuritis and strong glucocorticosteroid dependence.
- Treatment of CRION consists of three phases: restoring visual function in the acute phase with pulse IV glucocorticosteroids, stabilizing with oral glucocorticosteroids tapering down to minimal effective dose, and finally using steroid-sparing agents.
- Steroid-dependent ON typically has worse visual outcomes as compared to MSON and the treatment approach differs; hence, early recognition is critical.

# References

1. Kidd D, Burton B, Plant GT, et al. Chronic inflammatory optic neuropathy. Brain. 2003;126:276–84.
2. Petzold A, Plant GT. Chronic relapsing inflammatory optic neuropathy: a systematic review of 122 cases reported. J Neurol. 2014;261:17–26.
3. Petzold A, Plant GT, et al. Diagnosis and classification of autoimmune optic neuropathy. Autoimmun Rev. 2014;13:539–45.
4. Benoilid A, Tilikete C, et al. Relapsing optic neuritis: a multicentre study of 62 patients. Mult Scler. 2014;20(7):848–53.
5. Stiebel-Kalish H, Hammel N, et al. Intravenous immunoglobulin in recurrent-relapsing inflammatory optic neuropathy. Can J Ophthalmol. 2010;45(1):71–5.

# Chapter 41
# Neuromyelitis Optica Presenting with Bilateral Optic Neuritis

Carla Francisco and Emmanuelle Waubant

## Case Presentation

A 7-year-old female presented with acute vision loss in the right eye. She had been evaluated by an ophthalmologist 3 months prior to presentation secondary to poor visual acuity in her left eye and was found to have optic nerve atrophy on that side. At the time of her presentation with right eye vision loss, her neurologic examination was significant for optic nerve pallor on the left with acuity limited to light/dark perception on that side. Her right optic disk had hyperemia, and her visual acuity was 20/400. The rest of her general and neurological examination was normal. MRI of the brain and orbits with and without gadolinium demonstrated enlargement and contrast enhancement of the right optic nerve (Figs. 41.1, 41.2, and 41.3). MRI of the spine with and without gadolinium was normal. Cerebrospinal fluid analysis demonstrated 2 white blood cells, 0 red blood cells, normal glucose (62 mg/dL), and normal protein (28 mg/dL). IgG index was normal and there were no oligoclonal bands. She tested negative for serum aquaporin-4 (AQP4)-IgG antibody but was positive for CSF AQP4-IgG antibody. She received methylprednisolone 30 mg/kg/day IV for 5 days and was discharged on an oral prednisone taper beginning at a dose of 2 mg/kg/day. Following completion of intravenous methylprednisolone, her visual acuity improved to 20/200 on the right with no change on the left. She was treated with rituximab 750 mg/m$^2$ IV divided into four doses with additional booster

C. Francisco, M.D. (✉)
Multiple Sclerosis and Neuroinflammation Center, University of California,
San Francisco, San Francisco, CA, USA

E. Waubant, M.D., Ph.D.
Clinical Neurology and Pediatrics, Regional Pediatric MS Clinic at UCSF,
University of California San Francisco, 675 Nelson Rising Lane, Suite 221,
San Francisco, CA 94158, USA
e-mail: Carla.Francisco@ucsf.edu; Emmanuelle.Waubant@ucsf.edu

© Springer International Publishing AG 2017                                    321
E. Waubant, T.E. Lotze (eds.), *Pediatric Demyelinating Diseases of the Central Nervous System and Their Mimics*, DOI 10.1007/978-3-319-61407-6_41

**Fig. 41.1** MRI orbits T2
fat saturation sequence

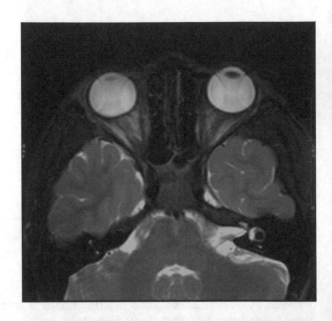

**Fig. 41.2** MRI orbits T1
fat saturation sequence
showing post-gadolinium
enhancement of right optic
nerve

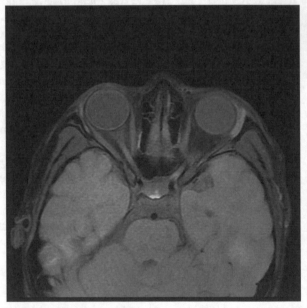

doses every 9 months. Visual acuity improved to 20/20 on the right but remained as light perception only on the left. She had no further relapses over the subsequent 3 years of follow-up.

**Fig. 41.3** MRI orbits T1 post-gadolinium showing enhancement of intracanalicular portion of right optic nerve and optic chiasm

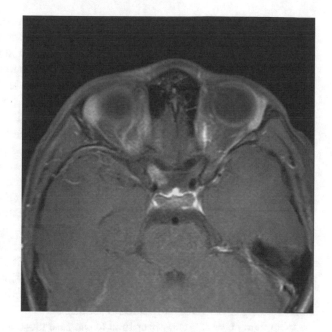

## Clinical Questions

1. What are the diagnostic criteria of neuromyelitis optica spectrum disease (NMOSD)?
2. What tests are recommended for the initial diagnosis and monitoring of NMOSD initially presenting with optic neuritis?
3. What are the best treatment options, both in the acute and chronic phase, for NMOSD initially presenting with optic neuritis?
4. What is the spectrum of the clinical course and outcomes in NMOSD initially presenting with optic neuritis?

## Discussion

### What Are the Diagnostic Criteria of Neuromyelitis Optica Spectrum Disease (NMOSD)?

Neuromyelitis optica (NMO or Devic's disease) was initially described in 1894 by Eugene Devic and Fernand Gault [1] when they reported a series of 16 patients with vision loss in one or both eyes followed by limb weakness and/or numbness and loss of bladder control. Diagnostic criteria for NMO were created in 1999 and included absolute criteria that required both optic neuritis and acute myelitis [2]. These criteria were revised in 2006 [2] after the discovery that many patients with NMO have detectable serum IgG antibodies to the water channel aquaporin-4 (AQP4-IgG). The 2006 criteria included seropositivity for AQP4-IgG as supportive criteria but continued to require both acute myelitis and optic neuritis upon presentation. Between 2011 and 2013, an international panel of physicians (International Panel on NMO Diagnosis or IPND) met to revise the diagnostic criteria for NMO and came up with a consensus that was published in 2015 [3]. The panel decided to unify the terms NMO and NMO spectrum disorders (NMOSD), a term that was introduced in 2007 to describe AGP4-IgG-positive patients with either myelitis or optic neuritis as well as patients with otherwise typical NMO but who also had cerebral, diencephalic, or brainstem lesions. The panel then developed diagnostic criteria for NMOSD with AQP4-IgG positivity as well as criteria for NMOSD without AQP4-IgG positivity or in whom the status of AQP4-IgG is unknown (Table 41.1).

In 2015, the United States Network of Pediatric MS Centers compared the sensitivity of the 2015 criteria to those proposed in 2006. Using data prospectively collected on pediatric patients clinically diagnosed with NMOSD between May 1, 2011 and December 31, 2013, it was found that 97% (36/37) met the 2015 criteria for NMOSD, whereas only 49% (18/37) met the 2006 Wingerchuk diagnostic criteria [4]. As such, it was concluded that the 2015 IPND criteria were more sensitive in identifying NMOSD in the pediatric setting.

In applying these diagnostic criteria to the case presentation, a patient who presents with optic neuritis can be diagnosed with NMOSD if he or she has seropositivity for AQP4-IgG. If the patient is seronegative for AQP4-IgG or if the status is unknown, the criteria are stricter (see Table 41.1) and require two of six core clinical characteristics and fulfillment of MRI criteria, if applicable. While not specifically addressed in these criteria, the prior history of unexplained optic atrophy in the presented case suggests that clinicians might consider testing for AQP4-IgG in such patients so as to initiate disease-modifying therapy in the setting of a positive result and prior to another clinical event.

## What Tests Are Recommended for the Initial Diagnosis and Monitoring of NMOSD Initially Presenting with Optic Neuritis?

Given that NMOSD with optic neuritis as the initial presentation can present in the same manner as other diseases, such as MS, but respond to different treatment, it is recommended that any pediatric patient presenting with acute vision loss undergo MRI of the brain and orbits with and without gadolinium. Depending on the rest of the neurologic examination and clinical presentation, MRI with and without gadolinium of the entire spine is also suggested, as silent asymptomatic lesions can be found in the spine in both NMOSD and MS [5]. A lumbar puncture should also be performed and includes cell count, glucose, and protein, oligoclonal bands, and IgG index. CSF pleocytosis (>50 leukocytes/ml) can be seen in 35% of patients with

NMOSD [3] and is more commonly seen in NMOSD than MS. In contrast, while oligoclonal bands and elevated IgG index can be transiently elevated in an acute attack of NMOSD, they are more commonly seen in MS.

While AQP4-IgG is highly sensitive and specific for an NMOSD diagnosis, patients who are seronegative should be further investigated for alternative etiologies. The diagnostic criteria suggest consideration for alternate conditions such as neoplasm and sarcoid. HIV and syphilis are also on the differential. While such

**Table 41.1** NMOSD diagnostic criteria [3]

*Diagnostic criteria for NMOSD with AQP4-IgG*
1. At least one core clinical characteristic (see below)
2. Positive test for AQP4-IgG using best available detection method (cell-based assay strongly recommended)
3. Exclusion of alternative diagnoses

*Diagnostic criteria for NMOSD without AQP4-IgG positivity or NMOSD with unknown AQP4-IgG status*
1. At least two core clinical characteristics (see below) occurring as a result of one or more clinical attacks and meeting *all* of the following requirements:
    (a)  At least one core clinical characteristic must be optic neuritis, acute myelitis with longitudinally extensive transverse myelitis (LETM), or area postrema syndrome
    (b)  Dissemination in space, DIS (two or more different core clinical characteristics): occurrence of two or more discrete clinical attacks in different CNS regions (optic nerve, spinal cord, brainstem, diencephalon, or cerebrum). NOTE: Recurrent, isolated optic neuritis (even if bilateral) and recurrent transverse myelitis (even if different cord regions involved) do not establish DIS. Acute myelitis with extension into the brainstem does not establish DIS
    (c)  Fulfillment of additional MRI requirements, as applicable
2. Negative tests for AQP4-IgG using best available detection method or testing unavailable
3. Exclusion of alternative diagnoses

*Core clinical characteristics*
1. Optic neuritis-nadir within 3 weeks of onset
2. Acute myelitis-acute sensory, motor, or sphincter dysfunction in pattern consistent with spinal cord lesion with nadir of deficit reached within 3 weeks of onset
3. Area postrema syndrome: episode of otherwise unexplained hiccups or nausea and vomiting occurring most of each day for at least 7 days not associated with other causes (2 days suffices if associated with new or acute lesion on MRI of area postrema/dorsal medulla)
4. Acute brainstem syndrome: acute brainstem symptoms such as ocular motor dysfunction, long tract signs, ataxia with nadir of deficits within 3 weeks of onset and associated with "NMOSD-typical"[a] lesions on MRI in area postrema/dorsal medulla or periependyma in brainstem
5. Symptomatic narcolepsy or acute diencephalic clinical syndrome with NMOSD-typical diencephalic MRI lesions: hypersomnolence or narcolepsy-like syndrome or other acute diencephalic syndrome such as anorexia with substantial weight loss or hypothermia with "NMOSD-typical" lesions on MRI in diencephalon, especially thalamus, hypothalamus, and peri-third ventricular region
6. Symptomatic cerebral syndrome with NMOSD-typical brain lesions: acute cerebral symptoms and signs such as encephalopathy, hemiparesis, and cortical visual loss with nadir of deficits within 3 weeks of onset and associated with cerebral "NMOSD-typical" lesions on MRI

(continued)

**Table 41.1** (continued)

*Additional MRI requirements for NMOSD without AQP4-IgG positivity and NMOSD with unknown AQP4-IgG status*

1. Acute optic neuritis: requires brain MRI showing (a) normal findings or only nonspecific white matter lesions or (b) optic nerve MRI with T2-hyperintense lesion or T1-weighted gadolinium-enhancing lesion extending over >1/2 optic nerve length or involving optic chiasm
2. Acute myelitis: requires associated intramedullary MRI lesion extending over ≥3 contiguous segments (longitudinally extensive transverse myelitis or LETM) OR ≥3 contiguous segments of focal spinal cord atrophy in patients with history compatible with acute myelitis. LETM optimally detected by MRI with gadolinium of entire spinal cord obtained within 1 month of clinical onset
3. Area postrema syndrome: requires associated dorsal medulla/area postrema lesions
4. Acute brainstem syndrome: requires associated periependymal brainstem lesions

a"NMOSD-typical" lesions: Brain lesion patterns are associated with NMOSD and include LETM or longitudinally extensive cord atrophy as described above as well as typical lesions noted on brain MRI. These include T2 hyperintense lesions: (1) involving the dorsal medulla and especially area postrema; (2) involving the periependymal surfaces of fourth ventricle; (3) involving the hypothalamus, thalamus, or periependymal surfaces of third ventricle; (4) large, confluent, unilateral, or bilateral subcortical or deep white matter lesions; (5) long (1/2 of length of corpus callosum or greater) diffuse, heterogeneous, or edematous corpus callosum lesions; (6) long corticospinal tract lesions, unilateral, or bilateral, contiguously involving internal capsule or cerebral peduncle; or (7) extensive periependymal brain lesions, often with gadolinium enhancement

etiologies are rare in the pediatric population, they should be checked if indicated. In children, comorbid rheumatologic diseases such as antiphospholipid antibody syndrome or systemic lupus erythematosus are a higher consideration in the differential diagnosis. Certain mitochondrial diseases, such as leukoencephalopathy with brainstem and spinal cord involvement and lactate elevation (LBSL) may also present with an NMOSD phenotype and might be given consideration in the setting of elevated CSF lactate. Various infections including *Bartonella henselae* and West Nile virus can produce optic pathway disease in childhood, and serologic testing might be considered if the clinical picture warrants.

Since the diagnosis of NMOSD presenting with isolated optic neuritis can be made with a positive AQP4-IgG result, it is imperative that serum be sent for AQP4-IgG. Current recommendations include cell-based serum assays for detection, as they have a higher sensitivity and a low false-positive rate compared to other methods. CSF analysis for AQP4-IgG should be pursued if there is high clinical suspicion of NMOSD, yet serum antibody results are negative. The presented case would be an example of such a circumstance, as the history of optic atrophy with a fixed vision deficit followed by an optic neuritis event would be consistent with the more severe morbidity associated with NMOSD attacks. Some patients who are initially negative for serum AQP-4 antibody later become positive, so retesting for up to 4 years after an initial attack is recommended if clinical suspicion is high [4]. In addition, testing prior to B-cell or antibody-targeted therapies such as plasmapheresis or immunosuppressive drugs is recommended. Other tests, such as visual evoked potential or optical coherence tomography, may be helpful but are not part of the current recommendations.

Finally, some studies have found that patients with clinical characteristics of NMOSD, but who are seronegative for AQP4-IgG, test positive for serum myelin oligodendrocyte protein (MOG); these patients may have different clinical characteristics than those who are positive for AQP4-IgG. In one study of NMOSD in adults, positive MOG antibodies correlated with a more favorable outcome compared to positive AQP4 antibodies [6]. However, the role of testing for MOG antibodies remains to be determined and is not done systematically, as there is no commercial test available at the time of this writing.

Of note, patients with autoimmune disorders such as systemic lupus erythematosus (SLE), Sjogren syndrome, juvenile rheumatoid arthritis, Graves' disease, and autoimmune hepatitis can also be diagnosed in a patient with NMOSD. These diseases may coexist, and underlying central nervous system (CNS) symptoms are thought to be due to the coexisting NMOSD rather than a complication of SLE or Sjogren syndrome [3]. As such, patients with NMOSD are more likely to develop other autoimmune disorders and may be screened for those as needed.

## What Are the Best Treatment Options, Both in the Acute and Chronic Phase, for NMOSD Initially Presenting with Optic Neuritis?

Treatment protocols for NMOSD with optic neuritis are essentially the same, regardless of the specific presentation. Acute therapy includes intravenous (IV) methylprednisolone 30 mg/kg/day up to 1 g/day for 5 days. When the clinical syndrome is severe or refractory to steroids, additional high-dose steroids can be given for up to 10 days. Given the antibody-mediated pathology, plasma exchange should be considered if there is poor response within 7 days of initiating steroids. Plasma exchange of one plasma volume is typically performed every other day for a total of between five and seven exchanges. This has been shown in a randomized trial to be associated with better outcomes in patients with initial poor recovery after high-dose steroids. If plasma exchange cannot be given, intravenous immunoglobulin (IVIG) 2 g/kg divided over 2–5 days can be considered [7, 8].

There is no standard treatment to prevent NMOSD relapses, as no medication is currently FDA-approved. Therapies include rituximab, azathioprine, and mycophenolate mofetil. Rituximab has been shown to be effective in populations of adult NMOSD patients, and one observational study recently suggested it is superior to azathioprine and mycophenolate mofetil. One study found that the majority of a series of 11 pediatric patients with MS or NMOSD treated with rituximab experienced fewer relapses and had no adverse events [9].

# What Is the Spectrum of Clinical Course and Outcomes in NMOSD Initially Presenting with Optic Neuritis?

Visual outcomes vary in pediatric NMOSD patients presenting with optic neuritis. In one study of 58 pediatric NMOSD patients followed for a median of 12 months (range 1–120 months), 48 (83%) presented with visual impairment. Of these, 25 (54%) had persistent visual impairment: 13 (27%) had binocular blindness with visual acuity of 20/200 or less in the better eye, 9 (19%) had monocular blindness, and 4 (8%) had milder visual impairments [7]. Another series compared visual outcomes in pediatric patients with monophasic or relapsing forms of either NMOSD or optic neuritis [10]. Patients with monophasic illness were defined as those with an absence of recurrent optic neuritis or transverse myelitis following the initial event. In 17 patients with NMOSD, 5 (29%) had normal vision, 8 (47%) had decreased vision but no limitation in daily activities, and 4 (24%) had severe impairment requiring visual aids. Of 13 patients with isolated optic neuritis, only 1 of the 13 was seropositive for AQP4-antibody. In those 13 patients, 9 (69%) had normal vision, 3 (23%) had decreased vision but no limitation in daily activities, and the only 1 (8%) who was AQP-4 IgG seropositive had severe impairment requiring visual aids. Pediatric NMOSD patients appear to have a higher number of attacks and higher vision disability than their pediatric counterparts with MS, indicating the need for prompt diagnosis and treatment of NMOSD [4].

Patients with poor visual recovery should be referred for supportive services including training for the visually impaired. The website, http://www.guthyjackson-foundation.org, provides further information for patients with NMOSD.

# References

1. Jarius S, Wildemann B. The history of neuromyelitis optica. J Neuroinflammation. 2013;10(1):8.
2. Wingerchuk DM, Lennon VA, Pittock SJ, Lucchinetti CF, Weinshenker BG. Revised diagnostic criteria for neuromyelitis optica. Neurology. 2006;66:1485–9.
3. Wingerchuk DM, Banwell B, Bennett JL, Cabre P, Carroll W, Chitnis T, de Seze J, Fujihara K, Greenberg B, Jacob A, Jarius S, Lana-Peixoto M, Levy M, Simon JH, Tenembaum S, Traboulsee AL, Waters P, Wellik KE, Weinshenker BG. International consensus diagnostic criteria for neuromyelitis optica spectrum disorders. Neurology. 2015;85:177–89.
4. Chitnis T, Ness J, Krupp L, Waubant E, Hunt T, Olsen C, Rodriguez M, Lotze T, Gorman T, Benson L, Belman A, Weinstock-Guttman B, Aaen G, Graves J, Patterson M, Rose JW, Casper TC. Clinical features of neuromyelitis optica in children: report from the U.S. Network of Pediatric MS Centers. Neurology. 2016;86(3):245–52.
5. Jacobi C, Hahnel S, Martinez-Torres F, Rieger S, Juttler E, Heiland S, Jarius S, Meyding-Lamde U, Storch-Hagenlocher B, Wildemann B. Prospective combined brain and spinal cord MRI in clinically isolated syndromes and possible early multiple sclerosis: impact on dissemination in space and time. Eur J Neurol. 2008;15(12):1359–64.

6. Kitley J, Waters P, Woodhall M, Leite MI, Murchison A, Chandratre S, Vincent A, Palace J. Neuromyelitis optica spectrum disorders with aquaporin-4 and myelin-oligodendrocyte gly-coprotein antibodies: a comparative study. JAMA Neurol. 2014;71(3):276–83.
7. Lotze T, Northrop JL, Hutton GJ, Ross B, Schiffman JS, Hunter JV. Spectrum of pediatric neuromyelitis optica. Pediatrics. 2008;122(5):e1039–47.
8. McKeon A, Lennon VA, Lotze T, Tenebaum S, Ness JM, Rensel M, Kuntz NL, Fryer JP, Hombruger H, Hunter J, Weinshenker BG, Krecke K, Lucchinetti CF, Pittock SJ. CNS aqua-porin-4 autoimmunity in children. Neurology. 2008;71:93–100.
9. Beres SJ, Graves J, Waubant E. Rituximab use in pediatric central demyelinating disease. Pediatr Neurol. 2014;51(1):114–8.
10. Banwell B, Tenembaum S, Lennon VA, Ursell E, Kennedy J, Bar-Or A, Weinshenker BG, Lucchinetti CF, Pittock SJ. Neuromyelitis optic-IgG in childhood inflammatory demyelinating CNS disorders. Neurology. 2008;70:344–52.

# Chapter 42
# Sarcoidosis with Optic Nerve Presentation

Sabrina Gmuca, Pamela F. Weiss, and Amy T. Waldman

## Case Presentation

A 15-year-old Caucasian male was diagnosed with idiopathic thrombocytopenic purpura (ITP) after developing petechiae, bruising, and thrombocytopenia. He was treated with rituximab (375 mg/m$^2$ intravenously weekly for four doses) after failing intravenous immunoglobulin (IVIg) dosed at 2 g/kg intravenously divided over 2 days and prednisone 2 mg/kg/day orally for 1 week followed by a taper. Six months later, he developed visual obscurations and impaired vision (right visual acuity of 20/200) with optic disc swelling unaccompanied by pain with extraocular movements. Magnetic resonance imaging (MRI) of the orbits revealed diffuse

S. Gmuca, M.D. (✉)
Division of Pediatric Rheumatology, The Children's Hospital of Philadelphia,
34th Street and Civic Center Boulevard, Wood Building, Fourth Floor, Philadelphia,
PA 19104, USA

Department of Pediatrics, Perelman School of Medicine, University of Pennsylvania,
Philadelphia, PA, USA
e-mail: gmucas@email.chop.edu

P.F. Weiss, M.D., M.S.C.E.
Division of Pediatric Rheumatology, The Children's Hospital of Philadelphia,
34th Street and Civic Center Boulevard, Wood Building, Fourth Floor, Philadelphia,
PA 19104, USA

Department of Pediatrics, Perelman School of Medicine, University of Pennsylvania,
Philadelphia, PA, USA

A.T. Waldman, M.D., M.S.C.E.
Division of Neurology, The Children's Hospital of Philadelphia, 34th Street and
Civic Center Boulevard, Wood Buildi ng, 6th Floor, Philadelphia, PA 19104, USA
e-mail: weisspa@email.chop.edu; waldman@email.chop.edu

© Springer International Publishing AG 2017
E. Waubant, T.E. Lotze (eds.), *Pediatric Demyelinating Diseases of the Central Nervous System and Their Mimics*, DOI 10.1007/978-3-319-61407-6_42

**Fig. 42.1** MRI of the brain with and without contrast (T1 with gadolinium): diffuse enhancement of the right optic nerve and the right aspect of the chiasm with swelling and enlargement of the optic nerve sheath on the right side. This process involves the retrobulbar fat that surrounds the optic nerves. There is slight tortuosity of the right optic nerve. The left optic nerve appears unremarkable

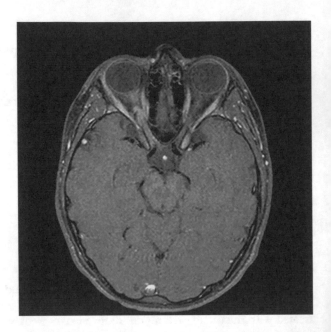

enhancement of the right optic nerve with enlargement of the right optic nerve and sheath and normal brain parenchyma (Fig. 42.1). Cerebrospinal fluid studies (including extensive infectious testing) were unremarkable. He developed hypogammaglobulinemia (initially attributed to rituximab) for which he has started on IVIg (400 mg/kg IV monthly).

Despite treatment with glucocorticoids (methylprednisolone 30 mg/kg IV daily for 3 days followed by prednisone 50 mg PO daily), he progressed to no light perception from his right eye with a relative afferent pupillary defect and disc edema. Optic neuritis was suspected; however, due to concern for a possible infiltrative process given his MRI findings, he had an optic nerve biopsy, which demonstrated an inflammatory infiltrate involving the dura and nerve. There were few axons and no granulomas. CD20 staining was negative for lymphoma, and the proliferative index was low, making an oncologic process unlikely. He had negative NMO-IgG (serum), normal positron emission tomography (PET) scan, and a normal bone marrow biopsy. The initial serum ACE level was obtained during corticosteroid treatment and was normal (45 U/L). However, 4 months after completion of corticosteroid treatment, the patient had two significantly elevated serum ACE levels: 151 U/L and 188 U/L. He was also noted to have neutropenia and thrombocytopenia. Further review of his medical history revealed that he had a glucocorticoid responsive erythematous facial rash that initially started 1 year prior. About 9 months after the onset of his ocular symptoms, he developed hyperpigmented nodules on his hands which raised suspicion for sarcoidosis.

Given the constellation of cytopenias, hypogammaglobulinemia (consistent with common variable immunodeficiency), inflammatory optic neuropathy, and elevated ACE he was diagnosed with sarcoidosis. Chest radiograph and high-resolution chest CT were unremarkable. At this time, he continued to have no light perception from his right eye. He started on methotrexate (25 mg subcutaneously weekly) and infliximab (10 mg/kg IV every 4 weeks) for disease control. His cytopenias improved and he has not had recurrence of optic neuritis. After 2 years of treatment with methotrexate and infliximab, he was transitioned to adalimumab 40 mg subcutaneously every 14 days. Three years later (and 6 years from his initial diagnosis), he continued to do well on adalimumab and was attending college.

## Clinical Questions

1. What is optic neuritis and what is the differential diagnosis?
2. What is atypical about this patient's presentation for idiopathic (demyelinating) optic neuritis?
3. How does pediatric sarcoidosis present and how is it diagnosed?
4. What are the possible neurologic manifestations of sarcoidosis?
5. What is the treatment and prognosis for sarcoidosis?

## Diagnostic Discussion

### *What Is Optic Neuritis and What Is the Differential Diagnosis?*

Idiopathic optic neuritis (ON), or inflammatory demyelination of the optic nerve, is the most common cause of acute unilateral visual loss in young adults with an incidence of 1–5 in 100,000 per year [1]. There is a female and Caucasian predominance, and most patients range between the age of 18 and 40 years old. Patients typically present with monocular subacute (often painful) visual loss and impaired color vision. Ninety-five percent of patients have demonstrable optic nerve inflammation on MRI. Symptoms develop over a few to several days, reaching maximum severity in about 2 weeks. ON may be an isolated syndrome in adults but often occurs in the context of a diffuse central nervous system neuroinflammatory disorder, such as multiple sclerosis or neuromyelitis optica.

Demyelinating ON is the most common cause of optic neuropathy [1] and is associated with multiple sclerosis (MS). Other non-demyelinating causes of optic neuropathies include autoimmune diseases (systemic lupus erythematous, sarcoidosis, Behçet's disease), infectious diseases (viral etiology, syphilis, tuberculosis, Lyme disease), tumors, and ischemic, hereditary, toxic, or nutritional neuropathies. Although these entities are less common, their clinical and therapeutic management differs dramatically. Therefore, a correct and early diagnosis of the underlying etiology of ON is crucial [1].

## What Is Atypical About This Patient's Presentation for Idiopathic (Demyelinating) Optic Neuritis?

Pediatric ON, similar to adult disease, presents with visual acuity loss, the presence of moderate pain during activity of the extrinsic eye muscles, dyschromatopsia, and visual field deficits. The neuro-ophthalmologic examination may reveal a relative afferent pupillary defect (RAPD) (in asymmetric disease) or papillitis (swelling of the optic nerve head). In children, there tends to be a relationship between age and monocular or binocular disease, with unilateral optic neuritis more common in older children (≥10 years of age) and bilateral disease in younger children [2]. The patient in our case had monocular symptoms, which is typical based on his age of 15 years. The visual acuity in idiopathic ON is variable at presentation (ranging from subtle deficits to no light perception). However, even with profound visual loss, most children with idiopathic optic neuritis, even in a patient with multiple sclerosis, demonstrate recovery (often to 20/40 or better) with steroids. Additionally, most patients have spontaneous recovery after 2–3 weeks regardless of glucocorticoid treatment [1] which was not the case for our patient. The vision loss in children with optic neuritis as a symptom of NMO may not respond to glucocorticoid treatment; however, our patient did not meet diagnostic criteria for NMO spectrum disorder.

An atypical presentation of ON should initiate a careful diagnostic search for other differential diagnoses. An atypical presentation would include lack of pain, marked visual loss, bilateral visual loss, or absence of spontaneous recovery after 2–3 weeks (Table 42.1) [1, 3]. Our patient did have ocular pain. He demonstrated transient, minimal recovery of his vision with corticosteroids, but upon corticosteroid withdrawal, he redeveloped complete vision loss; therefore, additional investigative studies were performed with sarcoidosis presumed to be the underlying etiology. The diagnosis, however, could not be confirmed as the patient did not have biopsy-proven granulomas.

**Table 42.1** Atypical Features of Demyelinating Optic Neuritis

| |
|---|
| • Bilateral involvement |
| • Absence of pain |
| • Insidious onset |
| • Younger than 15 years or older than 50 years of age |
| • Presence of systemic symptoms |
| • Isolated recurrent optic neuritis |
| • Normal brain imaging |
| • Atypical visual field abnormalities |

Adapted from *Martinelli V, Bianchi Marzoli S. Non-demyelinating optic neuropathy: clinical entities. Neurological Sciences. 2001;22(Suppl 2):S55–9*

## How Does Pediatric Sarcoidosis Present and How Is It Diagnosed?

Sarcoidosis is a chronic, granulomatous disorder of unknown etiology. It is multi-systemic and may involve any organ. Childhood sarcoidosis is rare with a higher incidence reported among African Americans and most cases occur between the ages of 13 and 15 years. No clear sex predominance exists in contrast to the female preponderance seen in adults. The clinical presentation depends on the affected organs and the age of onset with two distinct forms of pediatric sarcoidosis. Older children usually present with a multisystem disease similar to adult manifestations, with predominant lung involvement (including hilar lymphadenopathy and pulmonary infiltrations). Early-onset sarcoidosis is a unique form of the disease characterized by the triad of rash, uveitis, and arthritis in children presenting before 4 years of age.

There is no single diagnostic test for sarcoidosis. Laboratory findings may reveal elevated acute phase reactants (including sedimentation rate, C-reactive protein, and platelet count). Anemia, leucopenia, and eosinophilia are commonly seen. Hypercalcemia and/or hypercalciuria may also be found. The serum level of ACE is elevated in over 50% of children with late-onset sarcoidosis although the test is not specific for sarcoidosis. ACE serum levels have been shown to be useful in diagnosing sarcoidosis and following disease activity and the effect of therapy in older children with sarcoidosis. Chest radiograph is also useful and may reveal bilateral hilar adenopathy. Additionally, high-resolution chest computed tomography (CT) is useful for delineating the extent of parenchymal disease and hilar adenopathy. The definitive diagnosis of sarcoidosis is made when patients have (1) compatible clinical findings and (2) histopathological evidence of noncaseating granulomas in affected organs with the exclusion of other granulomatous diseases.

## What Are the Possible Neurologic Manifestations of Sarcoidosis?

Neurologic manifestations in sarcoidosis are varied and may mimic other diseases, making it additionally difficult to diagnose neurosarcoidosis (NS). The neurologic manifestations of sarcoidosis may affect virtually any part of both the central and peripheral nervous systems. Although up to 5–10% of all sarcoidosis patients present with neurological symptoms, those with isolated NS are exceptionally rare, and the exact prevalence is unknown. Among Caucasians, the incidence of isolated NS is estimated at less than 0.2 per 100,000 [4]. Granulomatous inflammation may result in meningeal or parenchymal lesions, including pituitary and hypothalamic involvement and myelitis, cranial neuropathies, peripheral neuropathy, and myopathy. In adults, cranial nerve palsies, especially facial nerve palsy, are the most common clinical feature of NS affecting up to 75% of patients. NS in children may present with encephalopathy including seizures, hypothalamic dysfunctions, and mass-like brain lesions. Another manifestation is Heerfordt syndrome (uveoparotid fever), consisting of ocular symptoms (uveitis and less commonly optic neuritis) associated with facial nerve palsy and swelling of the parotid gland.

Ocular involvement in childhood sarcoidosis is common. In fact, in one study in Louisiana, the most common clinical manifestations on presentation were constitutional symptoms (63%) followed by ocular complaints (37%). Visual symptoms including eye pain, blurry vision, photophobia, and redness may be present in 29% of patients. Notably, patients may present without associated eye pain, which is a common feature of idiopathic ON.

Sarcoidosis can affect all structures of the eye but most commonly results in anterior uveitis; therefore, ophthalmological slit lamp examination is mandatory in the evaluation of childhood sarcoidosis [5]. Anterior segment disease is the most common, consisting of chronic granulomatous uveitis, acute iritis, and conjunctival granulomas [5]. Posterior segment disease is less common. The uveitis of sarcoidosis is characterized by firmly edged keratic precipitates that most commonly develop in the lower part of the cornea but can also be seen in the limbus. Patients may also develop iris nodules and related focal synechiae; however, the majority of the synechiae are caused by adhesions between the iris and lens secondary to inflammation. Choroidal granulomas and peripheral multifocal choroiditis are very specific for ocular sarcoidosis. Conjunctival granulomas are the second most common ocular manifestation in sarcoidosis and may appear as tiny, translucent, pale yellow nodules. In addition, granulomas can occur either at the optic disc or in the retrobulbar portion of the optic nerve. Important clinical features of optic neuropathy due to sarcoidosis include poor visual acuity (no light perception), often with poor recovery, retinal vasculitis, and a thickened optic nerve on MRI of the orbits. Pain with eye movements is not as common as in idiopathic optic neuritis. Additional complications include cataracts, glaucoma, macular edema, retinal ischemia, retinal detachment, vitreous hemorrhage, and subretinal neovascularization.

Since there is no definitive test for NS, the diagnosis relies on clinical suspicion, along with associated laboratory, imaging, and pathological abnormalities. Zajicek et al. [6] established a diagnostic classification system for NS that distinguished definite, probable, and possible NS based on tissue evidence of noncaseating granulomas and supportive evidence of sarcoid pathology in laboratory and imaging studies (Table 42.2). MR imaging remains the study of choice for evaluation of optic nerve sarcoidosis. Mafee et al. note certain imaging features that should raise the possibility of optic nerve sarcoidosis. These include (1) enhancement of optic nerve associated with prominent enlargement of the intracranial segment of optic nerve, (2) enlargement of the intracranial segment of optic nerve associated with contrast enhancement, and (3) abnormal enhancement of optic nerve, associated with abnormal dural and leptomeningeal enhancement. Additionally, bilateral optic nerve enlargement along with abnormal enhancement was not seen in any cases of optic nerve sarcoidosis. Bilateral involvement therefore should favor optic nerve sheath meningioma, demyelinating disease, optic glioma, lymphoma, leukemic infiltration, and pseudotumor. A diagnosis of NS

**Table 42.2** Classification of neurosarcoidosis

| |
|---|
| Neurosarcoidosis can be diagnosed in patients with a clinical presentation suggestive of neurosarcoidosis with exclusion of other possible diagnoses as outlined: |
| Definite |
| *Histologic evidence from a biopsy of the central nervous system* |
| Probable |
| A.   *Laboratory evidence of CNS inflammation* |
| • *elevated levels of CSF protein and/or cells* |
| • *the presence of oligoclonal bands and/or* |
| • *MRI evidence compatible with neurosarcoidosis)* |
| B.   *Evidence for systemic sarcoidosis* |
| • *Positive histology and/or at least two indirect indicators from Gallium scan, chest imaging and serum ACE* |
| Possible |
| • *Above criteria are not met* |

Adapted from *Zajicek JP, Scolding NJ, Foster O, Rovaris M, Evanson J, Moseley IF, et al. Central nervous system sarcoidosis—diagnosis and management. QJM. 1999;92(2):103–17. By permission of Oxford University Press*

should prompt evaluation for additional organ involvement including a screening of chest radiograph and/or PET scan and basic laboratory studies to evaluate for cytopenias and hepatic involvement.

## What Is the Treatment and Prognosis for Sarcoidosis?

There are no evidence-based treatment guidelines for NS. First-line treatment consists of glucocorticoids with a proposed starting dose of prednisone 0.5–1 mg/kg/day for 6–8 weeks. This is then followed by a slow taper to 0.1–0.25 mg/kg/day which is continued while the patient is symptomatic. Repeat MRI helps determine steroid dose reduction. In patients with acute severe clinical deterioration, 30 mg/kg/day (maximum dose 1000 mg) methylprednisolone administered over 3–5 days is recommended.

In more severe cases, with insufficient therapeutic responses to steroids or adverse side effects secondary to glucocorticoids, various immunosuppressants and immunomodulators have been used, but there is no uniform treatment plan. Patients who continue to develop neurologic deficits or lack improvement of MRI findings while on corticosteroids or develop adverse side effects (hypertension, glucose intolerance, low bone mineral density) from glucocorticoids are considered glucocorticoid non-responsive, and their level of care should be escalated.

Methotrexate is commonly used as a second-line treatment and acts as a steroid-sparing agent. Methotrexate is recommended at a dose of 10–25 mg, orally or subcutaneously, weekly accompanied by folic acid 1 mg/day [7]. Alternatively, azathioprine (2–2.5 mg/kg orally daily) or cyclosporine (2 mg/kg orally twice daily) may be used in conjunction with steroids. More recently, rituximab and adalimumab have shown significant benefit in cases of neurosarcoidosis requiring immunosuppressant therapy and are considered third-line treatment [8, 9]. Mycophenolate mofetil, cyclophosphamide, and hydroxychloroquine have been reportedly used to treat NS, but the dosage and duration of treatment in the pediatric population is not well established. The course of the disease seems to be more severe in younger children, but approximately 2/3 will recover completely with corticosteroid treatment and the remainder will have a relapsing-remitting course [5]. Overall prognosis is dependent on the organ systems involved.

## Clinical Pearls

- Idiopathic (demyelinating) ON is the most common cause of optic neuropathy, typically presenting with subacute painful visual loss and is a common presenting symptom of multiple sclerosis or neuromyelitis optica.
- Atypical presentations of ON should prompt additional investigative studies to evaluate for other possible etiologies (including autoimmune disorders, infectious diseases, tumors or genetic neuropathies) because this affects clinical management.
- NS is a disorder of unknown etiology characterized by noncaseating granulomas and can affect any part of the nervous system. In pediatric NS, common manifestations include uveitis, optic neuropathy, hypothalamic dysfunctions, mass-like brain lesions, and encephalopathy, including seizures.
- Clinical features of optic neuropathy due to sarcoidosis include poor visual acuity (no light perception), often with poor recovery, retinal vasculitis, and a thickened optic nerve on MRI of the orbits. Pain with eye movements is not as common as in idiopathic optic neuritis.
- Prolonged course of glucocorticoids are the mainstay of treatment for NS, but in severe or refractory cases, other immunomodulating or immunosuppressant agents are used as adjuvant or steroid-sparing agents.

## References

1. Voss E, Raab P, Trebst C, Stangel M. Clinical approach to optic neuritis: pitfalls, red flags and differential diagnosis. Ther Adv Neurol Disord. 2011;4(2):123–34.
2. Waldman AT, Stull LB, Galetta SL, Balcer LJ, Liu GT. Pediatric optic neuritis and risk of multiple sclerosis: meta-analysis of observational studies. J AAPOS. 2011;15(5):441–6.
3. Martinelli V, Bianchi MS. Non-demyelinating optic neuropathy: clinical entities. Neurol Sci. 2001;22(Suppl 2):S55–9.
4. Nowak DAD. Neurosarcoidosis: a review of its intracranial manifestation. J Neurol. 2001;248(5):363.
5. Fauroux B, Clément A. Paediatric sarcoidosis. Paediatr Respir Rev. 2005;6(2):128–33.

6. Zajicek JP, Scolding NJ, Foster O, Rovaris M, Evanson J, Moseley IF, et al. Central nervous system sarcoidosis—diagnosis and management. QJM. 1999;92(2):103–17.
7. Hoitsma E, Faber CG, Drent M, Sharma OP. Neurosarcoidosis: a clinical dilemma. Lancet Neurol. 2004;3(7):397–407.
8. Bomprezzi R, Pati S, Chansakul C, Vollmer T. A case of neurosarcoidosis successfully treated with rituximab. Neurology. 2010;75(6):568–70.
9. Sollberger M, Fluri F, Baumann T, Sonnet S, Tamm M, Steck AJ, et al. Successful treatment of steroid-refractory neurosarcoidosis with infliximab. J Neurol. 2004;251(6):760–1.

# Index

Printed in the United States
By Bookmasters